The Obesity Fix

How to Beat Food Cravings, Lose Weight and Gain Energy

Dr James DiNicolantonio

Author of The Salt Fix

&

Siim Land

Author of Metabolic Autophagy

2022

DISCLAIMER

You agree to accept all risks of using the information presented inside this book. You need to consult a professional medical practitioner in order to ensure you are both able and healthy enough to participate in this program.

Jacket design by James DiNicolantonio and Siim Land

Table of Contents

About the Authors

Dr. James DiNicolantonio

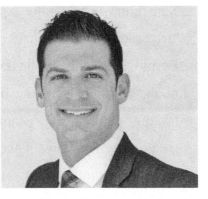

As a cardiovascular research scientist and Doctor of Pharmacy, Dr. James J. DiNicolantonio has spent years researching nutrition. A well-respected and internationally known scientist and expert on health and nutrition, he has contributed extensively to health policy and medical literature. Dr. DiNicolantonio is the author of 6 best-selling health books, The Salt Fix, Superfuel, The Longevity Solution, The Immunity Fix, The Mineral Fix and WIN.

His website is www.drjamesdinic.com. You can follow Dr. DiNicolantonio on Twitter and Instagram at @drjamesdinic and Facebook at Dr. James DiNicolantonio.

He is the author or co-author of more than 300 medical publications, including several high-profile articles related to nutrition, including a December 2014 opinion piece about sugar addiction in *The New York Times* that was the newspaper's most emailed article during the 24 hours following its publication. Dr. DiNicolantonio has testified in front of the Canadian Senate regarding the harms of added sugars and serves as the Associate Editor of British Medical Journal's (BMJ) Open Heart, a journal published in partnership with the British Cardiovascular Society. He is also on the Editorial Advisory Board of several other medical journals, including Progress in Cardiovascular Diseases and International Journal of Clinical Pharmacology & Toxicology.

Siim Land

Siim Land is an author, speaker, content creator and renown biohacker from Estonia. Despite his young age, he is considered one of the top people in the biohacking and health optimization community with thousands of followers worldwide. Siim Land has written books like Metabolic Autophagy, Stronger by Stress, The Immunity Fix, The Mineral Fix and WIN.

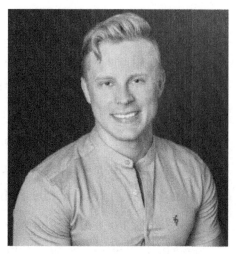

His website is www.siimland.com. You can follow Siim on Instagram @siimland and as Siim Land on YouTube.

Siim started researching and doing self-experiments with nutrition, exercise, and other strategies to improve his performance and health after high school when he enrolled in the military for a year. He then obtained a bachelor's degree in anthropology in Tallinn University and University of Durham in the UK. By now he has written several books about diet, creates content online, and keeps himself up to date with the latest knowledge in science.

Introduction: Consequences of The Obesity Epidemic

There are 1.9 billion overweight and 650 million obese people worldwide[1], which equates to 52% of adults globally being overweight or obese (body mass index $\geq$ 25 to < 30 and $\geq$ 30, respectively). In the United States, approximately 42% of adults are obese[2] and 34% have metabolic syndrome[3]. Those numbers are quite mind-boggling, but now it's more common to be overweight than in shape. However, this hasn't always been the case. Indeed, there has been a trend with obesity increasing with the rising affluence of developed countries.

"According to the surgeon general, obesity today is officially an epidemic; it is arguably the most pressing public health problem we face, costing the health care system an estimated $90 billion a year.

Three of every five Americans are overweight; one of every five is obese. The disease formerly known as adult-onset diabetes has had to be renamed Type II diabetes since it now occurs so frequently in children.

A recent study in the Journal of the American Medical Association predicts that a child born in 2000 has a one-in-three chance of developing diabetes. (An African American child's chances are two in five.) Because of diabetes and all the other health problems that accompany obesity, today's children may turn out to be the first generation of Americans whose life expectancy will actually be shorter than that of their parents.

The problem is not limited to America: The United Nations reported that in 2000 the number of people suffering from overnutrition--a billion--had officially surpassed the number suffering from malnutrition--800 million."

Michael Pollan, The Omnivore's Dilemma: A Natural History of Four Meals

It's estimated that since 1975, the worldwide incidence of obesity tripled[4]. Yet, it was only until 1997 that the World Health Organization (WHO) recognized obesity as a global epidemic[5]. By 2000, the number of adults with excess bodyweight surpassed the number of adults who were normal weight or underweight[6]. In 2013, an estimated 2.1 billion adults were overweight compared to the 857 million in 1980[7]. The rate of obesity in the United Kingdom (UK) has risen 4-fold since 1980, now characterizing 22-24% of the population[8]. In the United States, obesity has doubled since 1960[9,10]. More worrisome, the rate of overweight children has increased from 6% to 19% over the last 25 years[11,12]. According to 2019 Eurostat Statistics, the highest rates of obesity in the European Union (EU) can be found in Croatia (65%), Hungary (60%), Czech Republic (60%), Romania (59%), Slovakia (59%), Finland (59%) and Turkey (59%)[13]. Overall, 53% of people in the EU are considered overweight (BMI $\geq$ 25).

Obesity is linked to a higher risk of overall mortality[14,15,16,17]. **A severely obese person can expect to live anywhere from 5-20 years less.** Being obese increases the risk for diabetes, cardiovascular disease, neurodegeneration, cancer, and kidney disease[18,19,20]. Obese people are 3.5 times more likely to have hypertension and 60-70% of hypertensive cases in adults can be traced back to excess adiposity[21]. Bariatric surgery has been found to reduce overall mortality by 30.7% after a 15-year follow-up, compared to control subjects without surgery[22]. Furthermore, a 7.1-year retrospective cohort study saw a 40% mortality reduction in the bariatric surgery group compared to controls[23]. Mortality in the surgery

10

group decreased by 56% for coronary artery disease, 60% for cancer and 92% for diabetes. Lastly, gastric bypass surgery patients have been found to have an 89% lower rate of death compared to control subjects with a mean follow-up of 2.6-years[24]. In other words, losing a significant amount of weight can lower the risk of death as well as cardiovascular disease, cancer, and type 2 diabetes.

Obesity and Risk of Chronic Disease and Mortality:

1. Obesity = very high risk of hypertension and cardiovascular disease
2. Obesity = higher risk of cancer development
3. Obesity = higher risk of type 2 diabetes and insulin resistance
4. Obesity = shorter life expectancy (5-20 years less)

Excess adiposity promotes the creation of reactive oxygen species (ROS) that over the long-term damage the mitochondria[25]. Importantly, pro-inflammatory substances called cytokines rise and anti-inflammatory cytokines decrease, creating inflammation in the body[26,27]. Chronic inflammation promotes cancer, cardiovascular disease, atherosclerosis, diabetes, major depression, immunodeficiencies and autoimmune diseases[28,29,30,31,32,33,34,35,36,37,38,39]. Inflammation is considered the seventh hallmark of cancer[40]. Immune dysfunction and chronic low grade inflammation – a term called inflammaging – are a hallmark of many age-related diseases[41]. On the flip side, fat loss can cause a drop in those circulating pro-inflammatory markers, such as c-reactive protein (CRP) and interleukin-6 (IL-6)[42]. (below figure redrawn from Nakamura 2014)

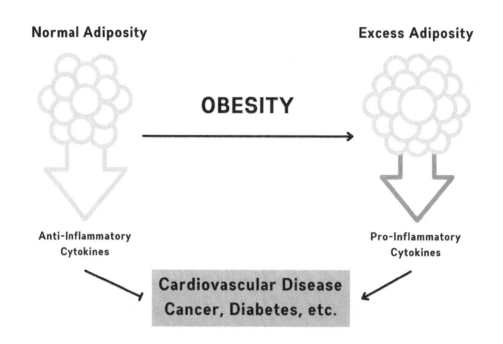

Normal Adiposity ... OBESITY ... Excess Adiposity

Anti-Inflammatory Cytokines → Cardiovascular Disease Cancer, Diabetes, etc. ← Pro-Inflammatory Cytokines

During the 2009 Swine Flu (influenza A H1N1) pandemic, many studies found that obesity was an independent risk factor for worse outcomes with the virus[43,44]. Similar findings were also observed with the coronavirus[45]. Obese humans and mice show reduced immunity and higher rates of death against influenza A virus[46,47]. Obesity also impairs wound healing and memory T-cell function and causes more lung damage from influenza A[48,49]. Furthermore, obesity is associated with increased severity of influenza A, increased viral replication, prolonged viral shedding, and a higher amount of exhaled viral load[50,51,52,53]. Studies also find obese individuals show greater declines in vaccine efficacy than non-obese individuals[54]. They also have reduced protection from vaccination over time[55]. Even worse, the pro-inflammatory environment in obesity may promote the emergence or mutations of novel virulent influenza strains[56].

Obesity and Viral Infections[57]

1. Obesity = delayed and blunted antiviral responses

2. Obesity = poorer viral outcomes

3. Obesity = reduced efficacy of antivirals and vaccines

4. Obesity = increased viral shedding, replication, and mutation

Obesity and metabolic syndrome are the biggest non-genetic risk factors contributing to the severity of COVID-19[58]. Metabolic syndrome is a condition in which at least three or more of the five are present: high blood pressure, central obesity, high fasting triglycerides, high blood sugar and low serum HDL cholesterol[59]. Metabolic syndrome is associated with cardiovascular disease and type 2 diabetes[60]. Metabolic syndrome doubles the risk of cardiovascular disease and increases all-cause mortality by 1.5-fold[61]. Diabetics have a 27.7% higher rate of mortality from COVID-19[62]. Chronic hyperinsulinemia is the most apparent underlying mechanism for this trend[63]. Obese individuals have a 50% greater chance of dying from COVID-19 and a 2x higher risk of being hospitalized from it[64]. Those with metabolic syndrome have a 4.5-fold risk of ending up in the intensive care unit (ICU) due to COVID-19 and 3.4-fold higher risk of dying[65].

All of this suggests that being obese has a major negative impact on your overall health and longevity. Obesity clearly impairs your metabolic health, immunity, cardiovascular function, and healthspan. If there's one thing that would make you healthier, it's avoiding obesity and establishing a normal body composition.

Defining Obesity

According to the World Health Organization, obesity is characterized as a waist to hip ratio above 0.90 for males and 0.85 for females[66]. People with more weight around the midsection are at a higher risk of heart disease, diabetes, and premature death than those who carry it around their hips and thighs[67]. You calculate this by taking your waist circumference and dividing it by your hip circumference (W/H). The optimal W/H ratio for women is < 0.80 and for men < 0.95. A waist circumference over 40 inches (men) or 35 inches (women) increases the risk of heart disease, diabetes, and premature death[68].

The most widely used tool to assess obesity for decades has been the Body Mass Index (BMI). BMI describes a person's bodyweight divided by their squared height[69]. It can be used as an epidemiological tool to assess an individual's weight status and categorize them as either underweight, normal, overweight, or obese. A BMI of 25-29 is considered overweight and $\geq$ 30 obese. By 2000, 65% of adults had a BMI above 25, and 30% above 30[70]. The BMI formulas are as follows:

- Formula: BMI = weight (kg) $\div$ height^2 (m^2)

- Imperial BMI Formula: BMI = weight (lb) $\div$ height^2 (in^2) $\times$ 703

Classifications of overweight and obesity by BMI[71]:

Classification	Obesity Class	BMI (kg/m^2)
Underweight	-	< 18.5
Normal	-	18.5–24.9
Overweight	-	25.0–29.9
Obesity	I	30.0–34.9
Severe Obesity	II	35.0–39.9
Morbid Obesity	III	40.0–49.9
Severe Morbid Obesity	III	>50

An analysis of prospective studies among 894,576 subjects found that **overall mortality follows a J-shaped curve, increasing at both above and below a BMI of 22.5-25**[72]. Other studies support the link between a BMI > 25 and higher mortality[73]. Survival is reduced by 2-4 years at a BMI of 30-35 and by 8-10 years at a BMI of 40-45. The higher mortality below a BMI of 22.5 is hypothesized to be caused by smoking-related diseases. Type-2 diabetes risk increases by 100% at a BMI between 27.2-29.4 and by 300% at a BMI of 29.4[74]. Deaths from mental health issues, neurological diseases, and behavioral disorders, as well as suicide and accidents, were found to be linked with a lower bodyweight (BMI < 18.5).

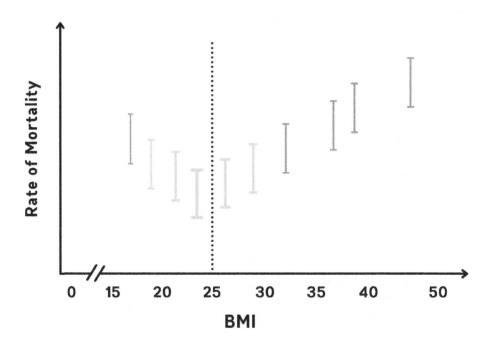

Lowest mortality is between 22.5-25 BMI

Source: Prospective Whitlock et al (2009)

Despite the epidemiological association between BMI and mortality, it can be misleading in some cases. For example, if you carry even a little bit of muscle, your BMI might tell you that you're overweight and thus at a higher risk of metabolic disorders. In reality, your BMI is fine and your body composition excellent. **There is a lot of evidence suggesting that muscle mass and strength are inversely associated with all-cause mortality**[75,76,77]. What's more, a 2014 meta-analysis found that fit individuals with good muscle strength (but categorized as overweight) had a similar odds of death as those in the normal weight range[78]. Thus, overall biomarkers, body composition and body fat percentages can be much more accurate and descriptive of a person's overall health than BMI.

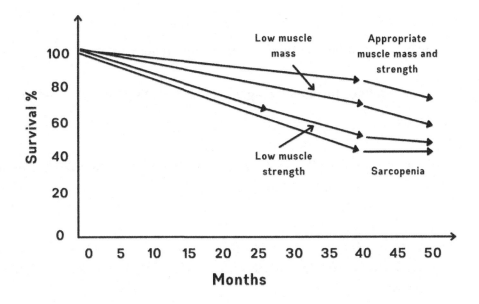

Redrawn From: Isoyama et al (2014)

Having a higher or lower BMI doesn't always predict the onset of metabolic disorders. Roy and Hulman coined the term 'personal fat threshold' in their 2015 paper investigating normal-weight individuals who develop type-2 diabetes[79]. According to this concept, every person has their own subjective capacity to store subcutaneous body fat and once that limit is exceeded, excess calories will be directed into visceral fat[80]. Exceeding your personal fat threshold makes it more likely to develop type 2 diabetes[81,82]. This has been seen in both overweight, as well as normal weight people.

Visceral adipose tissue, which is fat stored in and around the organs, is a very important trigger for the development of metabolic syndrome[83]. Whereas subcutaneous fat gets stored underneath the skin and is used for energy, visceral fat begins to continuously secrete pro-inflammatory cytokines, leading to inflammation and insulin resistance. Visceral fat accumulation, not total fat mass, is strongly linked with metabolic disorders, diabetes, cardiovascular disease, and type 2 diabetes[84,85]. In other words, losing liver fat is more important than losing subcutaneous fat. Everyone's threshold at which they begin to accumulate visceral fat is different, depending on genetics and lifestyle.

Here are guidelines for measuring your personal fat threshold and metabolic syndrome:

- **Fasting Insulin**: Normal range: 3-8 uIU/mL (18–48 pmol/L); moderate insulin resistance: 8-12 uIU/mL (48-72 pmol/L); severe insulin resistance: > 12 uIU/mL.

- **Fasting Blood Sugar:** Normal ranges: < 100 mg/dl (5.3 mmol/L), prediabetes: 100-125 mg/dl (5.6-6.9 mmol/L), diabetes: > 126 mg/dl (7 mmol/L).

- **Blood pressure:** Normal blood pressure is < 120/80 mmHg. 130-139/80-89 mmHg is considered stage 1 hypertension. Stage 2 hypertension is ≥ 140/90 mmHg.

- **Triglycerides**: Normal range: < 150 mg/dl (1.7 mmol/L); borderline-high levels: 150-200 mg/dl (1.8 to 2.2 mmol/L); high levels: 200-500 mg/dl (2.3 to 5.6 mmol); very high levels: > 500 mg/dl (5.7 mmol/L or above).

- **HDL Cholesterol:** Normal fasting HDL is between 40-60 mg/dl. Optimally, it should be between 50-80 mg/dl. HDL < 40 mg/dl can be problematic and a sign of either dyslipidemia or metabolic syndrome.

- **Triglyceride to HDL Ratio**: Normal range: 1.0 +/- 0.5; moderate insulin resistance: 2-3; severe insulin resistance: > 4.

- **A1C (average 3 month blood sugar):** Normal range: ≤ 5.6% (≤ 38 mmol/mol); prediabetes: 5.7-6.4% (> 39-46 mmol/mol); diabetes: ≥ 6.5% (> 47 mmol/mol).

- **HOMA-IR (Homeostatic Model Assessment for Insulin Resistance)**: Normal range: (0.5-1.5); moderate insulin resistance: 1.5-2.5; severe insulin resistance: > 3.0

- **Body Fat Percentage**: Normal range: 5-20% for men and 10-25% women. Anything above 20-25% is an excess amount of fat for men and women, respectively.

- **Waist to Hip Ratio**: Optimal ratio for women is < 0.80 and for men < 0.95. Moderate risk for women is 0.81–0.85 and for men 0.96–1.0. High risk for women is > 0.86 and for men > 1.0. A waist circumference over 40 inches (men) or 35 inches (women) is problematic and increases risk of heart disease, diabetes, and premature death[86].

Health risk with W/H ratio	Women	Men
Low	0.80 or lower	0.95 or lower
Moderate	0.81–0.85	0.96–1.0
High	0.86 or higher	1.0 or higher

Fortunately, no one is born obese, and losing weight can be easier than you think, if you have the right plan and you are consistent. Weight loss can be a long process with many trials and tribulations, but it doesn't have to be a miserable process. There are certain methods that make it easier to lose weight and we are going to provide you with the guide to to lose the weight and to keep it off for good. You may encounter some roadblocks along the way, such as physiological and psychological challenges, food cravings and occasional weight plateaus. Nevertheless, you shouldn't let that be an excuse to not start your weight loss journey. It doesn't matter what weight you are starting at, the only thing that matters is consistent measurable improvements each day.

Chapter 1 – What Caused the Obesity Epidemic?

Obesity has been depicted in art and sculptures throughout human history in one form or another[87]. In the past, being slightly more overweight was a sign of affluence and food abundance. That's why such figures were not that common to see – food was scarce and in its natural state[88]. The 'thrifty gene' hypothesis speculates that individuals who were predisposed to storing calories as body fat most efficiently would survive periods of famine, but such genes don't exist[89]. In the modern world, where most of the population is carrying a bit too much extra weight, it's actually more beneficial to be less efficient in gaining fat mass because now food is overabundant.

Hippocrates from Ancient Greece was first to realize the health dangers associated with being obese and that it shortened lifespan[90]. Co-morbidities of obesity, such as sleep apnea, diabetes, infertility, coronary heart disease and metabolic syndrome have been associated with being overweight since the 16th century and even Hippocrates' era[91,92,93]. Hippocrates said that consuming more food and wine than you can bear, without using it for physical activity, damages health, whereas perfect health is found in balance[94]. Ancient Egyptians were said to prevent themselves from getting too heavy by fasting and limiting their food or alcohol intake periodically[95]. Herodotus noted that Egyptians 'purged' themselves three times a month for the sake of health preservation, which they thought was caused by over-nourishment[96]. Pythagoras and Herodicus promoted moderate food consumption and sticking to plain temperate meals[97,98].

So, what happened that caused 2 out of every 3 adults living in the United States to be overweight or obese? Did we all suddenly decide to become gluttons and sloths? It turns out that there were several key changes in the food supply that helped drive the obesity pandemic in the United States. In this chapter, we're going to look at all of them.

Why Has Obesity Risen?

During the 19th century Industrial Revolution, industrialized societies saw an increase in the average height and weight of people, which boosted their industrial productivity[99,100]. This was due to better access to calories and nutrients that make the body grow. At the 20th century, most populations had reached their genetic limit for height, but this is when the average adult weight began to rise exponentially[101]. For example, in Texas in the 19th century, only 1.2% were obese,[102] which increased 35-fold, with now 42% being obese today [103].

In the 19th century U.S., there was a correlation between higher Body Mass Index (BMI) and lower socioeconomic status[104]. However, an increase in wealth is also associated with a rise in BMI due to access to more high calorie foods and a decrease in manual labor[105,106,107]. In recent decades, the most dramatic rise of obesity has been seen in developing countries[108]. Income inequality appears to be a driver of obesity and higher BMI even in the United States[109]. Parent education, household income and socioeconomic status also contribute to obesity risk[110,111].

The classic reasoning for the rise in obesity is an increased calorie intake, which follows the same rising trend as the increasing rate of obesity[112,113,114]. However, what caused the rise in caloric intake? Surely the entire population didn't decide to start eating more calories at the same time. It turns out that the consumption of highly palatable processed foods and beverages was the primary culprit. Indeed, fast food between 1977 and 1995 tripled and the calories obtained from those meals quadrupled[115]. Compared to 1977, the U.S. population in 1996 was consuming about 200 kcal/day more[116]. A major reason for this was a shift from consuming meals at-home to away-from-home, with large increases in total calories from snacks, soft drinks and pizza, and a large decrease in calories from milk, beef, and pork. Regarding soft drinks, sugar-sweetened beverages accounted for up to 25% of total daily calories in adults[117,118,119,120]. From 1977 to 1996 total caloric intake in those 19-39 years old increased from 1,840 to 2,198 calories (an increase of 358 calories/day). Global food production by 2002 reached roughly 2,600 kcal per capita and is predicted to reach 3,000 kcal by 2030[121]. That's almost double the calories compared to 1977. The biggest contributors to this increase in caloric intake are processed foods high in refined carbohydrates, sugars, and vegetable oils. Indeed, up to 20% of calories in the American diet comes from just soybean oil.[122] Other contributors to increasing daily calorie intake are easier access to calorie-dense foods and higher consumption of ready-made packaged foods that tend to be higher in calories than self-made whole food meals[123]. Those foods are consumed more often by low-income populations because they are cheaper[124]. U.S. counties with poverty rates > 35% have 145% higher obesity rates than wealthier counties[125].

High calorie foods (high in fat and sugar) tend to also be hyperpalatable, which promotes their overconsumption[126]. Ultra-processed food consumption results in roughly 500-600 more calories consumed per day, which results in significant weight gain[127]. Those additional calories come predominantly from fats (+230 ± 53 kcal/d) and carbohydrates (+280 ± 54 kcal/d) instead of protein (−2 ±12 kcal/d). Limiting processed food intake is common among most diets that are considered healthy and beneficial for weight loss[128,129]. Ultra-processed foods are typically refined, cheaper to produce, high in calories, with added sugars, fats and engineered to be hyperpalatable, which encourages overeating[130,131,132]. Examples include frozen pizza, chocolate, pastries, chips, etc. Semi-processed food, such as cottage cheese or olive oil, can be healthy as it's less processed and still provides nutritional value. Food processing itself isn't bad as it does help to lengthen shelf life, prevent waste and make things more convenient[133]. It's just that ultra-processed diets tend to make it harder to maintain a healthy body composition because they are high in calories, low in satiety and promote overconsumption.

Consuming Ultra-Processed Foods Increases Calorie Intake by 500-600 Calories and Leads to Weight Gain

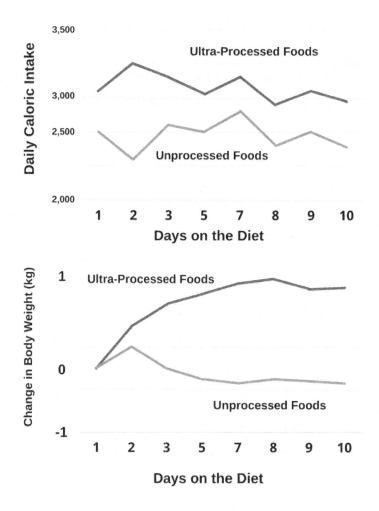

Redrawn From: Hall et al (2019)

Sedentary lifestyle is the second biggest reason for the rising prevalence of obesity in developed countries, which also contributes to a positive energy balance[134]. There has been a large shift from manual labor to desk work, which reflects in about 30% of the global population getting insufficient exercise[135,136]. In 2000, the Centers for Disease Control and Prevention estimated that less than 30% of the U.S. population meets adequate levels of physical activity, 30% are active but not enough and the remaining 40% are completely sedentary[137]. Physical activity from commuting has also decreased.[138] The number of children who walk or bike to school has dropped from 41% in 1969 to 13% in 2001[139]. In 2007, only 17% of 9-12th grade students claimed they were physically active for at least 60 minutes a day and only 30% said they attended physical education classes daily[140,141]. At home, the average American teenager watches over 30 hours of TV per week[142], which is associated with a higher risk of obesity[143,144,145]. A 2008 review of 73 studies found rates of childhood obesity rising in proportion to time spent consuming media[146]. TV viewing is also an activity that's associated with increased consumption of calorie-dense snacks and reduced intake of fresh fruit and vegetables[147,148].

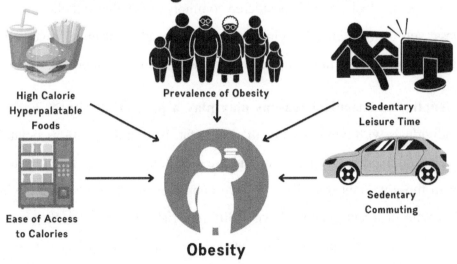

The Obesogenic Environment

High Calorie Hyperpalatable Foods

Prevalence of Obesity

Sedentary Leisure Time

Ease of Access to Calories

Sedentary Commuting

Obesity

A 2006 review outlined the 10 other possible contributors to the rise in obesity[149]:

1. Insufficient sleep[150,151]
2. Endocrine disruptors and pollutants that interfere with fat metabolism
3. Reduced rates of smoking (smoking suppresses appetite). Those who stop smoking have been found to gain on average 4.4 kg (9.7 lb) for men and 5 kg (11 lb) for women over the course of ten years[152].
4. Decreased ambient temperature variability (fat loss with cold exposure)
5. Use of medication that can cause weight gain, such as atypical antipsychotics
6. Pregnancy at a later age, which can increase susceptibility to obesity in children
7. Transgenerational epigenetic risk factors
8. Natural selection for higher BMI
9. Proportional increase in ethnic and age groups that tend to be heavier
10. Assortative mating (finding a partner with a similar body composition than yours)

In addition to that, certain personality traits are also associated with obesity, such as neuroticism, impulsivity, and reward sensitivity[153]. Self-control and conscientiousness, on the other hand, are less common in obese people[154]. However, the findings from such studies may be biased due to the social stigma obese people feel, i.e., it's considered common knowledge that obese people have less self-control etc. Loneliness appears to also promote overeating and gravitation towards high calorie, hyperpalatable comfort foods[155].

Genetics and medical reasons may play a part in obesity[156]. For example, individuals with two copies of the FTO (fat mass and obesity associated) gene weigh on average 3-4 kg more and are 1.67-times more susceptible to obesity than those without this allele[157]. Two people exposed to the same environment but with different genetics have a different risk of obesity[158]. Survivors of the Dutch famine during World War II show a higher incidence of obesity, cardiovascular disease, and diabetes due to nutrition-deprivation-induced intrauterine growth retardation[159,160]. This plays outs in animals too. For example, pups born undernourished show tendencies of overeating, which accelerates weight gain and increases adiposity[161,162]. There is also an association between low birth weight, early life malnutrition and adult obesity in humans[163,164,165]. However, your genetics don't have to determine your destiny and epigenetic lifestyle adjustments, such as eating whole nutritious foods, regulation of calorie intake and physical activity can still change your final result[166,167,168,169]. It's acknowledged that genetics are important, but they don't explain the dramatic rise in global obesity[170]. The more likely reason is the creation of an obesogenic environment that favors overconsumption of high calorie hyperpalatable foods while promoting sedentary behavior. That's why in this book, we focus on giving practical real-world steps for addressing the factors you can control.

Refined Sugars

It's quite common knowledge that eating too many sweets and desserts promotes weight gain. An increased intake of refined sugar can lead to weight gain, especially belly or visceral fat, fatty liver disease, insulin resistance, type 2 diabetes, high blood pressure, heart disease and more[171,172,173,174,175,176,177,178,179,180,181]. In the United States, more than 1 out of 10 adults consumes at least 25% of their total caloric intake per day from added sugars[182]. To give you an idea of how much sugar that equates to, one would need to consume between 24-47 teaspoons of sugar per day to reach this amount. However, we aren't consuming sugar by the teaspoon because it's already hidden in nearly every packaged food. Hidden sugar is a major problem and it's why we have such a high level of intake throughout the Western world because we are consuming sugar without even realizing it.

In the past, sugar consumption was very low or non-existent. For example, around 300 years ago, we only consumed a few pounds of sugar per person per year[183,184]. However, the average adult in the United States now consumes anywhere from 77-152 lbs. of sugar per year[185,186]. Certain individuals, especially children, consume abnormally high amounts of sugar, many consuming several times their body weight in sugar each year[187]. Indeed, in a study of over 1,000 American adolescents aged 14-18, the average daily intake of added sugars was 389 grams for boys and 276 grams for girls, which ended up being up to 52% of their total caloric intake[188]. Considering that there is no physiological requirement for refined sugar, this exorbitant intake is quite alarming.

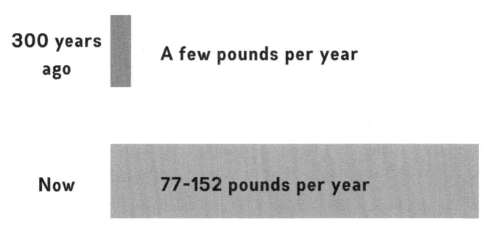

Sugar Consumption Then VS Now

300 years ago   A few pounds per year

Now   77-152 pounds per year

Redrawn From: DiNicolantonio and Lucan (2014); Storm (2012)

In the 1940s in the United States, the intake of sugar was only around 10 kilograms (22.5 pounds) per person per year[189]. However, by the 1970s sugar intake had doubled, to 20 kilograms (44 pounds) per person per year, which is when the intake of sugar really took off. From 1970 to 2000 the intake of sugar increased approximately 3-fold, going from 44 pounds per person per year to 120-152 pounds[190,191]. Essentially, we went from eating somewhere between 25-33% of our body weight in sugar per year, to eating our entire body weight in sugar per year. At the very same time the prevalence of obesity doubled in adults[192]. In men aged 60-69, the prevalence of obesity increased by more than 3-fold. Thus, the rise in the intake of sugar in the United States positively correlated with the rise in obesity. In fact, from 1950 to 2000, sugar intake increased nearly 4-fold, going from around 33 pounds per person per year to 121-154 pounds, while the prevalence of obesity in older men also increased 4-fold, going from 10% to 40%. Thus, **from 1950 to 2000, the 4-fold rise in the prevalence of obesity in older men correlated with a 4-fold rise in the intake of sugar.** It's true that correlation doesn't equal causation, however, there are many clinical studies in humans that show that the overconsumption of refined sugar leads to an increase in calories consumed and an increase in body weight/body fat, particularly if provided in liquid form[193,194,195,196].

Increase in the intake of sugar correlates with the obesity epidemic[197]

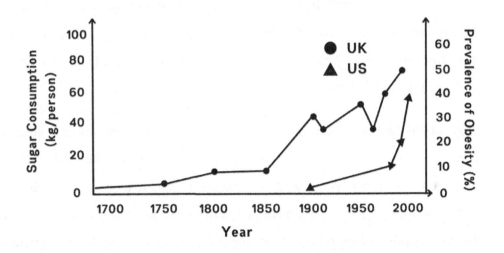

Redrawn From: Johnson et al (2007)

29

Sugar, also known as sucrose, is composed of equal parts glucose and fructose. We used to only get sugar from fruit, which came with fiber, water, and polyphenols and perhaps some honey. Moreover, as hunter gatherers, we would have had to seek out fruit and honey, which typically required walking long distances or expending significant energy climbing trees and fighting off bees to get some honey. Thus, to even be able to get something sweet we had to move our bodies.

Fruit and honey are whole foods. In other words, we don't do anything to them before we consume them. They are not processed in any way, they simply exist in nature and we consume them in their whole food form. In fact, many of the fruit that naturally occur in Africa are massive and contain large amounts of natural sugar. However, refined sugar goes through significant processing before it hits the grocery store shelf. Refined sugar comes from sugar cane or beet. The sugar from the cane is extracted as a liquid, which contains molasses and other vitamins and minerals. However, the liquid gets boiled down and all the nutritive value is removed, which leaves pure white crystals known as table sugar. This process of extracting sugar from the sugar cane is similar to what occurs with cocaine or opium. **Just like sugar, cocaine and opium are natural plant compounds that are extracted but the key is that they are all concentrated into fine powders**. And it is the concentration of plant compounds into powders/crystals that creates addictive substances.

Why would simply concentrating a natural plant compound make it addictive? The reason is because of the increased effects it has on the body once you concentrate it. When you consume pure white sugar, there is a much greater release of dopamine in the brain compared to consuming sugar from fruit[198]. With the consumption of pure crystalline sugar there is a large spike of dopamine in the brain which causes a dopamine crash later on. It's the dopamine spike, known as "the high", which then leads to a crash, known as "the low", which leads to constant sugar cravings. Additionally, there is also a concomitant blood sugar spike and crash when we overconsume refined sugar, which leads to cravings for more sugar to elevate low blood sugar levels creating a vicious cycle of high and low blood sugars and constant sugar cravings. This is what we call "the sugar spiral".

Just like alcohol is not addictive for everyone, not everyone will become addicted to sugar, but many will, especially when it's concentrated and placed into highly palatable foods like cakes, cookies, donuts, brownies, etc. The combination of added fats, refined carbs and refined sugar creates a very palatable substance creating the perfect addictive storm in the brain. When you consume these foods, the brain lights up like a pinball machine, similar to what occurs in those who use cocaine or other addictive substances and therein lies the problem.[199]

Liquid Sugar and Sugar-Sweetened Beverages

One of the easiest ways to increase someone's caloric intake is to give them sugar-sweetened beverages. Liquid sugar allows people to consume more calories faster and it doesn't provide the same amount of satiety. There is also zero fiber to slow down the sugar surge and stretch out the stomach to signal feelings of fullness. Consuming liquid sugar also creates larger spikes in blood glucose and larger blood sugar crashes. In other words, **consuming liquid sugar is one of the easiest ways to get someone to gain weight.**

In the United States, from 1955 to 1995, the intake of soft drinks increased nearly 5-fold, going from approximately 10 gallons to 47 gallons per person per year[200]. During this time, obesity rates in U.S. adults increased approximately 4-fold![201] Between 1970 and 1997 alone, the increase in soft drink consumption nearly doubled, going from 22 gallons per person per year to 41 gallons[202,203]. At the same time, the prevalence of obesity increased by over 2-fold[204]. In the United States, between 1965 to 2002, the caloric intake from sweetened beverages (soda/cola, fruit drinks, sweetened coffee, sweet tea, other sweetened beverages) more than quadrupled, going from 50 to 203 calories per day[205]. **The overconsumption of sugar-sweetened beverages, as well as other sugary beverages, is one of the biggest drivers of the obesity and Type 2 diabetes epidemic in the United States.**[206,207]

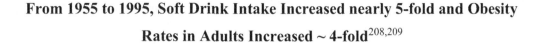

From 1955 to 1995, Soft Drink Intake Increased nearly 5-fold and Obesity Rates in Adults Increased ~ 4-fold[208,209]

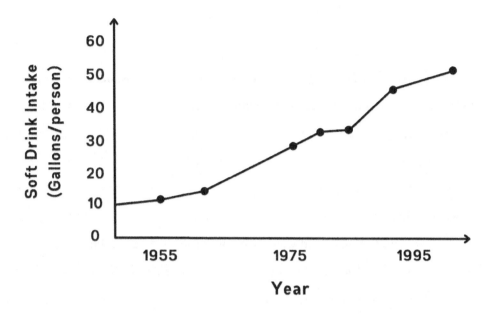

Redrawn From: Bray and Popkin (2014)

One prospective study followed 548 children and noted that for each additional serving of a sugar-sweetened beverage, body mass index and the frequency of obesity significantly increased[210]. Another study gave free-living, normal-weight subjects approximately 40 oz. of soda (sweetened with high-fructose corn syrup) per day for 3 weeks, which lead to a significantly increased intake of calories per day and an increase in body weight in both males and females[211]. In other words, when you provide free-living people with sugar-sweetened soda, they end up consuming more calories per day and gaining weight. This has been confirmed in other studies. For example, when subjects were instructed to consume a sugar-sweetened beverage during a 10-week ad libitum study, their total caloric intake significantly increased above baseline[212]. It also led to a significant increase in body weight (+3.5 pounds) and body fat (+ ~ 3 pounds) in just 10 weeks. Thus, **introducing sugar-sweetened beverages into the diet leads to an increase in**

33

calories consumed and an increase in body weight and body fat. These studies support the notion that the increased consumption of liquid sugar helped drive the obesity epidemic.

Additional data support this idea. Indeed, a meta-analysis noted that **in 12 cross-sectional studies, 10 reported a significant positive association between soft drink consumption and energy intake**, 1 reported mixed results and 1 reported no statistically significant effect[213]. A systematic review of systematic reviews found that when studies did not have a conflict to the food industry, **83.3% of studies showed a positive association with sugar-sweetened beverage consumption and weight gain[214]**. Ironically, the exact same percentage (83.3%) of studies found insufficient evidence for sugar-sweetened beverages increasing weight gain when looking at studies with conflicts to the food industry. In other words, ties to the food industry clearly biases the results of clinical studies in favor of sugar-sweetened beverages.

Sugar now goes by over 100 different names (e.g., evaporated cane juice, brown sugar, coconut sugar, agave nectar, fruit juice concentrate, etc.). **See the list on the next page for the different types of sugar to look out for in packaged foods**.

Over 100 names for sugar[215,216]

Least Refined Sugars

The processing of these sugars usually involves collecting cane juice but not removing the original cane molasses. Thus, these sugars typically have more nutrients in them (particularly iron, calcium, magnesium, vitamin B6 and selenium). They typically contain 8-14% molasses, giving them a strong flavor and brown color.

- Hand crafted cane sugar
- Unrefined cane sugar
- Whole cane sugar
- Light muscovado sugar
- Dark muscovado sugar
- Jaggery
- Ground jaggery
- Okinawa kokuto
- Piloncillo
- Panela
- Ground panela
- Sucanat
- Traditional cane syrup
- Original molasses
- Homestyle molasses
- Organic molasses
- Organic blackstrap molasses

Raw Sugars

These sugars are less refined than white sugar and typically retain around 2% molasses. This gives them a hint of flavor and color.

- Raw cane sugar
- Washed sugar
- Turbinado sugar
- Demerara sugar
- Evaporated cane juice
- Dried cane syrup
- Dehydrated cane juice
- Natural cane sugar
- Less processed sugar
- Golden sugar
- Golden syrup
- Organic sugar
- Organic powdered (confectioners)
- Organic light brown sugar
- Organic dark brown sugar
- Demerara sugar cubes
- Liquid cane sugar
- Agave nectar

Refined Sugars

Refined sugars are made from either cane or beet plants. They are highly processed and typically contain zero nutrition.

- Granulated
- Fine granulated
- Extra fine granulated
- Superfine

- Quick dissolve
- Ultrafine
- Baker's special
- Caster
- Powdered
- Confectioners
- Fondant & Icing
- Sparkling
- Sanding
- Decorating or decorative
- Swedish pearl
- Belgian pearl
- Light brown
- Golden brown
- Dark brown
- Pourable brown
- Sugar cubes
- Sugar tablets
- Gourmet sugar
- Sugar crystals
- Rock sugar
- Simple syrup
- Golden syrup
- Cane syrup
- Liquid cane sugar
- Invert (inverted) syrup
- Invert (liquid invert) sugar
- Light or mild molasses
- Baking molasses
- Full molasses
- Robust molasses
- Black treacle
- Barley malt
- Barley malt syrup
- Brown rice syrup

- Corn sweetener
- Corn syrup
- Corn syrup solids
- Dextrin
- Dextrose
- Malt syrup
- Maltodextrin
- Maltose
- Rice syrup
- High-maltose corn syrup
- Agave syrup
- Beet sugar
- Birch syrup
- Caramel
- Date sugar
- Dehydrated cane juice
- Castor sugar
- Carob syrup
- High-fructose corn syrup
- Sorghum syrup
- Yellow sugar
- Refiner's sugar
- Refiner's syrup
- Birch syrup
- Buttered syrup
- Grape sugar
- Non-centrifugal cane sugar
- Panela sugar
- Powdered sugar
- Icing sugar
- Glucose

Here is a list of the healthier natural sugars

- Raw honey
- Pure maple syrup
- Blackstrap molasses
- Jaggery

These more natural sugars are not nearly as bad as refined sugars, but they still need to be limited.

Refined Carbohydrates

The increased intake of refined sugar isn't the only thing that increased during the obesity epidemic. Indeed, an increase in the intake of refined carbohydrates, such as white flour, refined wheat, corn, and other grains also occurred. **Jean Anthelme Brillat-Savarin, a 19th century physician, wrote in 1825 that the second main cause of obesity is the excess consumption of starch and floury foods, which are also used to fatten up animals[217]. In the early 1900s, physicians considered refined carbohydrates to be the primary drivers of obesity[218].**

Prior to the invention of the steel roller mill in the late 1800s, grains were stone ground. However, when you take a grain and run it through a steel roller mill, this pulverizes the grain into very fine particles and it removes the bran, which is where the fiber resides. Thus, consuming refined grains leads to higher spikes in blood glucose and insulin and larger drops in blood sugar[219]. Consequently, refining grains makes them easier to overconsume, which can lead to continued cravings, insulin resistance and obesity. People with type-1 diabetes who inject insulin several times a day often gain weight rapidly[220]. A 1993 study took 14 diabetics and administered them insulin over a period of 6 months. The subjects' bodyweight increased on average by 8.7 kg-s (19 lbs), despite eating 300 fewer calories per day[221]. You can still lose weight with high levels of insulin when being in an energy deficit. However, if the body detects a state of constant nourishment and energy abundance, it becomes harder to reach a subjective negative energy balance.

Milled smooth grain leads to higher spikes in insulin vs. coarse grain

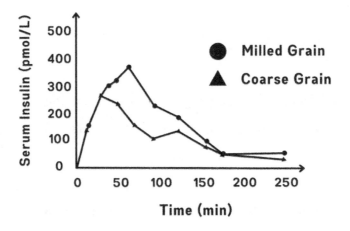

Redrawn From: Edwards et al (2015)

Milled smooth grain leads to higher spikes in glucose and higher risk for low blood sugar

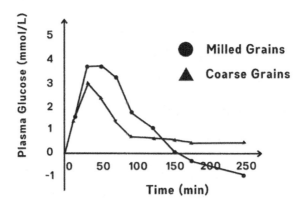

Redrawn From: Edwards et al (2015)

In the United States, the intake of refined carbohydrates, from flour and cereal products, went from 135.1 pounds per person per year in 1970-1974, to 200 pounds by the year 2000[222]. At the same, the prevalence of obesity doubled, going from around 14% to 28%. The overconsumption of refined carbohydrates is harmful to metabolic health but is not as bad as sugar. Indeed, in animals, replacing starch with sugar increases fasting insulin, worsens insulin sensitivity and leads to increased glucose concentrations[223,224,225,226,227,228,229]. There are also more detrimental effects on apolipoprotein B, triglycerides, fat storage and blood pressure. Studies in humans show that added fructose promotes impaired glucose tolerance versus other refined carbohydrates even when matched for total calories[230,231,232]. Men who replace wheat starch with sucrose have significantly higher mean fasting serum insulin levels, insulin to glucose ratio and insulin response to a given sucrose load[233]. The greater the amount of sugar that replaces wheat starch, even when calories stay the same, the worse the fasting serum insulin and insulin and glucose responses to a sucrose load[234]. Thus, refined carbohydrates are bad, but sugar is worse, even when matched for calories.

Prevalence of obesity in U.S. increased with increased refined carbohydrate intake[235]

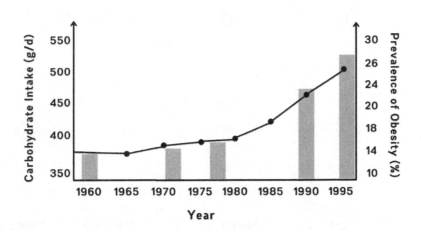

Redrawn From: Gross et al (2004)

Refined Omega-6 Seed Oils

Throughout our evolution we used to consume an omega-6:3 ratio of around 4-1:1[236,237]. The optimal ratio for health is somewhere around that balance. However, nowadays, we consume an omega-6:3 ratio of 20-50:1[238]. The increase in the intake of omega-6 primarily came from omega-6 seed oils, which were introduced into the United States in the early 1900s[239]. Indeed, cottonseed oil was the main ingredient in Crisco, which was invented in 1910. Other omega-6 seed oils followed, such as soybean, safflower, sunflower, corn, and canola. These omega-6 seed oils were created as a cheaper alternative to butter and tallow. Manufacturers of these omega-6 seed oils began promoting their toxic oils to the American public and it worked. In the United States, the intake of soybean oil increased by over 1,000-fold from 1909 to 1999[240]. The intake of linoleic acid, the omega-6 fat in industrial seed oils, went from making up just 2% of total caloric intake in the early 1900s, to 8-10% of total energy intake[241]. Furthermore, the level of linoleic acid stored in our fat tissue increased by ~ 2.5-fold, going from 9.1% to 21.5% from 1959 to 2008[242]. Thus, we started eating a tremendous amount these omega-6 seeds oils before and during the obesity epidemic.

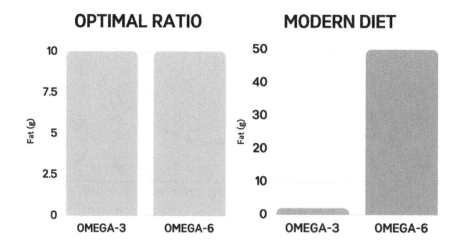

A diet high in the omega-6:3 ratio causes an increase in endocannabinoid signaling, leading to increased inflammation and obesity[243]. In animal studies, a high omega-6 intake decreases insulin sensitivity in muscle and promotes fat accumulation in adipose tissue, whereas dietary omega-3 reverses these issues[244]. A higher amount of linoleic acid (the omega-6 fat found in seed oils) in adipose tissue paralleled the rise in diabetes, obesity, allergies and asthma[245,246]. On the other hand, in mice, omega-3s promote fat burning and inhibit fat cell growth/proliferation[247,248,249,250]. It's been found that rats fed fish oil have lower visceral fat and less insulin resistance compared to those given corn oil or lard[251]. Even in the absence of these pro-inflammatory effects, added refined seed oils contribute a large percentage of extra unnecessary calories to an individual's diet. **Up to 20% of the total calories consumed by Americans comes from high linoleic acid soybean oil, which contributes to > 7% of the daily calories coming from omega-6 fats alone**[252]. Thus, an increase in the intake of omega-6 likely contributed to the obesity epidemic through various mechanisms.

% Caloric Intake from Linoleic Acid in the United States[253]

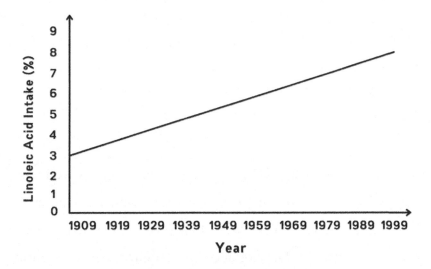

Redrawn From: Blasbalg et al (2011)

43

Linoleic Acid in Subcutaneous Adipose Tissue in the United States[254]

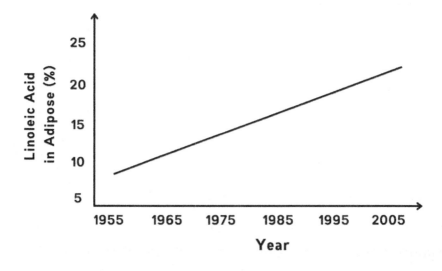

Redrawn From: Guyenet et al (2015)

It's important to remember that refined omega-6 seed oils have negative effects on metabolic health and are contributing to the rising rates of obesity through their prevalence in the food supply. Most processed foods and packaged meals have added canola oil, soybean oil or sunflower oil. This increases their overall calorie content, making it easy for individuals who consume those products to be in a caloric surplus. Whole foods rarely have added fats unless you use things like olive oil on your salad or other fats for cooking.

Trans-Fats

Trans-fats are created when solidifying industrial omega-6 seed oils. Trans-fats were originally introduced into the American diet with the creation of Crisco and then margarines. When World War II hit, the need to conserve animal fats increased, and between the shortages and required rationing during the war, people were forced to rely on these partially hydrogenated seed oils instead of animal fats[255,256,257]. Unfortunately, this switch has had a detrimental effect on people's health worldwide. Trans fat consumption has been linked to obesity, metabolic syndrome, heart disease, cancer, and Alzheimer's[258,259]. A Medical Research Council survey showed that men eating butter ran half the risk of developing heart disease as those using margarine[260]. Fortunately, in 2015, the FDA determined Partially Hydrogenated Oils (PHOs), which includes margarine and other trans fats, to no longer be Generally Recommended as Safe (GRAS)[261]. As of June 18, 2018, companies cannot add PHOs or other trans fats into their food products anymore.

Fats and Cheese

From 1970-1974 to 2000, the consumption of fats and oils increased from 55.7 pounds to 77.1 pounds/year[262]. Added fats (excluding naturally occurring fat in meats, milks, nuts, and avocados) went from 47.9 pounds per person in 1970-1974 to 65.3 pounds in the year 2000. This is reflected in the overall rise in total calorie intake. Red meat consumption, however, decreased from 177.2 pounds per person per year in 1970-1974 to 113.7 pounds in 2000. In other words, it doesn't appear that red meat is the cause of the obesity epidemic. The consumption of eggs also decreased during this time, from 285 eggs per year in 1970-1979 to 250 eggs in 2000[263]. Despite these reductions, obesity and Type 2 diabetes rates haven't decreased, in fact, they've increased. This doesn't mean that one couldn't become overweight if they ate too much bacon, butter, or burgers but they do not appear to be primary culprits of the obesity epidemic.

Cheese is high in fat and if overconsumed can promote weight gain, especially if eaten together with other high calorie foods, such as pizza, burgers, or fries. The intake of total cheese (excluding cream cheese) increased from 18.6 pounds in 1970-1979 to 30 pounds in 2000, a 61% increase[264]. Cottage cheese was down by

47% but mozzarella cheese was up by 365%! Cottage cheese is much higher in protein and lower in fat/calories than mozzarella cheese. It seems that we can't get enough of our refined carbohydrates combined with our favorite cheese and that is a recipe for weight gain. Cheese is often added to hyperpalatable foods like pizza and burgers to increase the palatability and lead to overconsumption.

Fruit and Vegetables

In the U.S., fresh vegetable intake rose by 35% from 1970-1974 to 2000 with an 82% increase in frozen potatoes. Typically, most "vegetables" consumed in the United States are corn, peas, and potatoes, which are starchy vegetables and aren't particularly high in fiber after prolonged cooking. **Epidemiological studies find that dietary fiber intake is associated with lower bodyweight, mostly because fiber promotes satiety and fiber-rich foods tend to be lower in calories**[265,266,267]. Fiber can also bind to fat, which reduces the amount of fat absorbed during digestion, helping to establish a greater calorie deficit[268,269].

The amount of fiber in starchy vegetables depends on how much you cook them. For example, consuming lightly cooked potatoes provides much more fiber and less starch compared to overcooked potatoes. Furthermore, potatoes provide a good amount of potassium and base-forming substances to help balance the acid load of animal foods. Thus, if you don't overcook your potatoes, they can be a good source of fiber and nutrients without providing too many carbohydrates. However, this is not the type of potatoes that we started eating. In addition to the higher intake of frozen potatoes, we started adding more fats, oils and cheese to the potatoes, which as discussed previously, is a recipe for obesity.

Many proponents of low carb diets say that the obesity epidemic is caused by eating too many carbohydrates. However, as we've seen by the evidence, total carbohydrate intake hasn't increased any more than the overall fat intake. It's the increase in ultra-processed foods that are high in calories from both fats and carbohydrates that is the main culprit. **Studies controlling for calorie intake have consistently found that low carb and low-fat diets work equally in terms of weight loss**[270,271,272,273,274,275,276]. A 2021 controlled-feeding trial on 20 adults discovered that a low fat plant-based diet resulted in about 500-700 fewer calories consumed than a carb restricted control group during 3 weeks of ad libitum food consumption[277]. This is probably due to fibrous vegetables providing more satiety with fewer calories ingested. In the real world context, where you're eating ad libitum, choosing more high fiber foods would generally lead to a spontaneous reduction in calorie intake. Thus, the obesity epidemic is not caused by eating too many low calorie fibrous vegetables. Quite the opposite, eating more low calorie fibrous vegetables, instead of other high calorie foods, would most certainly help individuals to lose weight.

The intake of fresh fruit only increased by 30% from 1970-1974 to 2000, going from 97.6 pounds to 126.9 pounds[278]. Fructose, which if consumed in a liquid in the form of added sugars, promotes less satiety than glucose and results in a smaller suppression of ghrelin (the hunger hormone) after a meal[279,280]. Sugar-sweetened beverages and high-fructose corn syrup may harm the body by stimulating the ghrelin receptor[281]. Fruit isn't inherently harmful for weight loss as it's still quite low in calories compared to sugar-sweetened beverages for example. However, fruit is generally much more easy to overconsume than broccoli or carrots. That's why an excess consumption of fruit, especially in those with baseline insulin resistance, may slow down attempts to lose weight by providing you too many calories. Sticking to berries (such as strawberries, raspberries, and blueberries) are a good way to get the polyphenols in fruit but a lower amount of sugar and calories. Eating unripe fruit is also a better way to get more fiber and less sugar. In other words, stick to eating hard fruit rather than soft fruit, or simply consume fruit in moderation.

Key Take-Aways

Sugar, whether it be added sugar in processed foods or liquids, was not the only driver of the obesity epidemic. There was also a dramatic increase in processed foods that were high in both fat and refined carbohydrates, resulting in an exponential rise in total daily calorie intake. In nature, we would have only consumed large amounts of fat and carbohydrates together when breast feeding, or if we consumed fresh liver (glycogen) plus organ fat. Furthermore, in ancestral times, the harms from a combined intake of fat and carbohydrates would have been alleviated by periods of food shortages, famines and by being more physically active.

Solving the obesity crisis requires addressing all the aforementioned factors and not simply advice to restrict caloric intake. Simply telling people to "eat less and move more" isn't addressing the root problem. Access to the current dietary guidelines has had little to no success in addressing overeating and poor dietary choices[282]. Thus, knowing what to do or being told what to do isn't enough to make any real positive changes. Ultimately, consuming whole nutritious foods (high in protein and fiber) and reducing the intake of processed junk food, is about the best advice that anyone could ever get for weight loss. However, there are other strategies that can take your fat loss to the next level, which we will cover in the following chapters.

Chapter 2: The Calorie Conundrum

You've probably heard about the concept of eating less calories when it comes to weight loss. Essentially, based on the second law of thermodynamics, you must be in a calorie deficit to lose weight and in a calorie surplus to gain weight[283,284,285]. At its core, this principle is true – the body needs to experience a negative energy balance to start withdrawing its backup fuel from stored fat. However, human beings aren't isolated systems with a stagnant metabolism. Our metabolic rate and energy balance are in constant motion and adaptation, which determine the rate of weight loss or gain. We wholly acknowledge the relevance of the calories in vs calories out model as the foundation to changes in one's body composition. However, we also need to stress the importance of additional factors that apply to weight loss.

There are many variables that change a person's energy balance and metabolic rate. For example, women who reported having more stress during the previous 24 hours have been found to burn 104 fewer calories than those who didn't experience any stressors[286]. This is hypothesized to be caused by higher levels of cortisol that suppress fat oxidation. People who used to be obese have also been observed to have a lower resting metabolic rate due to lower thyroid hormone output[287]. Prolonged periods of energy deficit lead to metabolic adaptations that decrease metabolic rate[288,289,290,291]. As a result, the body finds itself at a new threshold requiring greater effort to continue to lose weight. In this example, the second law of thermodynamics is still present, but the efficacy of remaining in calorie deficit becomes increasingly more difficult. Yes, a person needs to experience some sort of an energy deficit to lose weight but this does not mean it has to come from eating less or exercising more. For example, fixing nutrient deficiencies, adding supplements or getting better sleep can improve metabolic rate by enhancing hormone function, fat burning and/or muscle growth and thereby lead to more weight loss without eating less or exercising more. This is why two different people can eat the exact same diet (and the same amount of calories) and yet one person may lose weight and the other person may not (this happens all the time in nutrition studies, i.e., when placed on certain diets the weight loss of each individual in the study is all over the place, and only the average weight loss results are reported). It's not because of differences in calorie intake, it's because of differences in their physiology, which is ultimately driven by the quality of the food they eat and their lifestyle of the past several months. Everyone's weight loss threshold is different and it's possible to regulate where this threshold lies with what you eat (quality of your food), in what amounts, when you eat, how you exercise and what's the current state of your metabolic health.

To support some of the ideas we just mentioned, there are studies whereby simply giving certain supplements, such as sulforaphane, capsaicin/cayenne pepper, astaxanthin or berberine leads to fat loss despite no drops in caloric intake[292,293,294,295]. According to the "calories in vs calories out" model, weight loss should not have occurred because caloric intake did not drop. However, the reason why taking certain supplements can cause fat loss is because they can help improve metabolism, fat burning, hormone sensitivity, mitochondrial biogenesis (the growth of new mitochondria) and more[296,297,298,299,300]. These same differences in metabolism/hormones can occur when selecting different types of foods. Indeed, wild salmon is high in astaxanthin, and taking 8 mg of astaxanthin per day has been shown to significantly reduce visceral fat[301]. In other words, there are more important things that impact weight/fat loss in food than just calories. This doesn't mean calories don't matter – the energy balance is still the biggest determining factor. However, certain foods, habits and other factors regulate wherein that energy homeostasis lies and whether your body can achieve a negative calorie balance.

CALORIE BALANCE MODEL

Calories in < Calories Out = Weight loss

Adaptive Energy Balance Model

Weight Loss Inhibitory Factors

- Low muscle mass
- Insulin resistance
- Low thyroid
- Low fat oxidation
- Ultra-processed food
- Nutrient deficiencies
- Sleep deprivation

↓

Development of Obesity

Lifestyle change →

Weight Loss Supportive Factors

- Muscle mass
- Insulin sensitivity
- Normal thyroid
- High fat oxidation
- Nutritious food
- Adequate nutrients
- Adequate sleep

↓

Healthy Weight or Weight Loss

Thus, energy balance is as much dependent on your overall metabolic condition as it is on energy balance. If your body and hormones are geared more towards fat storage and low energy expenditure, as is seen in people who eat ultra-processed foods and/or have other metabolic ailments, it's going to be harder for your body to establish a calorie deficit and lose weight. The threshold at which your body begins to tap into its stored body fat has decreased so low that it feels impossible to lose weight. Thus, identifying and fixing the inhibitory mechanisms that counteract attempts to lose weight will make the process easier again. Calorie balance matters, but we shouldn't look at it in isolation, especially when talking about free-living humans who aren't willing or able to know exactly wherein their calorie balance lies at any moment. So, yes calories and energy balance matter, but we should also focus on improving the body's overall metabolic health in which weight loss and fat burning become an easier thing to achieve. We'll get back to that later but let's first understand your body's metabolic rate and calorie balance.

Basics of Calories

The U.S. Dietary Guidelines recommends women eat 1600-2400 calories per day and men 2000-3000[302]. In reality, overall caloric requirements vary greatly between individuals, depending on several factors. The Total Daily Energy Expenditure (TDEE) includes multiple variables that can be affected by gender, lifestyle habits, daily activities and current body composition. **Men tend to have a higher TDEE than women because of their higher muscle mass and testosterone levels which promotes muscle growth**[303]. Circulating levels of testosterone are positively associated with an increase in lean muscle tissue, strength and power[304]. Men also have a higher amount of androgen receptors that testosterone can attach to and trigger muscle protein synthesis[305,306]. Androgen receptors are located more on the upper body and shoulders in men, which is why they tend to have wider shoulders than women. Women, on the other hand, typically have weight accumulation around the midsection and hips[307]. Estrogen-dominant men with low testosterone may also develop this kind of pear-like body shape and gynecomastia (enlargement of breast tissue)[308]. Thus, hormones certainly play a role in weight loss or weight gain.

Here's what makes up your Total Daily Energy Expenditure (TDEE)[309]:

- **Basal Metabolic Rate (BMR)** refers to the number of calories your body is burning at rest when doing nothing. It includes breathing, heartbeat, brain function, circulation, and other maintenance physiological processes. The BMR makes up 60-70% of TDEE. **Muscle burns 2-3 times more calories than fat mass**[310], which means that having more lean tissue raises your BMR.

- **Exercise Activity Thermogenesis (EAT)** refers to calories burned during deliberate exercise. EAT typically contributes 0-10% of TDEE, depending on the duration and intensity of the exercise[311]. Exercise does increase your TDEE but most people only workout for about 30 minutes per day. For professional athletes and fitness enthusiasts, this number can certainly be a lot higher, but the average person doesn't typically dedicate a lot of time to exercise. Thus, one should certainly exercise frequently and build muscle but it's equally important to focus on creating an energy deficit through other less strenuous means.

- **Non-Exercise Activity Thermogenesis (NEAT)** refers to the number of calories burned while doing spontaneous non-exercise-like activities throughout the day, such as walking, taking the stairs, fidgeting, house chores, etc. NEAT contributes around 20% of TDEE, depending on your amount of spontaneous movement[312].

  o With low thyroid and chronic low-calorie intake, you may see a large reduction in NEAT, which does reduce your TDEE as well. This can make it seem that weight loss has plateaued but, you're just burning less calories due to moving less. To overcome this, you'd have to either move more or adjust your food intake accordingly. It's also possible to maintain high NEAT even during low calorie intakes but for that you would need to be getting all the necessary micro- and macronutrients that promote vitality and energy production. Maintaining high NEAT with a nutrient-deprived ultra-processed diet would be harder because the body lacks the necessary resources to function at its peak.

- **Thermic Effect of Food (TEF)** describes the number of calories spent on digestion. Protein has a TEF of 20-30%, carbs 7-15%, alcohol 15% and fat 2-4%[313]. Overall, TEF on a regular diet with mixed macros contributes about 5-15% to your total daily energy expenditure[314].

Energy Source	Thermic Effect	Calories Per Gram	Calories Stored Per 100 Calories
Alcohol	15%	7	85
Exogenous Ketones	3%	4	97
Protein	25-30%	4	70-75
Carbohydrates	7-10%	4	90
Glycogen Spillover	15-20%	4	80
Fat	3%	9	97

- o **High protein diets appear to be superior for weight loss because they burn more calories through TEF**[315,316]. Thus, when you get a large % of your daily calories as protein, you're going to be burning 20-30% simply trying to digest it, helping to create an energy deficit. In other words, 20-30% of the calories coming from protein are used to metabolize that protein. Thus, 1,000 calories of protein from a pork chop, is really like 700-800 calories. Furthermore, **protein is more satiating compared to carbohydrates and fat**. Additionally, protein provides prolonged satiety, and high protein foods (such as meat, fish, and eggs) are also the most nutrient dense, making protein the most nourishing macronutrient to target[317,318]. **When people are allowed to eat as much as they desire on a diet that consists of 30% protein, they end up consuming on average 441 fewer calories per day compared to eating only 10% protein**[319].

- o **Eating a high protein breakfast, such as eggs, increases satiety and reduces the calorie intake of subsequent meals compared to a cereal or bagel breakfast**[320,321]. The same effect is seen at lunch with an omelette compared to a jacket potato meal[322].

Different foods (and the calories they provide) have different effects on our hormones, satiety, fat storing/burning genes, metabolic rate, gut health, and a lot more. In other words, all calories are not created equal. For example, if you eat 1,500 calories from donuts you should not expect the same weight loss as eating 1,500 calories of broccoli. First, it's extremely challenging to eat 1,500 calories of broccoli because that would entail eating 5 kilograms of broccoli. A single donut, however, can provide you with up to 500 calories and eating 3 donuts is relatively easy, especially due to its hyperpalatable taste. It's not even a challenge to eat 3,000 calories worth of donuts in one sitting, whereas your satiety mechanisms will kick in much sooner with broccoli. Second, broccoli has a completely different TEF than donuts and it's higher in fiber, which results in a much larger proportion of the calories from broccoli being used for digestion.

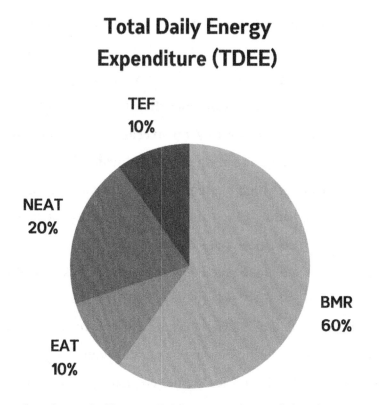

Total Daily Energy Expenditure (TDEE)

TEF
10%

NEAT
20%

EAT
10%

BMR
60%

BMR = basal metabolic rate, **EAT** = exercise activity thermogenesis, **NEAT** = non-exercise activity thermogenesis, **TEF** = thermic effect of food

It's difficult to precisely know your total daily energy expenditure. However, you can predict your BMR with sufficient accuracy. The most common formulas for measuring one's resting metabolic rate are the Cunningham equation, the Harris-Benedict equation, and the Mifflin St-Jeor equation. For non-obese people, the most used one is the Harris-Benedict formula[323]. However, it has been found to overestimate metabolic rate[324,325,326]. The Cunningham formula is based more on lean tissue, which makes it superior for those who are muscular[327,328]. Indeed, this formula has been found to be quite accurate in recreational athletes aged 18-35[329], which is why we suggest using this one for that specific group.

Here's the Cunningham equation for measuring your basal metabolic rate (BMR):

BMR = 22 x lean body mass (in kg) + 500

It has been argued that losing one pound of weight requires a 3,500-calorie deficit[330]. This would be true if one were to lose only adipose tissue[331,332]. However, weight loss isn't always the same as fat loss. For example, during weight loss you can lose primarily muscle and little fat[333,334]. During weight loss you also lose water, stored glycogen, and triglycerides[335,336]. Weight loss, at the expense of muscle, is unwanted and can lead to weight regain after dieting because one's basal metabolic rate drops due to the loss of lean tissue[337,338]. Skeletal muscle contributes about 15-17% to an average person's BMR[339,340,341]. It's also essential for preventing injuries, exercise performance and bone density[342,343,344]. Thus, you shouldn't be that focused solely on weight loss but more so on losing fat mass and maintaining or building lean muscle tissue. Building muscle improves your physique and makes weight loss easier. Thus, just being in a negative energy balance will indeed lead to a loss in bodyweight but whether the results are desired (fat loss and not muscle loss) depends on the way you go about establishing that deficit. That's why we encourage people to look beyond just calories in vs. calories out and consider the other variables we'll be discussing now.

It's also thought that your metabolism becomes slower with age, making it hard to lose weight. Although there is some truth to this idea, it's not as significant as you would think. A 2021 study found that an individual's metabolic rate stays relatively stable between ages 20 and 60, after which it begins to decrease 0.7% per year[345]. Your metabolism takes a steeper drop after 60 years of age and at 90 it's 26% lower compared to your midlife[346]. Thus, most adults in their 30s, 40s and 50s aren't gaining weight because of their declining metabolism. It's more so because of the overconsumption of ultra-processed foods that are creeping in additional calories into their diet and the harmful metabolic effects they cause.

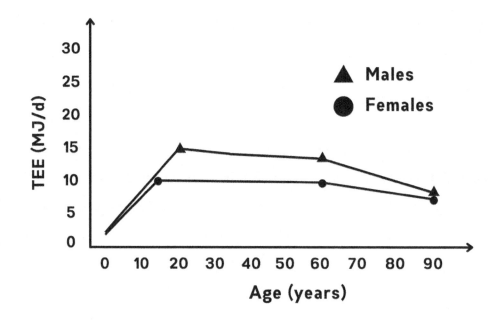

Total Energy Expenditure (TEE) across a lifespan
Redrawn From: Pontzer et al (2021)

Most people do not count how many calories they are eating in a day. Thus, the biggest factor that will help with weight loss is how satiating the diet is. Let's be honest, unless you literally weigh all the food you eat, you will not know exactly how many calories you're eating and whether or not you are in a calorie deficit. Thus, the easier and more logical solution is to leave your energy intake up to your body, let your body tell you when its full. This can be done by consuming whole nutritious foods that are satiating.

For sustainable weight loss focus on:

1.) **Consuming whole foods high in protein** (meat, eggs, fish) **and fiber/water** (berries, apples, broccoli, greenish bananas, potatoes).

2.) **Targeting your daily protein intake** (consume ~ 1-1.25 grams of protein per pound of lean body weight split between 2-4 meals per day)

3.) **Building muscle** (resistance exercise 3-4 times per week)

4.) **Intermittent fasting on non-work out days** (for most people this means skipping one meal, i.e., eating two meals per day instead of three meals)

These four above interventions will lead to greater weight loss compared to any other dietary or lifestyle intervention.

Does Over-Eating Calories Always Lead to Weight Gain

Many overfeeding experiments have shown that an excess consumption of calories usually results in less than expected weight gain[347]. That's because increasing energy intake increases energy expenditure, reflected in higher physical activity, increase in thyroid hormones and adaptive thermogenesis which is the increased production of heat in response to an increased caloric intake[348]. In other words, how much the body turns down heat production with calorie restriction or turns up heat production with calorie excess determines energy balance[349]. Some people may start to produce a lot of heat and use more ATP when they eat more calories, a phenomenon called ATP futile cycles, which buffers against weight gain from increased caloric intake. In other words, simply eating slightly more calories does not necessarily lead to weight/fat gain if it is offset by an increased heat production.

Several studies show that overfeeding leads to an increase in basal metabolic rate[350,351,352,353,354,355,356,357,358,359]. However, different diets have different effects on this outcome. Indeed, overfeeding mixed diets leads to different percentages of the excess energy intake that gets stored, ranging between 60-90%[360,361,362,363]. All overfeeding studies show a large inter-individual variation in weight gain[364]. Indeed, one study looked at 12 pairs of adult male twins and found that overfeeding of 1,000 calories per day, 6 days a week, for 84 out of 100 days caused a wide range of weight gain. Some individuals gained only 4.3 kilograms, whereas others gained 13.3 kilograms. If it's all about calories, then the weight gain should have been consistent across the individuals, however, there was a greater than 3-fold difference in weight gain. The range in visceral fat gain was also extremely variable, from essential zero to an increase of more than 200 percent. Importantly, the weight gain was similar among the twins, which suggests that hormonal and genetic differences is what primarily determines the amount of weight gain with overfeeding calories and not calories themselves. Indeed, the authors concluded: *"When the results for all 24 men were analyzed, the correlations between the total energy ingested during the 100-day period (including the 84,000-kcal surplus) and the gains in body weight (r = 0.26), fat mass (r = 0.26), sum of 10 skin-fold—thickness measurements (r = 0.25), and abdominal visceral fat (r = −0.31) were not statistically significant."*[365] In other words, the surplus of ingested calories did not significantly correlate with weight/fat gain.

The authors went on to state:

> *...the findings that some persons were more prone than others to store fat on the trunk, in the abdominal cavity, or both are of considerable clinical interest.*

The most likely explanation for the resemblance between identical twins in the response to overfeeding is that a person's genotype is an important determinant of adaptation to a sustained energy surplus. Since the excess energy intake involved the same composition of macronutrients and was fixed at 84,000 kcal for all the men, and since they kept the same relatively sedentary schedule during the period of overfeeding, differences in the efficiency of weight gain could result either from individual variation in the preferential storage of energy as fat or lean tissue or from variation in the components of energy expenditure during rest.

Our results strongly support the view that there are individual differences in the tendency toward obesity and in the distribution of body fat, and they suggest that these differences are partly related to undetermined genetic characteristics.[366]

Another study confirmed that a large variation in weight gain occurs with overfeeding calories[367]. This time however, the authors were able to pinpoint that a lot of this variation was due to non-exercise activity thermogenesis (NEAT). Indeed, 16 non-obese individuals were fed 1000 kilocalories per day more than weight-maintenance requirements for 8 weeks. During overfeeding there was an increase in total daily energy expenditure (TDEE), with two-thirds of the increases being due to NEAT, i.e., fidgeting, maintenance of posture, and other physical activities of daily life. Changes in NEAT accounted for the 10-fold differences in fat storage that occurred and directly predicted resistance to fat gain with overfeeding. These results suggest that certain humans will start to move more because they have overconsumed calories helping to preserve leanness. The reason they gained less weight from overfeeding was due to burning off more calories with their increased NEAT, which coincides with the second law of thermodynamics. It's just that individuals respond differently to overfeeding/underfeeding, depending on their metabolic condition and habits, which changes their results. **If you eat more calories, you tend to move more and you tend to gain less weight than originally expected. Those individuals who do not move as much end up gaining more weight.** This occurs on a subconscious level or due to other hormonal conditions, such as hypothyroidism. **In other words, your body determines calories in vs. calories out**[368]. If you have a good baseline metabolism and your hormones are working appropriately, you will likely move more when you overeat, whereas if you have a broken metabolism, you will probably not move more when overfed. Ultimately, this means that it's not always the result of just overeating calories that causes weight gain or the degree of weight gain but the response to those calories.

Differences in NEAT and adaptive thermogenesis may be the two biggest factors involved in whether someone gains weight with increased caloric intake. Importantly, these factors are determined by your baseline metabolic health. In other words, eating healthy foods and exercising improves adaptive thermogenesis and reduces weight gain with increased caloric intake. Essentially, a positive energy balance may not lead to obesity if someone is metabolically healthy and has good adaptive thermogenic responses to increased caloric intake. Studies conclude that adaptive thermogenesis does occur during overfeeding, considering that weight gain is less than expected and this can even be explained from what is called non-exercise activity thermogenesis (fidgeting, sitting, and standing). Obesity-prone people have a reduced capacity for adaptive thermogenesis compared to obesity-resistant people. For example, fat oxidation (burning) is greater in lean individuals vs. obese subjects during overfeeding[369,370].

Ultimately, if a body is healthy, it knows how many calories it needs, if you decide to acutely eat more than needed in one sitting, the body will do things

on a subconscious level to burn those extra calories off. Individuals who have a broken metabolism or dysfunctional hormones do not get the appropriate signals to increase their activity to burn the extra calories ingested. Thus, the goal isn't to tell someone to exercise more, because the body is supposed to do that for you! The goal is to fix the underlying biology and hormones so that their body automatically increases activity if it overeats. Again, calories matter, and yes you can be meticulous about the calories you eat vs. the calories you burn, but this isn't the point because we already showed you how different foods, regardless of increased calories, can lead to huge differences in weight gain. We also must eat to reach adequate nutrient intakes, so to think it's just about calories is only looking at half the picture. The calorie in vs. calorie out model of obesity assumes that the calories ingested is independent of calories burned. In other words, the model assumes that if you eat more, you will not increase activity. However, as the experiments previously mentioned so nicely demonstrated, calories in and calories out are highly dependent on each other (i.e., if you increase your intake of calories, you may start fidgeting more without realizing it because your body is telling you to burn the extra calories).

Why You Should Focus on More Than Just Calories

The second law of thermodynamics, that energy is neither created nor destroyed, doesn't consider changes in satiety, hormones, and metabolism with varying food choices. Thus, this law doesn't work in free-living humans who aren't counting calories. Here are some examples that challenge the myth that weight loss is solely determined by calories in versus calories out.

Take for example dietary fat. There are many different types of fats, such as medium chain triglycerides (MCTs), long-chain saturated fats, monounsaturated fat, polyunsaturated fat (omega-3s and omega-6 fats). Were you aware that each of these fats have different oxidation rates? In other words, matched for calories, different fats will get burned better for fuel vs. stored as fat in the body because their make-up is different.

- For example, **medium chain triglycerides (MCTs) are not as readily stored as fat as their oxidation rate is the highest among all the fats**[371]. MCTs are primarily turned into ketones and used as fuel. The increased liberation of energy with the consumption of MCTs can even increase the desire to perform physical activity[372]. In other words, **the quality and types of foods you choose can even affect your physical activity level!**
- **Long-chain saturated fats (e.g., cheese, heavy cream, full-fat milk, and butter) on the other hand have the lowest oxidation rates of all the fats and will be more readily stored as fat vs. burned for energy**, particularly if consumed with carbohydrate because glucose inhibits the oxidation of fatty acids further[373]. This isn't to say that consuming long-chain saturated fats are bad, far from it, but it shows that different foods have different effects on fat loss and physical activity that has nothing to do with differences in calories.

One study proved that weight/fat loss in humans is only minimally explained by differences in caloric intake, whereas most weight/fat loss is explained by the type of foods/fats that are consumed. Indeed, this group of authors took participants and had them replace long-chain saturated fats (e.g., full-fat milk, cream, and butter) with monounsaturated fats (MUFA) (olive oil, nuts, and avocado). This one change caused an ~ 6-pound fat loss in just 4 weeks without a significant difference in calories consumed![374] To be fair, those in the MUFA group did consume slightly less calories per day from a numeric perspective (i.e., 166.75 less calories per day) but this was not statistically significant. Even if we multiply the 166.75 calories less per day for the 28 days of the study, we get a total of 4,669 less calories consumed over the 4 weeks in the MUFA group vs. the long-chain saturated fat group. If we use the 3,500 calories equals 1 pound of body fat model, then this calorie deficit should have led to a 1.3-pound fat loss. However, the actual fat loss was 5.7 pounds. **In other words, the caloric deficit only explains 22.8% (less than one quarter) of the fat loss in this study. This study proves that eating less calories is not the most important factor for fat loss but rather it's the types of foods consumed that matters most.** Thus, when eating a diet moderately high in carbohydrates, replacing things like full-fat milk, cream, cheese and butter with extra virgin olive oil, nuts and avocadoes leads to significant fat loss that has very little to do with less calories consumed.

Focusing on calories also fails to consider the different levels of satiety of foods. This has been formally studied, where foods like potatoes (which are high in fiber and water) or steak (which is high in protein) have been found to be the most satiating[375]. This was measured by looking at how much calories the participants consumed at an ad libitum buffet after having eaten different types of only a single food. Some foods are easy to consume and are not very filling (think fries and chips), whereas foods high in water, fiber and protein are the most satiating (think potatoes and steak, respectively). In other words, eating 2000 calories from fries and chips will lead to completely different satiety signals and changes in metabolism/hormones, especially over the long run, compared to eating 2,000 calories from potatoes and steak.

Satiety Index of Common Foods

Food	Satiety Index
White Potatoes	———————————————— 323
White Fish	———————————
Porridge	———————
Oranges	———————
Apples	———————
Brown Pasta	——————
Red Meat	——————
Beans & Sauce	——————
Grapes	—————
Grain Bread	—————
Rye Bread	—————
All-Bran	—————
Popcorn & Butter	—————
Poached Eggs	—————
Cheddar Cheese	—————
Lentils & Sauce	—————
Crackers	————
Cookies	————
Bananas	————
White Pasta	————
Cork Flakes	————
French Fries	————
Ice Cream	———
Potato Chips	———
Chocolate Bar	——
Donuts	——
Cake	——
Croissant	— 47

Redrawn From: Holt et al (1995)

Ultra-processed foods have been found to override the body's satiety signals and dysregulate leptin, which is a satiety hormone[376]. Leptin gets secreted by fat cells and it regulates energy balance, food consumption and calorie expenditure[377,378]. Low leptin levels promote overeating and obesity in humans[379]. On the other hand, leptin therapy has been used to reverse obesity and improve biomarkers of health[380,381,382]. In obesity, you become leptin resistant and despite having enough energy in your adipose tissue, your brain doesn't get the message that you're full[383,384,385]. Leptin resistance, which leads to high leptin levels, is thought to be one of the biggest risk factors for obesity[386]. Thus, the types of food you eat determines your degree of leptin sensitivity and directly affects how many calories you end up being satisfied with.

How overconsuming highly processed foods leads to overeating

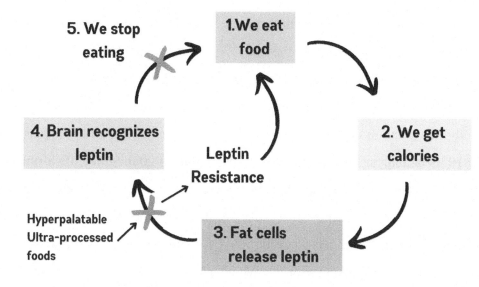

Another important point is that the human body requires vitamins and minerals to conduct various processes, such as fat burning, thyroid, and hormone function, all of which regulate your metabolic rate. For example, iodine and selenium are needed to create thyroid hormones.[387,388,389,390] The uptake of thyroid hormones into the thyroid gland itself depends on magnesium and sodium[391,392,393,394,395,396]. The activation of thyroid hormones depends on selenium[397]. Having low thyroid function can lower TDEE and result in weight gain. Thus, the root cause of a suppressed TDEE could be due to hypothyroidism caused by iodine, selenium, or sodium deficiency. Low thyroid function can also increase the risk of certain medical conditions, such as insulin resistance, cardiovascular disease, and metabolic syndrome[398,399]. What's more, you could have symptoms of hypothyroidism even with a low bodyweight, characterized by low testosterone, low libido, cognitive difficulties, intolerance to cold, joint pain, constipation, hair loss, brittle skin, depression, and high cholesterol levels[400,401,402,403]. In other words, simply **having suboptimal nutrient intake may lead to fat gain**.

Another example is magnesium, which helps bring glucose into the cell and improves insulin signaling in the body[404,405]. **Thus, consuming a diet deficient in magnesium may lead to insulin resistance and weight gain.** Another mineral involved with insulin signaling is chromium, which has been found to help with body composition and weight loss[406,407,408], but research is not conclusive[409]. A 2019 meta-analysis discovered that doses of 200-1,000 mcg/day of chromium for 9-24 weeks in 1,316 obese subjects lead to a weight loss of 0.75 kg compared to the placebo group[410]. In other words, weight loss isn't solely about calories but also constituents (in this case chromium). Chromium can also suppress appetite and reduce food consumption[411], which are the most important variables for weight loss. Keep in mind that most supplements haven't been shown to produce a weight loss any greater than 2 kg[412] and usually only work when combined with a calorie deficit. However, it does reveal that minerals and micronutrients are quite important in determining your metabolic rate and how your body reacts to a particular food. The objective number of calories you eat has only a fraction to do with what your body does with those calories.

The main take away is that **all calories are not created equal**! In other words, **the calorie in vs. calorie out model, as it pertains to obesity, has many shortcomings.** It's true that the total amount of calories consumed matters, but the quality of your food choices matters more. It's also true that you can overeat steak or salmon in a single sitting. However, after eating steak or salmon you tend to be full for a longer period compared to the same number of calories from highly processed foods. More importantly, steak/salmon doesn't wreak your metabolism and hormones, whereas overconsuming highly processed food does. **It's the damage to your body from overconsuming processed foods that is the primary driver of obesity. The quality of your food determines what your body does with the calories consumed and how many calories you ultimately end up consuming/burning.** Focus on quality not quantity. Your body will take care of the rest. This doesn't mean don't portion out your healthy food choices, or to eat as much whole foods as you want, it simply means eat real food to satiety.

Key Take-Aways

1.) Different individuals react differently to underfeeding or overfeeding, which determines how much weight they will gain or lose.

   a. This depends mostly on current body composition and metabolic health but also to a certain extent on genetics.

2.) Certain individuals will move more at rest, such as fidget more, if they overeat calories. This happens at a subconscious level.

   a. Just eating less and moving more may not always work because of inhibitory mechanisms from the body. Of course, you ultimately decide whether you are going to work out or not, however, there are certain signals from the body that will prompt you to move more, and you don't even realize it.

3.) Different people gain fat in different areas (subcutaneous vs. visceral) with the same amount of overfeeding.

   a. This clearly shows that there are biological differences to weight gain

People who fail to have an increase in non-exercise activities with increased caloric intake are at a greater risk of weight gain. This is likely due to hormonal issues that are inhibiting those subconscious signals to move more. We also know that people who do not have an increase in adaptive thermogenesis with increased caloric intakes are also at an increased risk of weight gain with overfeeding. However, these studies are forcing people to overeat, which again doesn't tend to occur in the real world when eating real food. **It's the people who are introducing highly processed foods into their diet that tend to overeat them, and at the same time, these processed foods damage their metabolism and hormones**. In other words, it's the quality of food that leads to hormonal and metabolism issues, overeating, lack of movement and increased fat storage. **Ultimately, fixing weight issues starts with removing the junk and bringing in real food.** When you fix your biology, you start to get the appropriate satiety responses and you also improve your metabolism and fat burning capacity.

Counterpoints to the calorie in vs. calorie out model of obesity

1. Calories in < calories out = weight loss
    a. This assumes calories in is independent of calories out. However, they are dependent on each other. In other words, when you eat less, you also tend to move less to conserve energy. Additionally, when you eat less calories, your basal metabolic rate drops. Your body is smart and needs a set number of calories to function, so metabolism, heart rate, body temperature, etc. will drop with reduced caloric intake. In this situation, you still need to be in a calorie deficit to keep losing weight, but the effort required to achieve that becomes increasingly more difficult.
2. Eat less and move more = weight loss

    a. This assumes that eating is a conscious decision. However, the body provides hunger and satiety signals. You don't tell someone to drink less water to lower their blood pressure. So why are we telling people to eat less when they are overweight. We should be telling people to focus on the quality of the food they eat, which will lead to natural satiety signals. Food, and the calories they provide, are not inherently bad. We need calories to live. It's when our metabolism is broken that our bodies can't process the calories correctly. Thus, **it's not about eating less, it's about eating the correct foods so you can eat the appropriate number of calories without storing an inappropriate amount of fat.**

3. Calorie deficits are not sustainable in the long run

    a. A 2016 study on the competitors of Biggest Loser found that 6 years after the show the participants had regained 70% of the weight they lost initially[413]. Their metabolism was also burning 700 fewer calories compared to when they started the show.

4. A calorie is a calorie

    a. This model assumes all calories are the same.

    b. This model does not consider the different effects that different foods have on satiety, hormones, and metabolism that is separate from the calories they provide.

    c. Clinical studies show that changing the types of foods consumed leads to significantly more weight/fat loss that can't be explained by caloric deficits[414]. In other words, caloric deficits only explain around 22.8% of weight/fat loss, whereas the changes in the quality of the food explains 77.2% of the weight/fat loss.

5. Overfeeding studies do not lead to the level of weight/fat gain that should occur based on the caloric surplus provided.

a. This is because of adaptive thermogenesis, where heat production and non-exercise activity thermogenesis increase.

6. Hormones don't matter, it's all about calories

    a. This assumes that body fat gain is not controlled by hormones but by a simple mathematical equation, calories in > calories out = weight gain. However, we know that body temperature is controlled by thyroid hormones, muscle mass by growth hormone and testosterone, sleep by melatonin, so why would fat gain not be controlled by hormones? Indeed, fat gain is controlled by things like leptin, insulin, ghrelin, peptide YY, adiponectin, hormone-sensitive lipase, lipoprotein lipase, adipose triglyceride lipase, fibroblast-growth factor-21, AMPK, etc.

7. Caloric deficits are safe

    a. When we go into a caloric deficit there are numerous side effects such as mood and cognitive declines, decreases in heart rate, body temperature, energy, thyroid hormones. There are also decreases in muscle mass, hair loss, brittle hair/nails, etc. In other words, eating less and moving more to induce a calorie deficit can be harmful to our overall health and is typically not sustainable.

So now you know that weight gain isn't all about calories, it's more about (1) baseline metabolic health because that's what determines, (2) baseline fat oxidation, (3) adaptive thermogenesis, (4) basal metabolic rate, (5) hormone function, (6) satiety signals, (7) physical activity responses to overconsumption of calories and more. People who are insulin sensitive, with a good amount of muscle mass, have a higher baseline fat oxidation rate compared to someone who is overweight. This means they will have less fat gain with the same caloric surplus compared to someone who isn't insulin sensitive. In fact, the former person will likely not gain weight because their body will compensate for the extra calories by burning the extra calories as heat (adaptive thermogenesis), increasing physical activity, decreasing food intake on the next meal, etc. Furthermore, the caloric surplus may not harm their hormones at all, whereas someone who is insulin resistant is much more likely to have a further decrease in insulin sensitivity with a higher caloric intake.

Chapter 3: The Hormonal Mechanisms of Obesity

As we showed in the previous chapter, weight loss depends on much more than just calorie intake. Although the final determinant is a negative energy balance, achieving that can be done through various means. What's more, several other factors, such as macronutrient ratios, micronutrient status, metabolic health, thyroid function, hormones, etc. determine energy production, energy partitioning, fat burning, satiety and how many calories someone needs to consume to lose weight.

The second law of thermodynamics is king but in free-living humans it's also important to pay attention to the dynamic variables that affect that process. That's why in this chapter we'll be looking in closer detail at the different ways your hormones and metabolic condition affects the calories in vs calories out equation. Beware, we are going to be going into deep science and human physiology, which may appear complex for the general reader who doesn't have a science background. **Warning, if you do not like heavy science, we recommend that you only read the bolded text, figures, and summary bullet points in this chapter.** We have added many graphs, images, and summaries to try and make it easier to comprehend. The remaining chapters will be much less science heavy.

Thyroid Function and Metabolic Rate

Your body's energy balance and metabolic rate are regulated by the thyroid gland located in your throat right below the Adam's apple. Thyroid hormones, called thyroxine (T4) and triiodothyronine (T3), get created when thyroid cells combine the amino acid tyrosine with the iodine absorbed from food. T3 is the active thyroid hormone that mediates most of the effects of thyroid hormones[415]. Thyroid hormones also influence your body temperature, heart rate and metabolic rate[416].

Hypothyroidism or low thyroid functioning increases the risk of weight gain and obesity[417,418]. Symptoms of hypothyroidism include fatigue, weight gain, cognitive decline, intolerance to cold, low body temperature, joint pain, inflammation, constipation, hair loss, dry skin, puffy face, water retention, high cholesterol, low resting heart rate, and depression[419,420,421,422]. It usually occurs in people with Hashimoto's thyroiditis or those who no longer have their thyroid. Hypothyroidism is typically diagnosed when thyroid stimulating hormone (TSH) is elevated or T4 or T3 levels are low. When TSH and thyroid hormones are in the normal range, the thyroid is working normally. Hashimoto's thyroiditis is diagnosed with a TSH between 5-10 mIU/L[423]. One study found that **supplementing with inositol and selenium (600 mg and 83 mcg, respectively) compared to selenium alone improved thyroid function (TSH and thyroid hormone levels), the auto-antibody anti-thyroglobulin and subjective symptoms in those with Hashimoto's thyroiditis**[424]. Thus, supplementing with myo-inositol plus selenium may be an important strategy for those with hypothyroidism, especially if due to Hashimoto's thyroiditis. Measuring body temperature can also quickly assess the status of your thyroid. If you're constantly cold or your body temperature is constantly below normal, even when in a warm room, then your body is conserving energy and not using it for heat production, which may suggest hypothyroidism.

Stress inhibits thyroid function and reduces the conversion of T4 into T3[425,426]. Inflammation also blocks T4 conversion into T3, which promotes hypothyroidism[427]. In healthy human subjects, raising levels of a pro-inflammatory cytokine IL-6 lowers serum T3[428,429]. Thus, being chronically stressed may suppress your metabolic rate by lowering thyroid output. To cope with stress, you need carbon dioxide (CO_2), which helps to release oxygen into the blood from hemoglobin, thus allowing tissue oxygenation via the Bohr Effect[430]. Hyperventilation that occurs during a panic attack promotes anxiety, high blood pressure and keeps the body stressed out by reducing CO_2 levels in the blood[431]. Hypothyroidism results in lower CO_2 production due to a lower respiratory rate[432]. Carbohydrate metabolism produces more CO_2 than fat[433] and ketogenic diets can reduce CO_2 production[434]. Thus, consuming some carbohydrates helps to increase CO_2 production and can reduce the overall stress on the body. In other words, don't completely cut out all carbohydrates from your diet.

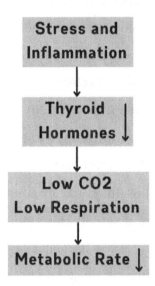

Hypothyroidism rates in iodine-sufficient countries are around 1-2%[435]. In Europe, the prevalence of hypothyroidism is between 0.2-5.3% and in the U.S. 0.3-3.7%[436,437,438]. The prevalence of undiagnosed hypothyroidism is 4.94% and hyperthyroidism 1.72%[439]. Thus, frank hypothyroidism is quite rare in developed countries. However, suboptimal thyroid functioning is much more prevalent. The average body temperature of U.S. people has declined by 0.03°C per decade since the 1860s[440]. Nowadays it's 36.6°C, compared to 37°C, which could reflect a general trend towards lower thyroid function among the general population. Decreased body temperature is associated with lower metabolic rates[441]. Thus, the drop in body temperature might indicate a rise in the prevalence of low thyroid functioning or thyroid dysfunction.

A 2009 cross-sectional study among 27,097 individuals discovered that **both overt and subclinical hypothyroidism were correlated with a higher BMI and a greater prevalence of obesity**[442]. Serum TSH (which increases in hypothyroidism to try and produce more thyroid hormones) is positively associated with BMI and obesity[443,444,445,446,447,448]. Increasing BMI is associated with lower serum free T4 levels, which is associated with fat gain[449,450,451]. In subclinical hypothyroidism, increased TSH could alter energy expenditure and thus lead to weight gain[452]. High circulating TSH levels in obese adults and children normalizes after weight loss[453,454].

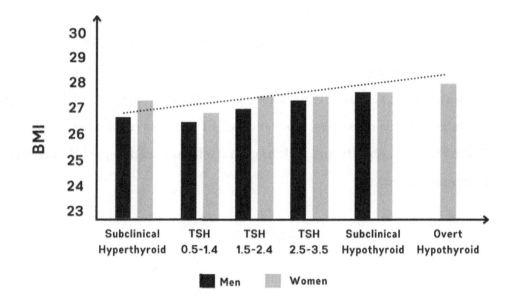

Redrawn From: Asvold et al (2009)

Leptin is a satiety hormone, which if elevated can induce leptin resistance, or vice versa. In other words, high leptin may lead to lack of a satiety signal. **Leptin gets stimulated by TSH in the adipose tissue**[455,456,457]. Furthermore, there is a positive correlation between serum leptin and serum TSH in obese subjects[458]. Leptin also increases the activity of thyroid deiodinase, which converts T4 into the active thyroid hormone T3[459,460]. Thus, leptin sensitivity is needed for optimal thyroid function. Obese subjects have been reported to have a modest increase in total and free T3, which may be a counter-mechanism against fat gain as a means to increase energy expenditure[461,462]. Increasing fat gain is associated with a parallel rise in TSH and free T3 independent of insulin sensitivity and other metabolic biomarkers[463]. Essentially, the body wants to start burning more energy and generate more heat to prevent the continuation of fat accumulation. Both the thyroid gland and the hormone leptin contribute to adaptive thermogenesis through mitochondrial uncoupling proteins and heat production[464,465]. However, obese individuals have a down-regulation of TSH receptor expression on fat cells, which further increases plasma TSH and free T3 levels, creating aspects of peripheral thyroid hormone resistance[466]. This normalizes after weight loss as weight loss reduces both TSH and free T3[467]. **Overall, weight gain down-regulates TSH receptor expression, which raises TSH, free T3 and leptin levels as counter measures, whereas weight loss decreases TSH, free T3 and leptin**[468]. **Thus, obesity and weight gain itself may lead to peripheral thyroid hormone resistance.**

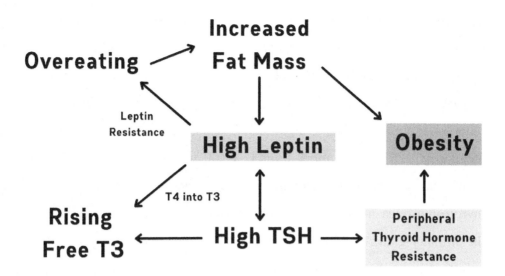

Here are the reference ranges for TSH[469]:

Age	Low	Normal	High
0–4 days	<1 mU/L	1.6–24.3 mU/L	>30 mU/L
2–20 weeks	<0.5 mU/L	0.58–5.57 mU/L	>6.0 mU/L
20 weeks – 18 years	<0.5 mU/L	0.55–5.31 mU/L	>6.0 mU/L
18-30	<0.5 mU/L	0.5–4.1 mU/L	>4.1 mU/L
31–50 years	<0.5 mU/L	0.5–4.1 mU/L	>4.1 mU/L
51–70 years	<0.5 mU/L	0.5–4.5 mU/L	>4.5 mU/L
71–90 years	<0.4 mU/L	0.4–5.2 mU/L	>5.2 mU/L

The connection between iodine intake and thyroid dysfunction is U-shaped[470,471]. Both too high, as well as too low iodine intake, can result in hypothyroidism or hyperthyroidism[472,473]. Excess iodine is a risk factor for thyroid autoimmune disease[474,475]. The RDA of iodine is 120 mcg in schoolchildren and 150 mcg in adults[476]. This increases to 220-250 mcg during pregnancy[477]. The safe upper limit is 1,100 mcg/d of iodine[478]. Nevertheless, iodine intakes of ≥500 mcg/d for several weeks can raise TSH's response to thyrotropin-releasing hormone (TRH), which stimulates the release of TSH from the pituitary gland[479]. Most people, except individuals with thyroid problems or iodine sensitivity, may be okay with an iodine intake up to 1 mg/day from the diet[480]. However, some data suggests that consuming > 300 mcg/day of iodine may increase the risk of thyroid issues (hyperthyroidism and Hashimoto's thyroiditis, especially if selenium intake is not optimized)[481]. Interestingly, the Japanese consume on average 1-3 mg/d of iodine[482]. The Standard American Diet (SAD) is usually low in iodine unless it includes seaweeds, shrimp, oysters, fish, pastured eggs, milk, yogurt, or cranberries[483].

Testosterone and Body Composition

There's a connection between low thyroid and low testosterone in men[484]. Low testosterone can promote obesity and weight gain, whereas testosterone replacement therapy can help obese men lose weight[485,486,487,488,489]. Testosterone not only promotes the increase of lean muscle mass but also suppresses fat gain[490,491,492]. Sleep and skeletal muscle are both important determinants of testosterone and your resting metabolic rate[493,494,495]. There's a relationship between low free testosterone and loss of muscle mass[496]. Patients who have hypothyroidism have reduced levels of free testosterone, whereas thyroid hormone treatment normalizes testosterone levels[497]. Thus, **having a low thyroid may promote weight gain through decreased testosterone levels**. Hypothyroidism is also associated with erectile dysfunction,[498] , which makes sense if testosterone levels are reduced.

The thyroid gland helps synthesize cholesterol, increasing pregnenolone, which then gets converted into either DHEA or progesterone[499]. DHEA, pregnenolone and progesterone are precursors to sex hormones[500,501,502]. Low DHEA and low pregnenolone levels are often seen in people with thyroid dysfunction or hypothyroidism[503]. In rats, pregnenolone increases the biosynthesis of thyroid hormones[504]. Under stress, cortisol steals pregnenolone from DHEA and progesterone, a process called 'pregnenolone steal', resulting in a decrease in sex hormones. Excess cortisol and stress also lower DHEA levels because DHEA is primarily produced in the adrenal glands and pregnenolone is the precursor to DHEA[505,506]. Thus, with high cortisol, all the sex hormones like testosterone become secondary, which if maintained for too long may lead to low sex hormones and thyroid dysfunction. Stress and cortisol will also lower thyroid hormones. Futhermore, low thyroid raises cholesterol levels and decreases the conversion of cholesterol into sex hormones[507,508].

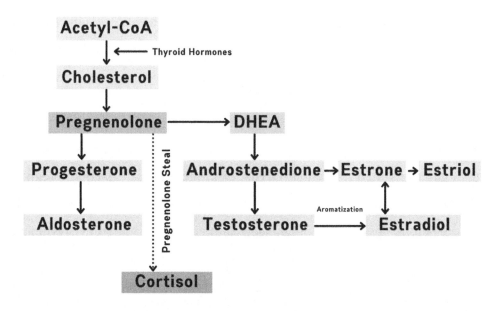

Average testosterone levels in men have been declining by about 1.2-1.3% every year since 1980[509,510]. This means men today have on average 20-30% less testosterone than their grandfathers did. That's quite astonishing! There are multiple reasons for why this is so, such as microplastics and xenoestrogens in the environment, chronic stress, low vitamin D levels, substance abuse and not enough exercise[511,512,513,514,515]. Alcohol, especially beer and spirits, boost aromatase, which converts testosterone into estrogen[516]. However, **obesity is one of the main contributors to low sex hormones (hypogonadism)[517].** Adipose tissue contains high levels of aromatase, which is reflected in the higher estrogen levels of obese men[518]. Aromatase and estrogen reduce the production of gonadotropin-releasing hormone (GRH), which lowers the levels of luteinizing hormone (LH) that is the precursor to testosterone[519,520]. Obese men have on average 30% lower testosterone than normal-weight men and more than 70% of men with morbid obesity have hypogonadism[521,522]. **Even modest obesity can lower testosterone due to insulin resistance[523].** Insulin resistance is linked to low testosterone beyond its link to visceral fat[524]. Visceral fat accumulation, which results in fat accumulating in and around your organs (primarily from insulin resistance[525]) secrets pro-inflammatory cytokines that reduce blood vessel function and promote erectile dysfunction[526]. Abdominal visceral fat is strongly correlated with insulin resistance and type 2 diabetes[527]. You can even be at a seemingly normal body weight but still have visceral fat that accumulates in and around your organs. This kind of fat deposition results primarily from insulin resistance and overeating highly processed foods.

A low carb high protein diet (44% protein, 35% carbs, 21% fat) has been found to lower testosterone by 28% in men compared to a high carb low protein diet (10% protein, 70% carbs, 20% fat) but these effects were reversed after increasing carb consumption[528]. The high carb intake also resulted in 14-64% lower cortisol. During the first 3 weeks of low carbohydrate dieting there is an increase in resting and post-exercise cortisol levels, but afterwards resting cortisol levels return to normal, whereas post-exercise cortisol still remains elevated[529]. The average reduction of testosterone in those on low-carb, high-protein diet is around 37%, whereas a low-carb, moderate-protein diet doesn't show those effects. That was probably due to the fact that excess protein keeps one out of ketosis, while simultaneously restricting carbs leads to a glucose-deprived state that can raise cortisol. By keeping protein moderate on a low-carb diet, you end up using fat for fuel (in the form of ketones) instead of glucose. Thus, if eating a high protein diet, it's probably best to consume a moderate amount of whole food carbohydrates, whereas you can get away with eating less carbohydrates when in a state of ketosis. A ketogenic diet has been shown to raise testosterone levels in obese men due to weight loss[530]. Nonetheless, a chronic low carb intake (< 50 grams/day) may not be advised for optimal thyroid and sex hormone function. Indeed, consuming just 50 grams of carbohydrates seems to be enough, even in caloric restriction, to maintain normal T3 levels[531]. Low levels of leptin are also associated with insulin resistance[532]. Thus, acutely spiking insulin and leptin may improve insulin sensitivity and weight loss[533]. Simultaneously, restoring leptin back to normal levels has been found to normalize blood glucose and insulin resistance[534]. The key is to consume whole food carbohydrates and raise insulin only at set times throughout the day without developing insulin resistance and chronically elevated insulin levels. For active healthy individuals, we recommend around 1 gram of protein per pound of lean body weight. For carbohydrates, we recommend ~ 1-2 g/kg of body weight on non-work out days, 2-3 g/kg on regular work out days and 3-8 g/kg on intense prolonged workout days.

Causes of low testosterone:

- Chronic stress[535,536]
- Low thyroid
- Overtraining
- Malnutrition, low calorie intake
- Chronic low carb intake
- Low fat diet
- Excess alcohol consumption
- Lack of sleep
- Exposure to xenoestrogens found in plastics, household chemicals and personal care products[537,538]
- Insulin resistance
- Obesity and excess body fat
- High estrogen
- High sex hormone binding globulin (SHBG)

Most of your daily testosterone gets released during sleep[539]. **Sleep apnea, fragmented sleep and sleeping disorders reduce testosterone levels**[540,541]. Simultaneously, low testosterone can also cause sleeping problems[542]. A 2011 study discovered that sleeping only 5 hours per night over the course of 8 days lowered daytime testosterone in 10 volunteers by 10-15%[543]. In elderly men, total sleep time is a predictor of morning testosterone levels[544]. Sleep deprivation also promotes insulin resistance and glucose intolerance. Just four nights of sleeping 4.5 hours reduces insulin sensitivity by 16% and makes fat cells 30% more insulin sensitive[545], which means the fat cells are more prone to storing energy. Blue light exposure at night from artificial sources also promotes insulin resistance, weight gain and diabetes due to circadian rhythm disruption[546]. There is a link between light exposure at night with obesity and type-2 diabetes[547,548]. Sleeping 5.5 hours instead of 8.5 hours reduces fat burning and increases the proportion of energy being burned to come from muscle protein[549]. This means that when you are sleep deprived, you are more prone to gain fat and lose muscle, creating a skinny-fat look. On top of that, not sleeping enough reduces leptin (the satiety hormone) and increases ghrelin (the hunger hormone). A study on 12 men noted that **if they slept only 4 hours a night, they ate on average 559 more calories the next day**, compared to sleeping 8 hours[550]. Generally, adults need about 7-9 hours of sleep per night and children 10-12 hours. Sadly, up to 40% of people report that they get less than 7 hours of sleep[551].

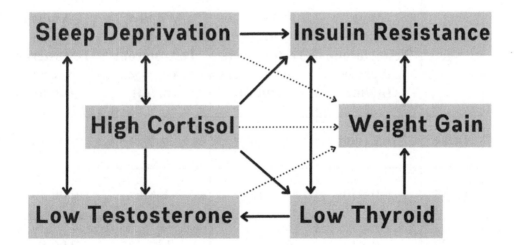

Thus, sleep deprivation promotes a whole cascade of things that puts you on the track for developing obesity. Fundamentally, it is rooted in being in a calorie surplus, but that positive energy balance is caused by various hormone changes that cause you to eat more than you burn.

How to increase testosterone levels:

- Fat loss
- Resistance training[552,553,554]
- Free weight exercises, such as squats, deadlifts, and bench press[555,556,557]
- High intensity exercise[558,559]
- High intensity interval training[560]
- Getting at least 35-40% of your calories as fat[561]
- Consuming foods with zinc and selenium[562]
- Eating a diet with carbohydrates[563]
- Sleeping at least 7-8 hours
- Reduce stress levels
- Boron supplementation 3 mg/day[564]
- Adequate vitamin D levels

Normal ranges for total/free testosterone levels in both men and women[565]:

Age	Men Total Testosterone Average (ng/dl)	Men Free Testosterone Average (ng/ml)	Women Total Testosterone Average (ng/dl)	Women Free Testosterone Average (ng/ml)
15-18	100-1200	5.25-20.7	7-75	0.06-1.08
19-40	240-950	5-18	8-80	0.06-1.00
40-49	250-910	4.46-16.4	13-63	0.06-0.95

50-59	210-880	4.06-14.7	10-54	0.06-0.90
60+	200-600	3.67-10	9-46	0.06-0.71

About 44% of your testosterone is bound to sex hormone binding globulin (SHBG) and 54% to serum albumin[566]. Only 1-2% of testosterone is free and biologically active. Thus, SHBG levels determine the bioavailability of sex hormones. Normal SHBG levels in adult premenopausal women are 40-120 nmol/L, in postmenopausal women it's 28-112 nmol/L and in adult males it's 20-60 nmol/L. Low testosterone from excess SHBG can also lead to metabolic syndrome[567].

Things that increase SHBG are high estrogen, pregnancy, cirrhosis or liver damage, anorexia, alcohol consumption, smoking, overtraining, stress, and elevated thyroxine (T4)[568,569,570,571,572,573]. Oral contraceptives or birth control pills are associated with higher SHBG[574]. This might explain why women on birth control tend to gain weight and have mood changes[575]. Prolonged calorie restriction of more than 50% increases SHBG while lowering free and total testosterone[576]. Anorexia or malnutrition also increases SHBG[577]. Protein intake is inversely associated with SHBG levels and weight gain in animal studies[578].

Estrogen and Weight Gain

As we stated just before, excess body fat can lower testosterone by aromatizing it into estrogen[579]. Estrogen does promote fat storage in certain body parts, such as the breasts, hips, buttocks, and legs but decreases abdominal visceral fat[580,581,582]. Men have significantly lower estrogen than women but both men and women have circulating estrogen levels at a lower level than androgens[583,584]. Both sexes need estrogen as it helps to regulate bone turnover and cholesterol levels[585,586]. Low estrogen can increase the risk of injuries, arthritis, and cardiovascular disease[587]. In men, estrogen affects libido, erectile function, and sperm production[588].

In women, low estrogen can result in weight gain, especially after menopause[589,590]. After menopause, women's reproductive hormones decline and many of them notice weight gain. These hormonal changes during perimenopause contribute to abdominal obesity[591,592]. Other reasons why a drop in estrogen may occur, even before menopause, include polycystic ovary syndrome (PCOS), low calorie intake, overtraining, stress-related adrenal disorders, removal of ovaries and lactation[593,594,595,596]. In PCOS, the female body is producing more male androgenic hormones and less estrogen, which is often caused by insulin resistance[597,598]. Insulin and hyperinsulinemia also increase aromatase activity, resulting in more testosterone being converted into estrogen, which is bad for men's sex hormones[599]. However, there's less aromatase activity in PCOS, which might contribute to the decline in estrogen levels and the subsequent weight gain[600]. Reducing insulin with metformin has been observed to also decrease aromatase activity[601]. **Inositol at 1-2 grams twice daily improves insulin resistance in PCOS women, gestational diabetes, pregnant women with a family history of type 2 diabetes and post-menopausal women[602].**

In mice, estrogen can inhibit binge-eating, which might explain why some women tend to eat more after menopause[603]. Binge-eating is found to be linked to decreased estradiol (E2) and progesterone[604]. This tends to be more the case with women who have had a history of binge-eating episodes[605].

Causes of low estrogen levels[606,607]:

- Chronic low calorie intake
- Anorexia, malnutrition
- Chronic strenuous exercise, overtraining
- Chronic stress
- Insulin resistance
- Thyroid dysfunction
- Pituitary gland dysfunction
- Autoimmune conditions
- Chronic kidney disease
- Removal of ovaries
- Family history of hormonal problems
- PCOS
- Aging
- Perimenopause

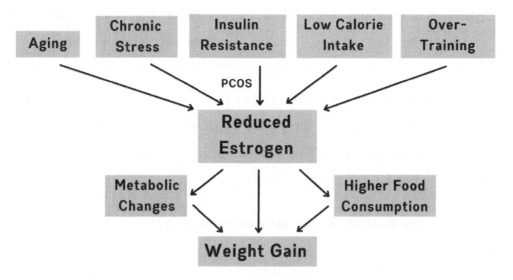

How to raise estrogen levels naturally:

- Consume sesame seeds and flaxseeds[608,609]
- Achieve normal vitamin D levels[610]
- Consume foods with B vitamins[611]
- Use evening primrose oil[612]
- Herbal supplements, such as red clover, chasteberry, black cohosh and dong quai[613,614,615,616]
- Maintain a healthy weight
- Boron supplementation 3 mg/day[617]
- Inositol at 1-2 grams twice daily (in men inositol compounds raise testosterone and lower estrogen)

Estrogen dominance describes a state wherein a person has more estrogen than progesterone, causing fatigue, mood disorders, weight gain and fibrocystic breasts[618,619]. In men, excess estrogen is implicated in gynecomastia or male breast tissue development. The most common causes of gynecomastia are obesity, alcohol consumption, hypogonadism (low sex hormones), and androgenic steroid use[620,621]. However, gynecomastia may even occur if both testosterone and estrogen levels are adequate but their ratios are imbalanced[622,623], meaning there's too much estrogen in relation to testosterone and other androgens. Estrogenic tea tree oils and lavender have been reported to cause prepubertal gynecomastia[624,625].

Causes of high estrogen and estrogen dominance[626,627]:

- Obesity and excess weight gain
- Low testosterone and androgens
- Lavender and tea tree oils
- Xenoestrogens found in plastics, household chemicals and personal care products
- Excess alcohol consumption and drug use[628]

- Certain medications, such as diuretics, statins, anti-depressants, NSAIDs, and contraceptives[629,630]
- Kidney disease or kidney failure[631]
- Liver cirrhosis or damage

There are 3 main estrogens the body produces endogenously: estrone (E1), estradiol (E2) and estriol (E3)[632]. Estetrol (E4) is made only during pregnancy. Estradiol is the most prevalent and potent estrogen.

Here are the normal E1 and E2 levels in both men and women[633]:

	Estrone (E1)	Estradiol (E2)
Women		
Prepubescent Female	Undetectable–29 pg/mL	Undetectable–20 pg/ml
Pubescent Female	10–200 pg/mL	Undetectable–350 pg/ml
Premenopausal Adult Female	17–200 pg/mL	15–350 pg/ml
Postmenopausal Adult Female	7–40 pg/mL	<10 pg/ml
Men		
Prepubescent Male	Undetectable–16 pg/ml	Undetectable–13 pg/ml
Pubescent Male	Undetectable–60 pg/ml	Undetectable–40 pg/ml
Adult Male	10–60 pg/ml	10–40 pg/ml

Here are ways to lower estrogen dominance:

- Moderate weight loss[634]
- Physical activity[635]
- Fiber intake[636]
- Eating cruciferous vegetables[637,638]
- Reduce alcohol consumption[639]
- Avoid xenoestrogens in plastics and household chemicals

Your hormonal status and metabolic health determine the underlying mechanisms that regulate your body's total daily energy expenditure, satiety, and thyroid function. **The biggest culprits to thyroid dysfunction and low involuntary energy expenditure are insulin resistance and excess cortisol.** Depending on the degree of one's metabolic health, it becomes increasingly easier to accumulate excess fat tissue once this condition is reached.

The Harms of Insulin Resistance

Insulin resistance (IR) is a medical condition in which the body's cells become irresponsive to the actions of insulin, denying the entry of glucose into the cells, leading to elevated blood sugar levels[640]. If fat cells become insulin resistant, they take up less lipids from circulation, resulting in elevated circulating fatty acids, which itself can promote insulin resistance further[641,642,643]. Even when skeletal muscle and the liver have become insulin resistant, the fat cells tend to still maintain their ability to store energy and form new fat stores, which accelerates weight gain[644]. Hyperinsulinemia is when there's more circulating insulin in relation to blood glucose, which is both the result and driver of insulin resistance[645]. Insulin resistance will eventually lead to type-2 diabetes and hyperglycemia[646,647]. Symptoms include increased hunger, thirst, elevated blood sugar, high blood pressure, lethargy, belly fat, elevated triglycerides and cholesterol levels. Hyperinsulinemia is associated with hypertension, diabetes, obesity and metabolic syndrome[648]. **Essentially, as with leptin, too frequent surges in insulin will eventually lead to the desensitization or resistance of cells to the actions of insulin, resulting in insulin resistance.**

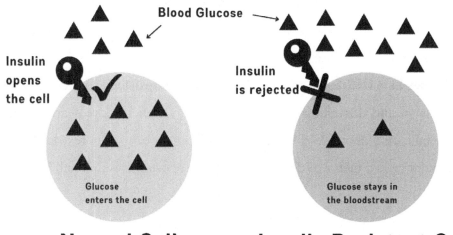

Normal Cell   **Insulin Resistant Cell**

A 1985 study in the journal *Diabetologia* took 12 non-obese men and injected them with increasing doses of insulin over the course of 40 hours[649]. By the end of the experiment, the men exhibited a 15% decrease in glucose tolerance, which means they became 15% more insulin resistant. Another study in 15 healthy non-diabetic men saw a 20-40% drop in insulin sensitivity when given normal doses of insulin over the course of 96 hours[650]. Thus, having high levels of insulin all the time will eventually make the body insulin resistant. Every person has a threshold at which this occurs but it's central human physiology that excess insulin will eventually lead to a pathological state in which the body is more geared towards storing energy.

Risk factors for developing insulin resistance include sedentary lifestyle, vitamin D deficiency, circadian rhythm mismatches and overconsumption of high fat and sugar foods[651,652,653,654,655,656]. Certain medications, such as corticosteroids, antipsychotics and protease inhibitors are also linked to insulin resistance[657,658]. Blunting of the diurnal cortisol rhythm is also associated with insulin resistance and type-2 diabetes[659]. It is healthy for the body to produce high amounts of cortisol after waking up to kick-start the daily circadian cycle and all the other hormones that are linked to that. However, excess cortisol may promote insulin resistance by counteracting the actions of insulin and downregulating the translocation of glucose transporters, such as GLUT4[660,661]. Pro-inflammatory cytokines like TNF-alpha can also lead to insulin resistance by reducing GLUT4 expression and disrupting insulin signaling[662]. Genetic issues are estimated to contribute only about 25-44% to the development of insulin resistance[663]. Thus, the major causal factor of developing insulin resistance is diet and lifestyle.

How to Reverse Insulin Resistance and Improve Thyroid Function

Insulin resistance is implicated in subclinical hypothyroidism, elevated TSH levels as well as hyperthyroidism[664,665,666]. Even minor increases in TSH are linked to subclinical hypothyroidism and insulin resistance[667,668,669]. Thyroid hormones and insulin production are interlinked, wherein a dysfunction in one can lead to a dysfunction of the other[670,671]. In humans with normal thyroid function, lower T4 levels (even within the normal range) are correlated with an increased prevalence of visceral fat and insulin resistance[672,673,674,675,676]. T3 improves glucose metabolism similar to insulin[677,678]. Metformin, a common diabetes drug, improves insulin sensitivity and TSH levels[679]. Hyperthyroidism, however, depletes glucose at an increasing rate, which raises the demand for insulin in peripheral tissues, eventually leading to decreased insulin sensitivity in the liver[680,681]. Hyperthyroidism also increases glucose absorption from the gastrointestinal tract, which causes hyperglycemia and further insulin secretion[682]. Hyperthyroid patients are also more susceptible to ketoacidosis due to excessive breakdown of fat[683].

The main transporter for thyroid hormones is the sodium-iodide symporter (NIS) [684]. To get iodine into the thyroid you need magnesium, ATP, and sodium[685,686,687,688,689,690]. This sodium-iodide symporter (NIS)-mediated delivery is the first step in synthesizing thyroid hormones[691]. Low salt diets cause insulin resistance in healthy subjects[692]. **There are at least 14 human studies showing how low salt diets worsen insulin resistance or elevate insulin after an oral glucose tolerance test**[693,694,695,696,697,698,699,700,701,702,703,704,705,706]. Salt restriction is harmful for other reasons, making the body release insulin to help retain the sodium and raises aldosterone, which increases oxidative stress and cortisol[707,708]. **Thus, not getting enough sodium can impair thyroid function in 2 ways: (1) inhibiting the transport of iodine into the thyroid gland and (2) causing insulin resistance that promotes thyroid dysfunction.** Being sensitive to salt's blood pressure-raising effects is driven primarily by insulin resistance and sympathetic nervous system dominance[709].

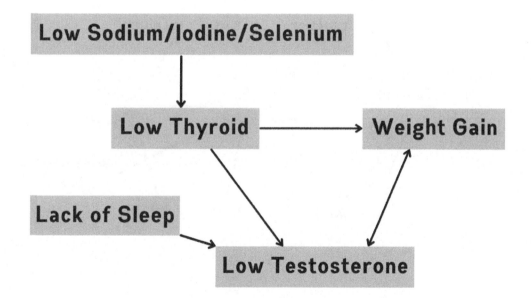

The modern diet's problem is also lack of potassium and bicarbonate. Potassium bicarbonate excretes sodium, reversing the blood pressure-raising effects of sodium chloride[710]. It's very well established that not getting enough potassium promotes hypertension and cardiovascular disease[711,712,713]. **Potassium deficiency impairs insulin production and leads to carbohydrate intolerance in humans**[714,715]. Producing insulin in the pancreatic beta-cells is potassium-dependent[716]. You also need potassium to activate pyruvate kinase, which is involved with glycolysis or producing energy from glucose[717]. A high potassium intake from the diet is associated with a reduction in diabetes and metabolic syndrome risk[718,719,720]. Serum potassium levels are inversely linked with fasting insulin[721]. The adequate intake for potassium in adult men is between 3,000 and 3,400 mg/day and for adult women 2,300-2,600 mg/day[722]. The World Health Organization recommends an intake of 3,150 mg/d[723]. To prevent hypertension, it has been recommended to get over 3,500 mg/d[724]. An average American adult gets less than 2,800 mg/d of potassium[725], which is why potassium is considered a "nutrient of public health concern" in the U.S. Dietary Guidelines[726]. **Thus, you should aim to get at least 3,500 mg/d of potassium.**

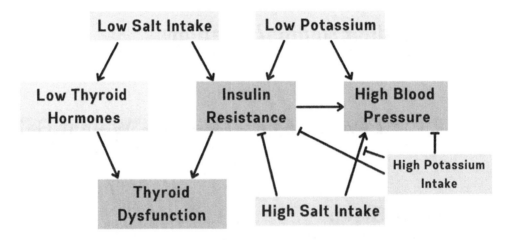

Being physically active for more than 90 minutes a day reduces diabetes risk by 28%[727]. Physical activity is the biggest determinant of how insulin sensitive you are[728]. Muscle contractions cause the glucose transporter GLUT4 to

96

translocate to the cell membrane, which improves glucose uptake into the cell[729]. The amount of muscle mass also increases your capacity to store glucose as muscle glycogen and working out facilitates this. Resistance training is effective for glycemic control in type-2 diabetes patients, especially in the early stages of glucose impairment[730]. **Thus, even if you have impaired glucose tolerance or insulin resistance, you can still see rapid improvements in your blood glucose levels simply by exercising – the glucose will get into the cell better thanks to GLUT4**[731,732]. Cortisol and chronic stress impair GLUT4, which can lead to insulin resistance[733,734]. Mindfulness-based stress-alleviating activities like meditation and yoga improve insulin resistance[735].

Here are the risk factors for developing hypothyroidism[736]:

- Pregnancy or lactation[737]
- Iodine deficiency
- Excess iodine intake
- Rapidly transitioning from iodine deficiency to sufficiency[738]
- Autoimmune conditions[739]
- Genetic risk factors[740,741]
- Smoking
- Selenium deficiency[742]
- Certain drugs and pharmaceuticals
- Infections[743]
- Insulin resistance

Here are things that decrease thyroid hormones or reduce their uptake:

- Low ATP/magnesium
- Low sodium, selenium, or iodine
- Chronic calorie restriction
- Prolonged starvation
- Extended fasting
- Severe illness[744]
- Kidney damage[745]

- Liver damage
- Chronic stress
- Excess fructose consumption
- Chronic sleep deprivation

How to balance your thyroid hormones:

- Moderate weight loss
- Fix insulin resistance
- Get enough sodium
- Get enough iodine
- Get enough selenium
- Get enough magnesium
- Reduce stress and cortisol
- Manage inflammation
- Avoid added sugars
- Eat a well-structures whole foods diet
- Supplement with inositol at 1-2 grams twice daily

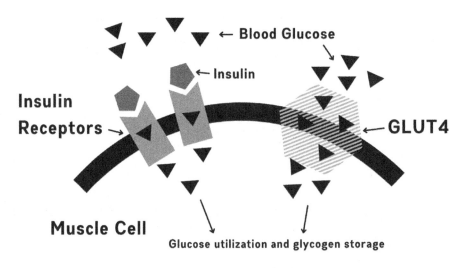

How insulin drives glucose into the cell

Redrawn From: Ishiguro et al (2016)

It was discovered in 1963 by Randle et al that glucose and fatty acids compete for oxidation via what's called The Randle Cycle or the 'glucose fatty acid cycle'[746,747,748]. This process controls the selection of fuel sources in different bodily tissues and is implicated in type-2 diabetes and insulin resistance[749,750]. You're always burning a mixture of everything (glucose, ketones, fatty acids, protein, lactate, etc.) but the body prefers to burn the most readily available one. Muscles and adipose tissue interact with each other via hormones that regulate fuel partitioning and utilization. Hormones that control fat oxidation affect circulation of fatty acids, and fatty acids, in turn, control fuel selection in muscles[751]. **Insulin and glucose uptake inhibit the burning of fat[752].** When you eat carbs or spike insulin, you slow down fat burning due to an increase in the insulin to glucagon ratio. **An excess break down of fat, and the subsequent rise in free fatty acids, is implicated in insulin resistance[753].** Elevated levels of triglycerides are associated with insulin resistance as well[754].

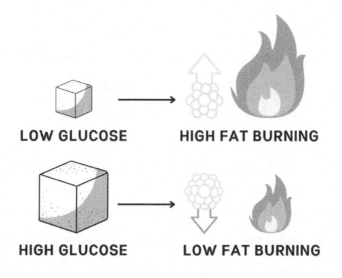

LOW GLUCOSE   HIGH FAT BURNING

HIGH GLUCOSE   LOW FAT BURNING

Burning glucose inhibits fat oxidation in the adipose tissue, whereas burning fatty acids in the muscle inhibits glucose oxidation in muscle tissue

Redrawn From: Hue and Taegtmeyer (2009)

Fast food that's high in both sugar and fat raises blood glucose, insulin and triglycerides, which promotes insulin resistance[755]. Trans fats are another culprit promoting insulin resistance[756]. Added fructose and sugar-sweetened beverages are one of the primary sources of diet-induced insulin resistance and type-2 diabetes in the Standard American Diet, much more than starch[757]. Fructose promotes obesity and insulin resistance by raising cortisol, visceral fat accumulation and triglycerides[758,759]. Thus, ultra-processed food that is high in fat and sugar is more likely to promote insulin resistance and hyperglycemia because it disrupts The Randle Cycle. There are some situations where rules of the glucose-fatty acid cycle are altered. Stress overrides the inhibition of glucose oxidation by fatty acids in muscle[760]. During physiological stress or exercise, the demand for fuel increases but the supply decreases. This activates AMPK, which is a fuel sensor that mobilizes the body's fuel sources. With activated AMPK, you can use both glucose and fat for energy production because there's an increased demand for ATP. That's why positive stressors that activate AMPK, such as exercise, fasting and calorie restriction can help to prevent the onset of insulin resistance caused by The Randle Cycle. It also means that you can tolerate eating high-carb, high-fat foods together better. When in a calorie surplus this will be harder to do. The take-away? Try and build muscle, practice intermittent fasting and have a daily exercise routine. This will allow you to burn fat and glucose better, even if a meal contains both macronutrients at the same time.

Insulin resistance also occurs in pregnancy, wherein the mother's muscles becoming less insulin sensitive to spare the glucose for the brain of the child and for her own needs[761,762]. Placental hormones can also promote insulin resistance[763]. Chronic insulin resistance caused by diet and lifestyle are pathological, but it also has a beneficial adaptive mechanism under certain conditions. **Under various metabolic states, such as pregnancy, fasting, ketosis or starvation, muscles become insulin resistant as to preserve the**

available glucose for the brain[764]. Insulin resistance is also a normal physiological response to overeating and energy excess as to protect the body from accumulating too much fat[765]. Animals who are overfed develop insulin resistance quite rapidly and become obese very fast[766].

Omega-3 fatty acids have anti-inflammatory effects and alleviate insulin resistance[767]. In rats, insulin resistance can be reduced with fish oil supplementation partly due to the anti-inflammatory effects of omega-3s[768]. Rats fed fish oil also have less visceral fat and insulin resistance compared to those fed lard or corn oil[769]. Long-chain Omega-3s in mice promotes fat burning and inhibits fat cell survival[770,771,772,773]. On the other hand, oxidized omega-6 PUFAs are implicated in various human diseases, such as insulin resistance, cardiovascular disease, cancer and neurodegeneration through a process called lipid peroxidation[774,775,776]. You can get omega-3s from foods, such as salmon, fish roe, grass-fed beef, sardines, mackerel, herring, krill oil, algae and various nuts and seeds. However, avoid consuming the omega-6 seed oils, such as corn, soybean, cottonseed, canola (rapeseed), safflower, sunflower, rice bran, grapeseed, etc.

To summarize, low thyroid hormone, stress, low sex hormones and low sodium, iodine and potassium may all lead to increased fat gain. If you optimize your thyroid, stress, sex hormones and nutrient intake, this can lead to improved weight loss.

Here are the main drivers of insulin resistance and glucose intolerance:

- Obesity and weight gain
- Visceral fat accumulation
- Hyperinsulinemia and hyperglycemia
- Excess consumption of refined carbohydrates
- Excess consumption of added sugar and fructose
- Ultra-processed foods high in calories, fat, and carbs
- Refined omega-6 seed oils
- Trans fat consumption
- Lack of exercise, especially resistance training
- Sedentary lifestyle
- Sleep deprivation
- Circadian rhythm mismatches[777]
- High inflammation and cortisol levels
- Smoking[778,779]
- Excess alcohol intake[780,781,782]
- Vitamin D deficiencies[783]
- Low salt and potassium intake
- Magnesium deficiency[784,785]
- Lack of vitamin C[786]
- Lack of chromium[787]

A fasting plasma glucose of 100-125 mg/dL indicates prediabetes and ≥ 126mg/dL diabetes[788,789]. Insulin resistance is measured with a fasting serum insulin of greater than 25 mU/L or 174 pmol/L[790]. The most common method of assessing insulin sensitivity and/or resistance is to take the oral glucose tolerance test, during which you consume 75 grams of glucose orally. After 2 hours, normal blood glucose levels are < 140 mg/dL, impaired glucose tolerance is between 140-199 mg/dL and diabetes starts at or above 200 mg/dL[791]. However, the oral glucose tolerance test may give misleading results if you take it in deep ketosis as your body will be less effective at clearing the blood stream from glucose. For greater accuracy, it is recommended to take the test after having consumed a moderate intake of carbohydrates for 2 weeks.

	Fasting Glucose Levels	Oral Glucose Tolerance Test
Normal	< 100 mg/dL	< 140 mg/dL
Prediabetes	100 mg/dL-125mg/dL	140-199 mg/dL
Diabetes	≥ 126mg/dl	≥ 200 mg/dL

Having insulin sensitivity and low insulin levels is important for health but it doesn't mean that you can't gain weight if you are in a caloric surplus. However, it does mean that you can eat the same or more calories than someone who has chronically elevated insulin levels and gain less weight. It's true that you will typically gain weight if you consistently eat more calories than you burn. No big shock factor there. However, you can induce weight loss without being in a calorie deficit. Indeed, if you take someone who eats 3,000 calories of junk food per day, and have them eat 3,000 calories from whole foods, even if they are in a caloric surplus, they can lose weight. In other words, **you don't have to be in a caloric deficit to lose weight. It depends on a person's baseline weight and what dietary pattern they are consuming.** If a high intake of processed foods led to weight gain, with some of this due to hormonal changes such as insulin/leptin resistance (and not just a higher intake of calories) then fixing the hormone issues by switching them to a healthier dietary pattern, even if they are in a caloric surplus, can lead to weight loss. This is what most people fail to realize. Yes, calories matter, but calories aren't everything.

If you are overweight, you can **take our Obesity Fix challenge**. Start by

- Adding up your current caloric intake for the day.

- Replace or remove all the highly refined/processed foods in your diet with whole nutritious foods.

  - For example, replace ice cream with fruit, pizza with greenish bananas, take-out burgers with grass-fed burgers, and stop or significantly reduce your intake of refined carbohydrates (don't eat burger buns, muffins, cereal, cakes, cookies, etc.).

- Consume the exact same number of calories that you did before each day but with your diet being composed of mostly whole nutritious foods.

This advice has led to significant weight loss for many overweight/obese people that we have worked with. All they had to do was reduce their intake of refined carbohydrates, take-out food, processed food, etc. and start eating whole nutritious foods. This is the key to weight/fat loss.

The next step in your weight loss journey should be to:

1.) **Portion out your meals**, yes even if you eat whole nutritious foods, you may gain weight if you are overeating them. Eat until you are 80% full (not hungry but not stuffed).

2.) **Practice intermittent fasting**, which is essentially skipping one meal (only eating two meals for certain days of the week). However, intermittent fasting does not have to be done in those who are physically active or have a lot of muscle mass.

Take our Obesity Fix Challenge

1.) Eat whole nutritious foods

2.) Drop the highly refined, processed foods

3.) Practicing intermittent fasting on non-work out days

4.) Resistance train at least 3-4 times per week (body weight movements, weightlifting, resistance bands, etc.)

5.) Perform some form of cardio 2-3 times per week (depending on where you are starting this could mean walking, jogging, interval sprinting, etc.).

6.) Fix hormonal imbalances (strategies discussed in this chapter)

Chapter 4: How Sugar Drives Obesity and Fat Gain Around the Stomach

Sugar cultivation dates back to ancient times in the Indian subcontinent[792,793]. Back then sugar was difficult to come by and most people just chewed raw sugar cane to obtain the sweetness. The technology for sugar refinement was discovered around the 5th century BC in the Gupta Empire[794]. From there, crystallized sugar or *khanda* in Indian (derivative for the word *candy*) spread to the Middle East and China[795]. Europeans first became aware of sugar around the 4th century BC during Alexander the Great's military campaigns to India[796].

Widespread sugar cultivation started during the mid-15th century after Europeans settled on the Canary Islands, Madeira, and São Tomé[797]. Initially, sugar was used a little for culinary purposes and considered to help with colds, stomach problems and lung issues[798]. Sugar cane from the Canary Islands was brought and introduced to the Caribbean Sea by Cristopher Columbus at the beginning of the 16th century where it was harvested extensively[799,800]. **Until the 19th century, sugar was a luxury good in Europe, which changed after sugar began to be extracted from beets in mid-18th century Prussia**[801,802]. After the establishment of the first beet sugar production facility in Prussia in 1801[803], sugar became extremely popular and spread to every household in Europe. By 1880, beets were the main source of sugar in Europe. From 1850 to the year 2000, global sugar consumption increased by over 100-fold[804].

Nowadays, sugar has been isolated and refined to such a degree that it is added into almost all packaged foods in unnaturally high amounts[805]. High-fructose corn syrup (HFCS), pure crystalline sugar and other sugar-based sweeteners found in processed foods and drinks create a supraphysiological glycemic load, which overwhelms the body's ability to deal with it and leads to high blood sugar and insulin levels and oxidative stress[806]. Since sugar is so highly refined, it acts similar to drug-like substances[807,808]. Indeed, sugar is more like a drug than a food because it provides you nothing but calories, which depletes vitamins and minerals in order to liberate those calories[809,810]. For example, thiamine (B1), riboflavin (B2) and niacin (B3) are required for glycolysis or glucose oxidation. Unlike refined sugars, whole foods like sweet potatoes or berries contain critical vitamins and minerals that are needed for breaking down the sugar and turning it into energy. In fact, it takes at least 22 micronutrients to turn the food you eat into energy[811]. Thus, when you consume empty calories, such as refined sugar, you reduce the body's ability to convert those calories into energy and at the same time increase oxidative stress in the mitochondria.

The popularity of low carb diets has resulted in a large segment of people, including many healthcare professionals, to demonize an entire food group. Although many insulin resistant or type-2 diabetic individuals may improve their glucose and insulin levels quite successfully by reducing carbohydrate intake[812,813,814], it's not carbohydrate-rich foods per se that lead to weight gain or disease. Rather, carbohydrates stripped of their natural micronutrients and fiber, which places a large metabolic burden on the body, especially in the form of added sugars found in soft drinks, breakfast cereal, bread, granola bars, etc. In this chapter, we're going to be looking deeper into how these added sugars drive obesity and fat gain.

How Added Sugars Deplete Energy and Promote Weight Gain

To metabolize sugar, phosphates are stripped from ATP, which can cause ATP depletion[815,816,817,818]. Metabolizing high amounts of fructose also damages the mitochondria through oxidative stress, causing ATP depletion in the liver[819,820]. Higher fructose consumption is associated with impaired ATP homeostasis in the liver where fructose is metabolized[821]. This can result in increased appetite and hunger due to lower energy levels[822]. The average American consumes 83.1 grams of fructose per day, with 20% of the population exceeding 100 grams a day[823]. Soft drinks with HFCS can contain up to 65% fructose, which is especially concerning[824,825,826]. Consuming large amounts of added fructose, particularly in beverage form, can lead to weight gain through reduced physical activity and higher energy consumption[827,828,829,830]. Consuming high amounts of added sugar in humans also promotes the development of metabolic syndrome, which includes elevated triglycerides, low HDL, high blood pressure, hyperglycemia and weight gain around the midsection[831,832,833,834,835]. The overconsumption of added sugars also contributes to early mortality, cardiovascular disease, non-alcoholic fatty liver disease (NAFLD) and atherosclerosis[836,837,838,839,840,841,842].

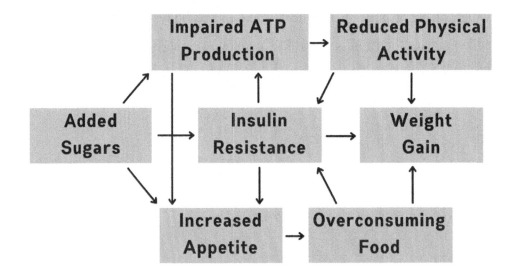

Thus, overconsuming sugar has a net negative effect on your health – as liberating the calories from added sugars depletes many essential nutrients while being a non-essential nutrient itself. It's estimated that the average person consumes 400-800 calories worth of added sugars per day, which on a 2000 calorie diet equates to 20-40% of empty calories with no nutritional benefit[843,844]. Cutting sugar consumption to a more reasonable intake of 5-10% total calories would yield massive improvements in public health as suggested by the World Health Organization[845]. We're not referring to natural sugars found in honey or fruit, which are whole foods that provide nutrients and polyphenols. Instead, the problem is refined industrial sugar and its derivatives (evaporated cane juice, high-fructose corn syrup, etc.). Animal experiments have shown that adding refined sugar to a nutrient-adequate diet leads them to malnourish themselves to death[846]. Numerous animal studies indicate that replacing starch with sugar shortens lifespan, which tells us that it's not that all carbohydrates are harmful, but instead, refined and nutrient-void sugars[847,848,849]. Added sugars in processed foods like refined sucrose and high fructose corn syrup (HFCS) do not even meet the criteria for being a food because they contain zero essential nutrients to sustain life[850]. These refined sugars also replace other nutrient-dense foods in a person's diet, promoting nutrient deficiencies and obesity. For example, consuming soft drinks is associated with lower intakes of calcium and other nutrients[851].

Insulin that gets released when you consume added sugars or refined carbohydrates inhibits hormone-sensitive lipase, which keeps fatty acids in adipose tissue, decreasing their availability to be burned for energy and ATP production[852]. This results in what's called 'internal starvation' or 'hidden cellular semistarvation' because you can't access your stored energy due to high levels of insulin[853]. Elevated insulin also increases energy requirements, leading to a larger net energy loss. People who are obese with hyperinsulinemia or insulin resistance fit the description of 'overfed but undernourished'. Essentially, they are carrying thousands of stored calories in their fat tissue but on a cellular level their body is starving of energy, which is why they keep overconsuming food.

Fructose and glucose both favor the growth of bacteria and yeast[854,855]. Sugar can promote metabolic disorders, endotoxemia and systemic inflammation through modulation of the gut microbiota by proliferating pro-inflammatory gut bacteria[856]. High amounts of refined carbs and sugar don't appear to promote the colonization of Candida in healthy subjects, but it does increase levels in those with already elevated amounts of Candida[857,858]. Importantly, *Candida albicans* competes with host cells for nutrients, further depleting the body of nutrition, and glucose promotes Candida albicans resistance to oxidative stress[859,860,861], making it harder to kill. This may be an additional concern regarding valuable nutrient loss due to consuming added sugars. Sugar can also lead to gut dysbiosis and damage the intestinal lining, which compromises digestion and assimilation of nutrients[862,863,864,865,866,867].

How added sugars promote weight gain through energy depletion[868]:

- Reduces appetite for nutritious foods
- Replaces nutrient-dense foods
- Depletes nutrients from the body
- Promotes the growth of pathogens and bacteria that steal nutrients from host cells
- Provides zero micronutrients
- Promotes insulin resistance
- Reduces nutrient absorption by damaging the intestinal lining
- Damages the mitochondria
- Causes ATP depletion
- Increases hunger
- Increases the accumulation of visceral fat
- Increases cortisol

A lack of almost any micronutrient (mineral or vitamin) can lead to an increased susceptibility to insulin resistance, elevated blood sugar and visceral fat gain. The main nutrients involved in glucose tolerance are vitamin B1 (thiamine), magnesium, sodium, chromium, and vitamin C. Vitamin B1 is an essential cofactor in carbohydrate metabolism and magnesium is required to activate vitamin B1. Clinical studies show that thiamine deficiency can lead to diabetic glucose responses and thiamine supplementation can improve blood glucose levels[869,870,871,872]. In other words, simply being deficient in vitamin B1 can lead to insulin resistance and the harmful effects that come along with it (prediabetes, type 2 diabetes, etc.). Similar evidence has been shown with magnesium, sodium, chromium and vitamin C[873,874,875,876,877,878,879,880,881,882,883,884,885,886].

In diabetic animal models and human subjects, primary sites of diabetic microvascular complications are depleted of intracellular myo-inositol and accumulate intracellular sorbitol[887,888]. **Diabetic humans and animals also excrete more myo-inositol from the urine**[889,890]. Myo-inositol or just inositol is carbocyclic sugar with half the sweetness of table sugar found throughout the body and synthesized from glucose. Myo-inositol makes up every cell membrane as phosphatidylinositol and thus is important for cell membrane structure, function, and for hormones to work[891]. Inositol is considered a non-essential nutrient, but we do not make nearly enough for optimal health[892]. Excess glucose in the bloodstream inhibits myo-inositol uptake by competing with myo-inositol transporters because glucose and myo-inositol have similar structures[893,894,895,896]. Myo-inositol depletion plays an important role in the development of diabetic nephropathy[897]. Thus, diabetes and glucose disorders contribute to myo-inositol depletion, while your demand for myo-inositol under those conditions increases. Impaired Na+/K+-ATPase (sodium–potassium pump) activity, which is usually caused by magnesium deficiency, directly causes myo-inositol deficiency as

99.8% of ingested free myo-inositol is absorbed from the gastrointestinal tract via the Na+/K+-ATPase[898].

Benefits of myo-inositol[899,900,901,902,903,904,905,906,907]:

- Improves glucose oxidation
- Drives glucose into skeletal muscle
- Improves glycogen synthesis and formation in skeletal muscle
- Drives creatine into skeletal muscle
- Drives calcium into bone
- Maintains cell membrane potential
- Improves insulin signaling
- Breaks down fat and improves cholesterol
- Improves TSH (Thyroid Stimulating Hormone) signaling
- Improves energy - ATP production increases from better glucose utilization for energy and inositol compounds provide the phosphate needed for ATP production
- Improves sleep (deep sleep can increase by 1-3 hours)
- Has a calming effect
- Regulates chromatin modeling, which affects circadian gene expression[908]

Many factors deplete the body of inositol including[909]:

- Magnesium deficiency
- Manganese deficiency
- Coffee/caffeine
- Elevated glucose levels
- Insulin resistance
- Lack of salt

Inositol supplementation has been shown to improve polycystic ovary syndrome (PCOS) and metabolic syndrome thanks to its insulin-sensitizing effects[910,911,912]. Studies have shown that myo-inositol supplementation can restore spontaneous ovarian activity (spontaneous ovulation, menstrual cyclicity) and fertility in most women with PCOS[913,914,915,916]. After myo-inositol, PCOS women have improved hormonal patterns, such as decreased testosterone and increased estrogen and progesterone levels[917]. Markers of cardiovascular disease risk factors have also been found to improve, such as cholesterol and lipids[918,919]. Some studies also find a reduction in BMI and circulating leptin[920], which indicates better weight loss.

Inositol is found in some foods, such as fruit, nuts, and seeds. In animal and plant sources, myo-inositol is stored as inositol-containing phospholipids or as phytic acid[921]. All living cells contain inositol phospholipids and phytic acid is the main stored form of phosphorus in most plant tissue. Thus, the greatest amount of myo-inositol is in nuts, grains, and beans[922]. However, inositol from phytates is generally not bioavailable to non-ruminant animals. Among fruit, citrus and cantaloupe are high in myo-inositol. For example, 120 grams of grapefruit juice contains roughly 470 mg of myo-inositol. The amount of myo-inositol in common foods ranges from 225-1500 mg/d per 1800 calories, depending on the diet[923].

Food	Myo-Inositol Content mg/100 g
Grapefruit Juice	376
Peanut Butter	300
Bran Flakes	271
Whole Grapefruit	117

Bologna	92
Navy Beans	65
Green Beans	55
Brussel Sprouts	40
Whole Wheat Bread	40
Lima Beans	44
Roast Beef	25
Ham	13
Skim Milk	10

An optimal dose of myo-inositol for improving insulin sensitivity is 2-4 grams a day[924]. However, **inositol can have a mild laxative effect, hence, some individuals prefer taking 500 mg-1 gram of inositol four times daily or just 1-2 grams an hour prior to bedtime.** Inositol can also dramatically improve mood and deep sleep. Most people find that inositol gives them consistent energy throughout the day, less need for caffeine or coffee and helps with sleep. Depending on how inositol affects you, you can take inositol several times per day, or an hour prior to bedtime. Many people find that their deep sleep increases by 1-3 hours after taking inositol.

How Fructose Makes You Fat on the Inside

It's been noted that people have a very different threshold for developing metabolic syndrome and obesity. Some are able to become very obese before developing metabolic syndrome, whereas others tend to develop metabolic syndrome even at relatively low bodyweights. This is refered to as the Personal Fat Threshold Theory (PFTT) as outlined by Roy Taylor and Rury Holman in their 2015 paper titled *'Normal weight individuals who develop type 2 diabetes: the personal fat threshold.'*[925] According to PFTT, **people get sick from excess bodyweight after they exceed their limit of storing subcutaneous adipose tissue underneath the skin and they begin to store calories into the visceral adipose tissue**[926].

Visceral adipose tissue (VAT) is associated with diabetes, insulin resistance, inflammatory diseases, and obesity more than subcutaneous adipose tissue (SCAT)[927,928,929,930,931,932,933,934,935,936,937]. Neck fat accumulation is also linked to greater mortality[938]. Visceral fat in low amounts can protect internal organs but in excess it begins to promote the spread of pro-inflammatory cytokines and oxidative stress[939]. Visceral fat also generates higher amounts of fatty acids and is more involved in glucose uptake, whereas subcutaneous fat is more involved with absorbing circulating fatty acids and triglycerides[940].

People with more weight around their midsection are at a higher risk of heart disease, diabetes and premature death than those who carry their fat around their hips and thighs[941]. Even someone who looks skinny on the outside may have a lot of visceral fat underneath – a term that's called 'TOFI – thin on the outside, fat on the inside' or just skinny fat[942,943]. These 'metabolically-obese but normal-weight' individuals represent 12-14% of the population[944,945,946,947]. The reason these people are TOFI is because they have a large amount of visceral fat deposited in and around their organs as opposed to subcutaneous fat underneath the skin.

The biggest drivers of visceral fat gain are excess cortisol and insulin levels[948,949]. People with higher urinary cortisol levels have higher waist to hip ratios[950]. Among patients with hypothalamus–pituitary–adrenal (HPA) axis dysfunction there's an association between visceral adiposity and glucocorticoids[951,952]. Insulin resistance and poor glucose control pre-dispose you to weight gain and metabolic syndrome, which increase visceral fat gain[953]. Visceral fat itself also contributes to insulin resistance[954,955,956]. Excess fructose consumption promotes visceral fat and fatty liver more than glucose, which primarily increases subcutaneous fat tissue[957,958,959,960].

Here are the mechanisms by which added fructose promotes visceral fat:

- Excess fructose consumption causes a secretion of glucocorticoids and cytokines that promote lipogenesis and visceral adiposity[961,962].

- Fructose decreases insulin sensitivity, which subsequently leads to insulin resistance[963,964].

- Fructose induces inflammation, and increases 11B-hydroxysteroid dehydrogenase-1, which raises intracellular cortisol inside the subcutaneous adipocytes[965,966,967,968]. As a result, they become insulin resistant and less fatty acids enter the subcutaneous fat cells and they get stored as visceral fat instead around the organs[969,970].

- Fructose can also promote fat storage in the liver and muscles instead of the adipose tissue[971,972]. Intracellular lipids in the liver and muscle cause insulin resistance[973].

Although fructose has a lower glycemic index compared to glucose, it's now known that fructose is deleterious in respect to diabetes, obesity, and atherosclerosis[974,975]. Thus, overconsumption of fructose and added sugars promotes the accumulation of visceral fat, which is much worse for metabolic health than subcutaneous fat.

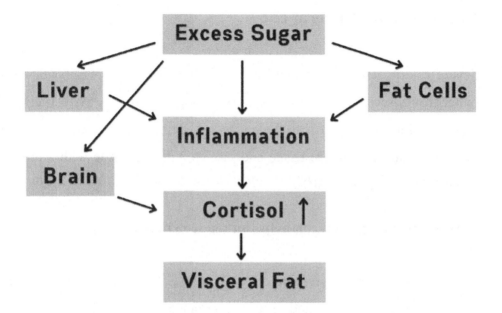

Redrawn From: DiNicolantonio et al (2018)

Added fructose is found in many industrial food products and its consumption from liquids started to increase around the 1950s[976]. In 2004, the average American was estimated to consume 50 grams of fructose per day[977]. A 2013 systematic review found that 83.3% of studies that have no conflict of interests to the food industry show a positive association between sugar sweetened beverage consumption and weight gain or obesity[978]. You can also get fructose from natural sources, such as honey, berries, fruit, and vegetables. These foods are not associated with metabolic dysfunction and obesity because they contain much lower amounts of fructose and also contain polyphenols that reduce oxidative stress. In fact, fruit and vegetable consumption is associated with better health and reduced risk of obesity[979,980].

How to Reduce Visceral Fat

Severe calorie restriction generally causes you to lose more subcutaneous fat rather than visceral fat[981]. However, combining modest energy restriction with either aerobic exercise or resistance training results in significant reductions in both subcutaneous adipose tissue and visceral adipose tissue with a preference towards loss of visceral fat[982].

Here are the things that can help you reduce visceral fat:

- **Avoid added sugars and added fructose.** These are the direct culprits of visceral adiposity and insulin resistance. People who consume more added sugars are found to have more visceral fat[983,984,985]. Excess fructose in the form of high fructose corn syrup can easily be converted into visceral fat[986,987]. Replacing fructose with starch has been found to decrease liver fat by 3.4% and visceral fat by 10.6% in just 10 days[988].

- **Avoid alcohol.** Consuming alcohol promotes visceral fat storage[989,990]. Even modest alcohol consumption is linked to having more visceral fat[991,992].

- **Avoid trans fats.** Trans fats can cause many health problems, including visceral adiposity[993,994]. A 6-year study on monkeys discovered that those monkeys on a trans fat diet gained 33% more visceral fat than those getting monounsaturated fat, despite being on the same calorie intake[995].

Trans fats can be formed during high heat cooking of vegetable oils. Thus, avoid or limit your intake of fast food and restaurant foods, which almost always cook in vegetable oils.

- **Exercise** has a more direct impact on visceral fat loss compared to dietary restriction[996]. At least 10 hours of aerobic exercise per week, such as brisk walking, jogging, or cycling, is required to get a reduction in visceral adipose tissue[997]. **High intensity exercise, specifically, is one of the most effective ways to decrease abdominal visceral fat**[998,999]. However, **aerobic exercise** should also be central to exercise programs targeted to reducing visceral fat because it **preferentially targets visceral fat even without calorie restriction**[1000,1001,1002].

  - Both resistance training and calorie restriction reduce visceral fat but their effects are not cumulative[1003]. Meaning, resistance training combined with calorie restriction isn't more effective in reducing visceral fat than resistance training alone. Strength training has been shown to improve insulin sensitivity[1004].

- **Get adequate sleep.** Inadequate sleep increases visceral fat gain[1005,1006,1007,1008]. Sleep apnea is also linked to higher visceral fat[1009,1010,1011]. On the flip side, **sleeping more can help to reduce visceral fat**. A 6-year study on 293 people found that sleeping 7-8 hours instead of 6 hours decreased visceral fat by about 26%[1012].

- **Intermittent fasting** helps to burn visceral fat and makes you more insulin sensitive[1013,1014]. It decreases visceral fat by 4-7% in just 6-24 weeks[1015].

- **Carbohydrate restriction** and low carb diets have been shown to be more effective in reducing visceral fat compared to low fat diets[1016,1017,1018]. An 8-week study among 69 overweight men found that those who followed a low carb diet lost 10% more visceral fat than those on a low fat diet[1019].

- **Fiber intake** reduces the risk of gaining visceral fat by up to 3.7%[1020]. The short chain fatty acids created from digesting fiber also promote fullness and satiety[1021,1022,1023]. In epidemiological studies, dietary fiber intake is associated with lower bodyweight because it's very filling and is low in calories[1024,1025,1026]. Fiber also binds to fat during digestion, helping to achieve a greater calorie deficit through reduced fat absorption[1027,1028].
  - Some probiotic strains from the *Lactobacillus* family reduce visceral fat[1029,1030]. In a study on 210 healthy Japanese women, taking *Lactobacillus gasseri* for 12 weeks resulted in a 8.5% reduction in visceral fat and after they stopped the supplement they regained all the visceral fat lost[1031].
- **Higher protein intake** is associated with less visceral fat and lower waist circumference[1032,1033]. Protein also increases energy expenditure, which helps with preventing excess fat gain in the first place[1034,1035].

Added sugars are one of the main culprits of obesity and weight gain. They promote fat storage through various ways besides just an excess intake of calories. High amounts of added fructose, specifically, promotes the accumulation of visceral adiposity, which leads to insulin resistance and central obesity. Given the fact that these refined sugars provide no nutritional value to your body besides calories, they actually deplete the body of micronutrients and ATP. It's hard to consider added sugars as food and when battling fat loss, it's wise to avoid their consumption.

Sugar Cravings and Addiction

Besides the physiological mechanisms by which added sugars drive obesity, they also have a psychological component that encourages overeating and addiction. **Studies suggest that added sugars are as addictive as cocaine, nicotine, alcohol, tobacco, and caffeine**[1036,1037]. In fact, smokers report increased sweet cravings after giving up smoking[1038], which accounts for the typical weight gain after cessation of smoking[1039]. Oral glucose administration may even reduce tobacco cravings[1040]. One study found that cocaine-addicted individuals liked and wanted food more than cocaine[1041]. Animal studies find that sweetness is preferred over addictive drugs like cocaine[1042,1043,1044]. So, what is the mechanism? Sugar produces similar drug-like psychoactive effects to that of cocaine[1045,1046,1047,1048]. This has an evolutionary reason – foods high in sugar help with survival and are available only during a very short window of time in nature[1049]. The fat-storing mechanisms are also beneficial as a surplus of adiposity enabled humans to get through times of scarcity. Some individuals are genetically more predisposed to preferring sweetness than others, which explains why not everyone becomes addicted to sugary substances (just like not everyone who consumes alcohol becomes an alcoholic)[1050,1051,1052,1053].

But is sugar a drug? Refining sugar leaves you with pure white sugar crystals, which is a similar process to other addictive white crystals, such as cocaine from the coca leaf and opium from poppy seeds[1054]. All three are refined crystals/powders from plants. It's the refinement and purification that makes them addictive. **Furthermore, the same increase in dopamine D1 receptor binding and decreased D2 receptor binding in the striatum of the brain that happens during cocaine intake also occurs during intermittent sugar intake**[1055]. In animals, access to sugar causes numerous symptoms of addiction, such as bingeing, cravings, tolerance, and withdrawal, which is beyond the necessary number of categories to be considered an addictive substance[1056,1057,1058,1059,1060]. There may even be an 'addiction transfer' from sugar to other drugs of abuse as seen among certain overweight individuals[1061]. Sugar causes similar withdrawal symptoms as other substances of abuse and creates a dependence on the body's endogenous opioids that get released when consuming sugar[1062]. From the standpoint of the brain's neurochemistry and behavior, there are many parallels between sugar and addictive substances.

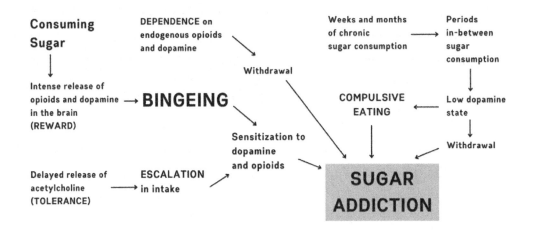

Redrawn From: DiNicolantonio and O'Keefe (2017)

Here's how sugar behaves like an addictive drug[1063]:

- Habit-forming like alcohol, tobacco, cocaine, nicotine, tea, coffee, and chocolate
- Creates a feeling of reward and cravings comparable to drugs
- Alters mood, induces pleasure, and motivates to seek out more sugar
- Produces drug-like psychoactive states
- Causes cravings comparable to cocaine and cigarettes

- Promotes dependence and addiction, which includes bingeing, withdrawals, and cravings

Thus, sugar not only increases your body's need for nutrients and promotes the accumulation of visceral adiposity, but it also makes you want to keep consuming it. That's a vicious loop that so many people find themselves in. No one gets obese overnight. However, a genetically predisposed individual may lead themselves down a dark path of dependence and addiction to hyperpalatable sugary foods quite easily. It won't happen with eating one treat, but it's the constant craving and consumption of these highly palatable foods loaded with added sugars that causes a slow accumulation of fat. Unfortunately, in our current obesogenic environment added sugars are hidden in almost all packaged foods and this conditions your brain to prefer a sweeter taste at the expense of other essential nutrients, while causing you to gain weight and visceral fat.

A Lack of Salt May Lead to Sugar Addiction

Sugar addiction may be partly caused by not getting enough salt[1064]. Salt depletion caused by exercise, diuretics or being on a low salt diet enhances the appetite for salt by activating the dopamine reward centers in the brain[1065,1066,1067]. If this weren't to happen, we wouldn't start to seek out this essential nutrient when we became deficient in it[1068]. The problem is that salt deficiency doesn't just sensitize the brain to salt, but it also increases the addictive potential of drugs (cocaine) and medications (amphetamines, such as Adderall) and opiates (such as morphine) through cross-sensitization[1069,1070,1071,1072]. Thus, sodium depletion stimulates an increased appetite for salt, but it can also make substances that stimulate the dopamine reward center in the brain, such as sugar, cocaine, and opiates, more addictive.

Salt is an essential mineral, not an addictive poison. In fact, humans used to consume up to 10x more salt than they do today[1073,1074]. Periods of greater liking towards salt lasts only until you've corrected the salt depletion, shifting from 'liking' signals to 'aversion'[1075]. Thus, your body has a 'salt thermostat', which regulates your salt intake based on how much salt are you consuming and how much you need. Excess consumption of salt typically only occurs if you're eating hyperpalatable processed foods that promote overeating.

Hunter-gatherer tribes are estimated to consume about 1,131-2,500 mg of sodium and 5,850-11,310 mg of potassium a day[1076,1077]. However, this number does not take into account sodium consumed from blood, salt licks, seafood and salty waters. For example, blood contains around 3,200 mg of sodium per liter and sea vegetation has 500x more sodium than plants on the land. The potassium:sodium ratio of human ancestors likely sits around 2-3:1 or even 1:1[1078,1079]. Conversely, industrialized societies sit at a K:Na ratio of 0.7:1 and get about 2,100-2,730 mg/day of potassium and 3,400 mg of sodium[1080,1081,1082]. On an ultraprocessed food diet consisting of canned foods, pre-packaged meals, and junk food you may get up to 10,000 mg of sodium, which may be a problem when potassium intake is low.

The Optimal
Potassium to Sodium Ratio

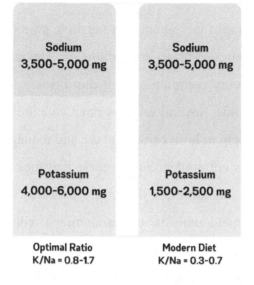

Sodium 3,500-5,000 mg	**Sodium** 3,500-5,000 mg
Potassium 4,000-6,000 mg	**Potassium** 1,500-2,500 mg
Optimal Ratio K/Na = 0.8-1.7	**Modern Diet** K/Na = 0.3-0.7

Salt also does enhance the flavor of what you eat and can promote satiety[1083]. Consuming a salty food to satiety leads to a decrease in the pleasantness of that food, resulting in cessation of eating, a term called sensory-specific satiety[1084,1085]. Sensory-specific satiety applies to other flavors as well – a food that has only a single predominant flavor eventually leads to satiety whereas changing things up, i.e., eating salty, sweet, and savory foods interchangeably, promotes higher calorie consumption[1086,1087]. "There's always room for dessert", is a common phrase to describe this phenomenon. You might be completely full and satiated from the main course but when they bring out the dessert you experience a new desire and craving for that novel taste. Thus, if you're struggling to control your appetite and calorie intake, you may not want to combine a whole range of different flavors and instead stick to a limited selection.

Non-Nutritive (Zero or Low Calorie) Sweeteners

It's worthwhile to also talk about non-nutritive sweeteners or sugar substitutes, such as aspartame, sucralose, acesulfame K, stevia, erythritol and countless others. They are very common among diet drinks, supplement powders, food bars, and other foods. Several reviews have concluded that use of zero calorie sweeteners does help to limit calorie intake and manage body weight[1088,1089,1090]. There is no consistent evidence to suggest that these non-nutritive sweeteners cause metabolic syndrome, diabetes, cancer, or obesity[1091,1092,1093,1094]. Furthermore, a meta-analysis of randomized controlled trials on steviol glycosides found no harms on metabolic or type 2 diabetic biomarkers compared to placebo[1095]. If having a diet soda or a drink with artificial sweeteners satisfies your sweet tooth and enables you to not overeat so many calories, then arguably it's perfectly fine and it can be a useful tool. Truth be told, you may still enjoy the sweet taste but at least it's not making you overeat calories and gain weight. Non-nutritive sweeteners should still not be overconsumed, particularly saccharin and aspartame, the former of which has data showing it can harm the human gut microbiome and cause glucose intolerance[1096].

Brown Fat vs White Fat

Evolutionarily, having some body fat is beneficial for obvious reasons. Your adipose tissue can contain hundreds of thousands of calories to withdraw during times of food scarcity. However, the type of fat you carry is also vital for survival and metabolic health. As we've shown with the differences between visceral fat and subcutaneous fat, some types of fat are worse for your health than others. This goes a level deeper when we're talking about the functional effects of various adipose tissue types. The main ones are brown adipose tissue (BAT) and white adipose tissue (WAT)[1097].

- **Brown Adipose Tissue (BAT) or just brown fat helps with thermoregulation and heat generation[1098].** BAT produces heat through shivering muscles called shivering thermogenesis and non-shivering thermogenesis[1099]. Newborn babies and hibernating animals have a lot of brown fat for this reason[1100], but you can also have it as an adult[1101,1102]. Brown fat has the potential to counteract obesity and metabolic diseases thanks to its higher contribution to energy expenditure and insulin sensitivity[1103,1104]. Activating brown fat has been seen to improve insulin sensitivity, glucose tolerance, weight loss, triglycerides, and cholesterol levels[1105,1106,1107,1108]. The amount of brown adipose tissue is inversely correlated with BMI, which indicates it's important for maintaining leanness[1109]. Unfortunately, brown adipose tissue decreases with age due to dysfunctional stem/progenitor cells[1110].

- **White Adipose Tissue (WAT) or white fat has a main role in energy storage.** It is also a thermal insulator that helps to regulate body temperature. Both visceral and subcutaneous fat are white adipose tissue. White fat produces leptin, the satiety hormone, and asprosin, which is a protein that releases glucose into the bloodstream[1111,1112]. Obese humans have elevated levels of asprosin which is thought to contribute to the development of metabolic syndrome and insulin resistance[1113,1114]. Bariatric surgery has been shown to decrease asprosin levels[1115]. Thus, an excess of white fat instead of brown fat could contribute to the pathology of obesity.

o **White adipose tissue can be converted into beige adipose tissue that resembles both white and brown fat[1116].** This conversion is stimulated by the sympathetic nervous system and adrenergic signaling. Asprosin decreases browning-related genes and proteins that would help to convert white fat into beige fat[1117].

The remarkable difference between white and brown fat adipocytes is the number of mitochondria in them. White adipocytes contain very few mitochondria and large lipid droplets, whereas brown adipocytes have a lot of mitochondria and very small lipid droplets[1118]. Hence the names brown and white fat – the more mitochondria the browner the fat cell. Beige fat has a bit more mitochondria than white fat but still holds some lipid droplets, which is why it looks light brown or beige[1119]. This is the biggest reason why brown fat increases your energy expenditure and white fat is mostly used as calorie storage. Brown fat also has more capillaries that can provide the tissues with more oxygen and nutrients. Brown adipose tissue is located around the trachea, spinal cord, pancreas, kidneys, scapula, neck, and upper chest[1120] to protect and heat the vital organs. Beige fat, on the other hand, can be found throughout the body where there's white fat.

White Fat Cell	Beige Fat Cell	Brown Fat Cell

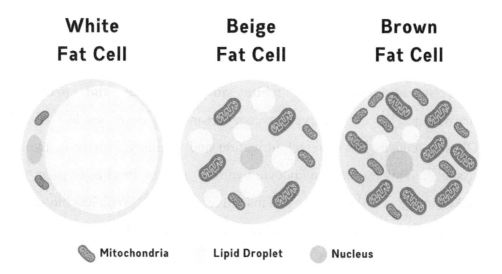

Mitochondria   Lipid Droplet   Nucleus

Redrawn From: Cedikova et al (2016)

The fastest way to activate brown adipose tissue is cold exposure, which improves mitochondrial function, thermoregulation, increases energy expenditure and metabolic rate[1121,1122]. Coldness stimulates fat oxidation, burns white fat, and decreases triglycerides[1123]. Cold exposure also promotes the browning of white fat into brown fat[1124]. A 10-day experiment found that sitting in a cold room at 58°F or 14°C for 6 hours per day increased the metabolic rate of obese men by 14%[1125]. Another study took 11 lean men and put them into a cold room at 67°F or 19°C while wearing a cooling vest at a temperature of 62°F or 16°C for 90 minutes and their metabolic rate increased by 16.7% and fat burning rose by 72.6% after just 30 minutes[1126]! Being immersed in 58°F or 14°C water for 1 hour raises metabolic rate by 350%[1127]! Immersion in 68°F or 20°C water for 1 hour increased metabolic rate by 93%, whereas 90°F or 32°C water didn't. Thus, exposure to cold water at 68°F or 20°C is going to burn a significant amount of calories trying to keep you warm. Granted, it's not an easy task and sitting in cold water is definitely not comfortable but the metabolic effect is there. Cold exposure also increases adiponectin levels, which is a protein that helps with blood sugar regulation and promotes glucose uptake via GLUT4 activation[1128,1129].

Exercise also modulates white adipose tissue and promotes its browning[1130,1131]. It can even reverse diet-induced decreases in brown fat[1132]. Obesity reduces blood vessel formation and capillary density in the adipose tissue[1133]. This results in adipocyte hypoxia or a low level of oxygen, which is linked to higher inflammation and insulin resistance[1134]. With less blood flow into the fat cells, it becomes harder to burn them. Exercise has been shown to prevent this and promote capillary density[1135].

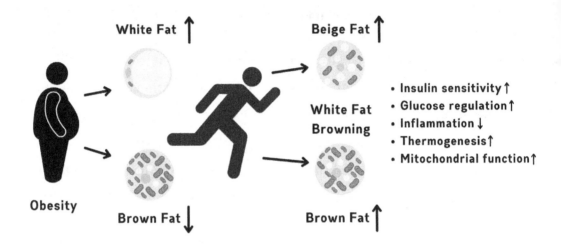

Redrawn From: Garritson 2021

Chapter 5: Flour Enrichment: How Getting our B-Fix from Refined Flour Drove the Obesity Pandemic

Food Enrichment and Fortification – Where Did They Begin?

Most of the processed and packaged food we buy today carries labels listing ingredients, nutritional values and percentages designed to monitor our daily performance against government approved targets for salt, fat and other nutrients. Some packaging makes a feature of particular contents, almost as if they were advertising slogans, i.e., gluten-free, GMO free, organic, but the words 'enriched' and 'fortified' are the ones which have been present on labels the longest. The two terms mean something similar, but they are not quite the same.

- **Enriched food tells us that nutrients which have been removed because of the manufacturing process have been replaced, as is the case with white flour**. In the interest of your health, since refined flour has been stripped of its nutrients, the FDA has mandated that certain B vitamins (B1, B2, B3 and folate) and iron be added back[1136].

- **Conversely, fortified foods have extra nutrients added to them, vitamins and minerals that were not necessarily found in the original raw product or in the list of ingredients, often as the result of public health concerns[1137]**. Salt has been fortified with iodine to prevent goiter since the 1920s[1138] and beginning in 1933, vitamin D was supplemented in all U.S. milk[1139], with the intention of reducing the incidence of rickets, a debilitating disease that weakens the bones of children[1140,1141,1142]. Iodine insufficiency was quite predominant worldwide before 1990 but this has been greatly improved upon with salt iodization[1143].

o The practice continues to this day, and we find it quite normal to find breakfast cereals fortified with all sorts of vitamins and minerals, orange juice that may be fortified with calcium, and even eggs fortified with omega-3 fatty acids – that is achieved by feeding omega-3 rich flaxseed to the mother hens. Another area for fortification is the numerous milk substitutes that have become popular in recent years with almond, rice and soy milk often featuring added calcium plus vitamins A and D[1144].

The hot debate over the years has been between those who have generally supported fortification and enrichment as being sensible public health measures, and those who have been suspicious of the benefits of adding synthetic vitamins and minerals, as if nutrition was just a matter of simple mathematics. If you hit your daily targets by consuming factory-made white bread to which some fiber, vitamins and iron have been re-added, is that the same as eating whole grain bread? If you eat fortified bread and cereal as well as taking a daily multivitamin pill, are you perhaps getting an effective overdose of certain substances?

The First Vitamin Additives

Wherever you stand on the issue, by the 1950s, attractively packaged vitamin pills in small medical bottles had become all the rage and today, it is reported that about 50% of Americans regularly consume multi-vitamin tablets[1145]. In daily life, we get our regular dose of vitamins from fresh, frozen, and canned food, from processed food and drinks which have been enriched and or fortified, but in many cases, also from the little pills we take each day. So, are we getting too much of a good thing? Are we getting insufficient quantities, just enough, or may be too many daily vitamins? And how long have we known about all this? We owe the discovery and the origin of the word 'vitamin' to a Polish-born chemist named Casimir Funk who in 1912, shortly before the outbreak of World War I, correlated the incidence of the disease beriberi (vitamin B1 or thiamine deficiency), with Asian communities consuming large quantities of refined, polished rice[1146]. It was originally thought that there was something toxic about the rice itself, but Funk isolated a compound in the rice husk which was found to be missing in the prepared rice. He named it 'water-soluble B' and coined the word vitamine (from, life-giving amines) for what he assumed would be a growing set of such compounds to be found in other foods. He was right, and with that discovery, the idea of deficiency diseases was born. Thirteen different vitamins were discovered in the following thirty-five years including eight forms of vitamin B, vitamin C, and the four fat soluble vitamins A, D, E and K[1147]. Incidentally, the very first vitamin pill to be approved by the American Medical Association (AMA) and launched in the early 1920s was named Oscodal, a vitamin A and D concentrate[1148].

Soon afterwards during the 1930s, the fortification of milk began, while Kellogg's best-selling Pep cereal started to feature added vitamins D and vitamin B1 (thiamine) from 1938, but it was particularly the supplementation of the various B vitamins which gained interest. Vitamin B1 is known as thiamine, B2 as riboflavin, B3 as niacin, B5 as pantothenic acid and B6 as pyridoxine – and all were isolated and synthesized before the outbreak of World War II. Vitamin B7 (biotin), B9 (folic acid) and B12 (cobalamin) were not synthesized until 1943, 1945 and 1972, respectively. Thiamine developed the nickname, the morale vitamin, because of the positive effect it can have on our nerves and in combating stress. With the imminent outbreak of war and President Roosevelt concerned about levels of under-nourishment in post-depression America, we saw the first list of recommended dietary allowances published in 1941 and after widespread voluntary measures introduced by the food industry, the enrichment of flour across the country was officially mandated in 1943[1149]. However, only 3 out of the 8 B-vitamins (B1, B2, B3) were added to flour at the time. Although technically, flour no longer has to be enriched in the U.S. today, practically all breads and flour are enriched according to FDA guidelines, although there are a growing number of un-enriched options, particularly in the organic area. Notably, Canada and the United Kingdom followed suit, but in those countries, minimum levels of vitamins and minerals in all the flour and bread sold are mandatory. Nevertheless, there are still many other countries who choose not to enrich or fortify their flour. This can lead to quite idiosyncratic situations. There is, for example, a growing artisanal trade in French flour (a country that forbids such additives) imported into the UK, but bread made from that flour has to be clearly labeled as passing European Union regulations but not British ones.

Vitamins Are Good for Us, so Enrichment Must Be a Good Thing, Right?

All the enriched flour that you buy today has also been fortified. In 1998, that was extended to include folic acid fortification for all enriched cereal grain flour, a measure fully implemented in both the U.S. and Canada, but interestingly not followed through within the UK. The addition of folic acid was designed to protect pregnant women from the potential dangers of neural tube defects such as spina bifida. It has as such been generally considered an effective measure, although opposing voices have expressed concern at the use of mandatory additives for the whole population when they are of importance to only about 2% of the population at any given time[1150,1151].

From a situation in the earlier half of the 20th century when we were getting vitamins from whole foods, times have changed dramatically, and now, many of us take in most of our nutritional requirement in the form of packaged fortified foods. Primary sources of nutrients used to come from fruit, vegetables, meat, and dairy, at least that's how it was at the start of the 20th century, but by the beginning of the 21st century, more than half (59%) came from enriched and fortified grain sources. This may not seem bad on the surface, but what if our simple and natural desire to eat vitamin rich food is being tampered with by vitamin fortifications. **What if our instinctive urges to prefer healthier food are being influenced by well-intentioned fortification programs, leading us to eat more junk food?**

Consider this animal study that has since been replicated by other researchers. Twenty-three lambs were intentionally fed a diet that was low in vitamin E (known for its anti-inflammatory properties) over several weeks[1152]. They were then given a choice of food; orange flavored food pellets, something lambs would never usually eat, or more of their regular unfortified feed. Unbeknown to them (of course), the orange flavored feed had also been fortified with vitamin E, and guess what, they much preferred it. *"Animals have an extraordinary ability to seek out nutrients that are essential to survival,"* said Fred Provenza, a behavioural ecologist who has studied animal eating habits for over 40 years[1153]. **In humans, it's known that less processed whole foods lead to higher satiety and reduced food intake compared to the same whole foods after processing (i.e., regular white potatoes vs French fries)[1154].** Diets high in ultra-processed foods result in 500-600 more calories consumed per day[1155].

Could it be that as humans, we are losing the natural ability to identify healthy food because our processed food is now loaded with synthetic vitamins? Certainly, a disturbing thought and it may be a pivotal reason behind our growing dependence on ultra-processed, hyperpalatable junk food. For those twenty-three lambs, the addition of one single vitamin got them selecting and eating food that was quite foreign in taste to them. Fortifying their largely carbohydrate-based feed with a greater palette of vitamins can fatten up animals too. As counterintuitive as that may sound, farmers have known this simple fact for more than a century. They knew that by adding corn and barley to their feed, they could fatten up animals in the short term, but that if their pigs and chicken were fed exclusively on that, over time, they would get sick[1156]. However, letting them run around outside to eat insects and forage was enough to protect them, while adding kitchen scraps and green feed (mostly veggies) proved even more effective, helping them to get all the vitamins they required. By being both observant, clever, and cost-effective, these early livestock farmers found that by adding nutrients to cheaper, carbohydrate rich animal feed, they would thrive by eating greater quantities, putting on more weight and avoiding disease. They were encouraged by the support of the scientific community, although as time went on, it became clear there was one potential downside. Allen Williams, livestock expert and former Professor of animal science at Louisiana State University explains:

> *If you supplement them with vitamins and minerals, they get lazy and have no desire to go out and graze. You can actually have an effect on their (animal) behaviour.* [1157]

This raises an interesting and provocative question. Is it possible that our human behavior is being manipulated in a similar way? 'Manipulated' is a strong word and implies that certain people, interest groups or institutions have deliberately promoted the addition of vitamins and certain other minerals to be able to sell more food which is based on the use of refined ingredients. Deliberate manipulation would also mean that selected information has been withheld or suppressed to promote the interests of processed foods manufacturers, just as happened in the tobacco and sugar scandals[1158]. There's no clear evidence of malicious intent but looking at the scientific catalogue from the last fifty years you can find one potential red flag and it is a large one. There is surprisingly little research material that explores the relationship and effect of food fortification on humans.

However, there is substantial research coming from studies using animals, mostly rats. Early tests focused on the effects of eating refined carbohydrates without sufficient amounts of other nutrients. Feeding studies in Germany demonstrated that rats who got half their diet from fresh, stone-ground wholemeal flour or the bread made from it, survived healthily, but that those fed with 15-day old milled flour or bread as well as those eating refined white flour all became infertile over four generations (assumed to be something like 100 human years)[1159]. In view of such results, it would normally be considered unethical to run extensive tests lasting many years on humans but no worries, the test is running – the experiment on us began in western economies around seventy to eighty years ago, albeit with selected added vitamins. Let's get back to the rats - further research, run in the early 1950s by Estelle Hawley of Rochester University showed how those rodents fed primarily commercially enriched white bread with the addition of a little margarine became ill, produced stunted offspring, and became extinct after four generations[1160]. The famous nutritionist, Dr Roger Williams, whose elder brother Robert was the first to synthesize Thiamine (B1), demonstrated the effect of eating bread made from enriched flour when compared to those eating whole grain bread. Most (rats again) died at a younger age while the rest exhibited stunted growth on the bread made from enriched flour[1161]. Earlier in 1933, Harris et al revealed another aspect, namely how rats sought out vitamin B-enriched food and preferred it to unfortified flour, even though there was of course, no taste difference[1162]. He even demonstrated that to speed up that process, they could be 'educated' to prefer the enriched food but added that generally, they ate enriched and non-enriched diets indiscriminately, until they first began to suffer from the vitamin deficiency. That is when they began to exhibit a clear preference for the enriched food. Could this be a relevant indicator for what can happen to us?

Of greater concern is perhaps that the FDA's recommendations on the levels of food fortification for Americans have not been updated since 1968 and currently conflict with the levels considered safe by the Institute of Medicine of the National Academies[1163]. We used to eat more food in its naturally occurring form back in 1968 when those recommendations were drawn up. **Today, Americans get most of their essential nutrients by eating highly processed food in the form of enriched bread, fortified sugary cereals and a mix of protein packed bars and vitamin drinks**. Gary Beauchamp, the former director of the Monell Center which is a hub for research on the science of taste and smell puts it like this.

> *The fact that we no longer need to get micronutrients via a wide range of plants is one of many ways that the current food system in humans no longer fits our evolutionary history.*[1164]

Humans are thought to prioritize protein intake when eating[1165]. This theory is called The Protein Leverage Hypothesis – that satiety is mostly determined by protein consumption. Protein intake promotes satiety and fullness by decreasing ghrelin aka the hunger hormone[1166,1167,1168]. A sufficient amount of protein that leads to satiety is considered to be around 20-30% of total calories. Unfortunately, the average Westerner only gets 11-18% of total energy as protein, which leads to food cravings and an overconsumption of calories. Whereas in the past, our natural cravings may have led us to eat a steak for example, guided not just by the fine cooking smells but also by the body's need for protein, fats, minerals, and vitamins, now, the nutrients in junk food may well be reinforcing our desire to eat more of them. Quoting Fred Provenza again:

> *People are being conditioned to want to eat them. And when they do, they wind up overconsuming calories in an attempt to obtain necessary nutrients.*[1169]

The analogy to what happens with animals is all too transparent. **Much of the high calorie food we eat today is very similar to the animal feed designed to fatten up livestock**. And just as with the animals, we eat a lot more of it, if it has been fortified. The processed food industry loves this situation, being able to use cheap, refined sugar and other starch-rich ingredients, loaded particularly with added B vitamins to stimulate your appetite. Keeping you alive just enough to come back for more. Such a blend, combined with a mix of preservatives, emulsifiers and taste enhancers contributes to creating that perfect bliss point which optimizes palatability… and leads so many down the pathway towards chronic disease and obesity.

It does not have to be this way. If we were to stop fortification and help people back towards their natural instincts, those cravings which lead to an increased desire for fresh foods and those which really supplement our body's natural urges would take over. In a very different world, so many years ago, during a period of peace between two world wars yet still deeply affected by the Great Depression, food policy decisions were implemented which still impact our lives today. Maybe more so. Let's not forget that the degree of fortification has increased over the years, and this is also the case for iron, another food additive which is supplemented in various different forms. By 1983, iron fortification in wheat flour and bread accounted for ~ 20% of the iron intake in the United States and the implications are worth careful consideration[1170].

The Harms of Iron Fortification

At first glance, it is all too rational to make the decision to fortify, where possible with added iron. After all, iron is a nutritionally essential trace element crucial for both optimal physical and cognitive performance. Furthermore, iron deficiency anemia is one of the top nutrient deficiencies in the world, affecting ~ 25% of the population[1171]. Despite advances in the nutritional sciences and the development of worldwide economies, iron deficiency continues to be the most prevalent single micronutrient deficiency disease in the world, affecting billions of people. You can imagine early meetings of the iron-supplementation committee. A summary might read like this: *topping up food with just a little iron will surely raise iron levels across the country and that must be good, particularly for children*. The irony is that today, those who are most exposed to the additives, overweight American children who get their iron from eating a lot of processed food, have been found to be twice as deficient in iron compared to normal weight children[1172,1173]. How can this possibly be?

The first study linking obesity and iron deficiency, published in 2003, described a greater prevalence of iron deficiency, in overweight and obese Israeli adolescents and children, than in the general population[1174]. The research team blamed 'unbalanced nutrition' or 'short-term diets' but a growing number of scientists now believe in an association between inflammation and increased adiposity, which cannot be solved by taking in more dietary iron[1175]. According to the European Union, in recent decades, iron-enriched breakfast cereals became the principal source of iron in young children's diets in the UK, replacing meat which was the main source of iron in the 1950s[1176]. And yet they note, levels of iron deficiency are no different in the UK from the rest of the EU where food is not fortified, and the habit of eating breakfast cereals is less common. Could the way different forms of iron get absorbed by the body play a role in this? One of the more intriguing theories is that since iron enrichment disrupts the gut flora, particularly impacting our ability to digest wheat, this could also lead to gluten intolerance (or increased gluten sensitivity) being more prevalent in countries such as the U.S., Canada and the UK with their iron fortification programs[1177,1178,1179].

It is widely accepted that the two forms of nutritional iron, heme iron, mostly from animal food sources, and non-heme iron, the only form found in non-animal food sources, are absorbed differently. Iron coming from animal foods like meat, fish and poultry is much better absorbed than that coming from vegetables. For example, the bioavailability of iron from steak is 20% but only 2% from spinach[1180,1181]. Yet when iron is added as a fortificant, it takes the form of non-heme iron, which is not well absorbed. There are ways to increase the absorption of this type of iron, such as eating fruit rich in vitamin C, especially when combined with animal protein, but who is considering that when they eat fortified bread or cereal?

Most African countries now state that in-home iron fortification for infants is recommended for the control of anemia, yet Kenyan research has shown that low absorption typically results in more than 80% of the iron passing straight into the colon[1182]. Studies from the Ivory Coast showed even higher levels, and overall fortification brought about no significant improvements in iron levels[1183]. Mostly ingested in the form of micronutrient powders, this was shown to adversely affect the infant gut microbiome and cause intestinal inflammation, which as we know, can also be a precursor for increased adiposity.

What's more, iron absorption, transportation and transformation into hemoglobin requires copper[1184,1185,1186,1187,1188,1189,1190]. Copper deficiency reduces iron absorption, impairs heme synthesis, and promotes iron accumulation in the body[1191]. What's worse, excess iron intake can inhibit copper absorption, which causes copper deficiency[1192]. It's been known since the 1930s that copper supplementation can help treat iron deficiency anemia[1193]. Low levels of copper in the blood are linked to a greater prevalence of anemia[1194,1195,1196]. Thus, cramming your system with more iron, especially the less bioavailable forms, does little to no good to your overall iron status, especially if you are not getting enough copper. For some, too much iron is positively dangerous. This is the case for those suffering from hemochromatosis, which is characterized by an inappropriate increase in the intestinal absorption of iron and its accumulation in organs and tissues including the liver, spleen, heart, pancreas, endocrine glands, skin, and joints. Although comparatively rare, it still affects over 1 million Americans and many more around the world. The disorder means that your body literally loads too much iron, which can eventually be fatal. **Iron overload is associated with many diseases like arthritis, cancer, tumor growth, diabetes, heart failure, and liver damage[1197,1198].** When copper deficient, iron overload is increased.

Unlike with many vitamins, the body is unable to get rid of excess iron, so in the case of hemochromatosis, where you can absorb as much as four times as much iron as others do, your organs become diseased. Too much ferritin (stored iron) promotes lipofuscin formation, which is one of the main age-related pigments that accelerates aging and oxidative stress[1199]. Not surprisingly, a healthy diet means avoiding iron rich food, but inevitably that now means staying away from much processed food, including bread which is fortified. In the U.S., cereal rich products like bread and breakfast cereals make up 45% of the daily iron intake for an average American[1200], so if you are suffering from an overload, you really need to be careful. In a 2012 paper on the topic, the haematologist José Martins wrote:

> *We are against mass food fortification, because we believe that one cannot correct one problem (iron deficiency) and exacerbate another condition (acceleration of cases of hemochromatosis) which is as severe as the first.* [1201]

It has been argued that decades of pill popping and food fortification have led many of us to ingest more iron than may be good for us, and unless you do a lot of your cooking from raw ingredients at home, iron-rich food can be difficult to avoid. Many other important self-interest groups such as diabetics, or those with celiac disease have the possibility to eat foods without sugar or gluten, yet if you have hemochromatosis, you must be very careful, not just with some natural foods such as red meat but increasingly because of all the iron fortification. Unless you live in France of course.

The French and many European countries sell flour and bread without the additional vitamins or minerals that are omnipresent in American food. Yet iron deficiency anemia is no greater in France. In his book, '*Iron, the Most Toxic Metal*', Jym Moon argues that we are over-simplistic with our western approach to fortification. It is simply not a nutritional deficiency disease, there being so many other factors at play, and that as a medical problem, anemia is improved by a whole variety of potential remedies[1202]. When the Food and Nutrition Board upped the level of iron fortification in 1981, Moon thinks that they should have admitted failure rather than adding what he considers to be a risk factor to the diet of many people. After all, iron, like certain other metals, accumulates with age in the body, and needs the counterbalance of copper, manganese, and zinc to avoid oxidative stress, which are nutrients that most of us are deficient in[1203].

For our body, iron is very much a double-edged sword because when found in moderate quantities and leashed to protein, it is an essential element in all cell metabolism and growth. Problematic though is the way in which iron can switch back and forward between its ferrous and ferric oxidation states, at times functioning as a strong biological oxidant and at others as a reductant. With a mineral imbalance in your body and iron being one of the most reactive metals, the tendency is always going to be towards oxidation. Put bluntly, just like with an old car left out in the rain, it rusts.

What Is Too Much Fortification Doing to Us?

The comments in this chapter have been all to do with eating fortified foods, but when you consume whole foods, unless you suffer from a disease such as hemochromatosis, there should be no worry. Eating animal meat, plants or seeds means eating organisms that were naturally in balance – let's face it, they have to be or they would not have thrived in the first place - but selectively refining food or fortifying it promotes an imbalance. Even the most well-intentioned shoppers who prefer to select organic foods pay scant attention to what's in their bread or flour. Even grocery stores that are considered to contain more natural and organic items have most of their aisles and bakeries full of enriched product.

So, putting this all together, if you have good access to fresh and only lightly processed foods (after all, even cooking and canning tomatoes is a mild form

of processing) including good sources of protein and fat, you certainly don't need your staple foods to be fortified. But Franklin Roosevelt in the 1940s and even George McGovern whose Select Committee on Nutrition and Human Needs authored the first U.S. Dietary Guidelines in 1977 had as their primary concern, the intent to once and for all, stamp out malnutrition[1204]. In that context, the American Bakers Association (ABA) lobbied hard and consistently to maintain or increase enrichment, while the Food and Drug Administration (FDA) considered it to represent the *"needless and irrational consumption of added vitamins and minerals"*[1205]. As late as 1980, the FDA's official policy was that the widespread fortification of food was unnecessary, but since Congress had recently passed a law which meant that natural and synthetic vitamins and minerals were no longer to be considered as drugs, the FDA's hands were tied. They could still express a strong opinion, but not provide a tight regulatory framework, so that the increases in the levels of B vitamins such as niacin, riboflavin and thiamine were as much down to industry influence as to the FDA. The same goes for the increases in iron that were agreed in 1973 but reversed (by the FDA) five years later, before being increased again in 1981. The problem for the FDA's interpretation was that their policy did not specify that deficiencies be present in a significant proportion of the population; rather that as long as some kind of deficiency existed, it would be okay for everyone to be dosed with the enrichment in question. It is not necessarily that the extra dose of B-vitamins is harmful, it's that the inclusion of them leads to an increased consumption of highly processed foods. It's the inclusion of B-vitamins that breaks our natural hunger signals to eat whole nutritious foods because we are now obtaining nourishment from milled flour. If milled flour did not have these B-vitamin enrichments, we would likely eat less of them, and seek out natural foods to obtain our needed nutrients.

Regarding iron, its addition to flour must be considered highly questionable and many doctors and iron toxicologists over the years have expressed their concern[1206]. Unfortunately, these concerns have been sidelined by the grain lobbyists who promote further iron enrichment[1207]. In 1975, William H Crosby, one of the founding fathers of modern hematology – the treatment and study of the blood – wrote that data was being manipulated to suggest a national catastrophe, especially concerning anemia. A nutritionist involved in discussions at the time informed Crosby that despite the constructive criticism, such fortification was simply what McGovern wanted. And so, he got his wish. Nearly forty years later, as we pass the second decade of the 21st century, where does this leave us? As written in an excellent review of the topic:

> *A single slice of enriched white bread now has as much appetite-stimulating B vitamins as a medium sweet potato and more riboflavin and niacin than a cup of beans. These enrichments are specifically designed to enable people to eat refined foods as staples, which are rapidly digested and lack the satiating fiber and phytonutrients that are found in whole grains and complex carbohydrates. Moreover, a diet that lacks fermentable fiber promotes diet-induced adiposity.[1208]*

The American Bakers Association's successful lobbying efforts helped position enriched grains as the substantial underpinning of the U.S. Dietary Guidelines and the original Food Pyramid which was first published in 1992. Even today, a look at the Bakers' website shows the pride associated with their successful lobbying activities since their formation in 1897[1209], and how closely linked they are to the current 'Choose MyPlate' nutrition guidance. Only three major countries, the U.S., Canada, and the UK insist on such broad food fortification programs. **Notably, the French, who consume a lot more flour per capita annually than Americans, have always banned enrichments in their traditional French**

bread. They also show much lower rates of obesity than the three countries who do use intensive fortification, but this also raises the question as to why we continue to fortify food at all, particularly wheat? It may sound cynical, but these days, probably the most important reason is to keep up our growing appetite for refined, highly processed food. To sustain that hunger, we must consume B vitamins, and if processed food is rich in those vitamins, we want more of them. You may well be thinking that sugar is surely the number one culprit for obesity today and yet, **without the presence of B vitamins in all those sugary cereals, cookies and energy bars, our natural selves would seek out real food, which is naturally rich in those B vitamins**. John Yudkin, an early proponent of the idea that too much sugar is harmful, showed that Vitamin B1 (thiamine) deficient rats who initially loved the taste of sweet sucrose even went so far as to avoid sucrose completely as their vitamin deficiency progressed[1210]. It seems that given the choice, **vitamin rich food is innately preferred to sweet food**.

To best support our lives as humans, we should only seek out unrefined whole grains (although most "whole grains" are highly refined), meat, eggs and dairy, legumes, nuts, seeds, and green vegetables to get our vitamin B fix, but the thing is, we no longer need to. Additives are everywhere. Many of America's favorite processed snacks are based on highly processed corn meal containing ferrous sulphate (iron), thiamine mononitrate (B1), riboflavin (B2), niacin (B3), and folic acid (B9) – a bold mixture of enrichment and fortification[1211]. This type of processing is like boiling an apple until it loses its red or green color and then using food coloring to make it look just like it did before. That's what the added vitamin/mineral powders do in replacing the natural ingredients which have been processed out of the original constituents.

During the mid-to-late 19th century as the consumption of refined carbohydrates in the form of white flour and sugar increased, dyspepsia or

indigestion became a widespread complaint. Dyspepsia affected the masses but not the rich or the well to do who still got plenty of meat in their diet, but apart from the digestive unpleasantness that went with it, the other major symptom was loss of weight. If they had known about the role of vitamins back then, and how to add B vitamins to their flour and bread, they would almost certainly have put on weight, cured short-term dyspepsia, and lived longer – but not necessarily heathier - lives. That is again why farmers to this day use fortified animal feed to fatten up their livestock, because they know how it works and what consistent results it brings. It is disheartening to accept, but what the processed food industry is doing to us humans today is very much the same thing. By feeding nutrient-fortified junk food to humans, they are fattening us up like livestock and creating similar patterns of chronic disease as found in rapid growing obese chickens, cows and by default, our pets.

Our desire for calorie-rich, sugar-loaded, junk food which has been enriched, and in many cases fortified, is driving up levels of obesity. Our natural cravings for specific whole foods have been dulled as an ever-greater percentage of the food we eat is ultra-processed and supplemented with synthetic vitamins and minerals. Speaking to Men's Journal magazine, Dr David Katz, director of the Yale University Prevention Research Center, sums the situation up like this:

Throwing nutrients into junk food does not produce good food. It produces nutrient-fortified junk.[1212]

Making Sense of Counterintuitive Information

Which came first, the chicken or the egg? Was he pushed, or did he jump? Riddles of causality lie deep in our psyche, and they serve to remind us that getting to the root cause of an issue or discovering the main reason that two events are connected can be very, very difficult. Conspiracy theories add to the complexity in an era of alt-news and alleged fake news, so our analysis of all this enriched nutrition information may be considered a step too far but there is a fair amount of evidence to support our view. Perhaps obesity and chronic disease are just accidents of civilization, the inevitable result of too many humans on a small planet, but perhaps not. It appears to us that **today's obesity epidemic was at least in part engineered by a super-enrichment policy**, and that very few were aware of the true consequences of the big decisions taken all those years ago. In all likelihood, certain vested interest groups still want to preserve our new 'fortified' status quo, when what we should now be having is a discussion about the removal of highly processed junk foods from our diet.

Of all the enticing B vitamins that we eat, vitamin B1 (thiamine) is the dominant hunger vitamin. Too little and we will suffer from disease. Our bodies, when left to their own devices, will crave such vitamin rich food, the brain associating appetite with healthy eating. It is true for rats and mice, as well as sheep and other animals and it is just as true for humans, having served as the foundation for all traditional cooking. Or it would be, if the highly processed junk foods of today were not loaded with such a high level of these additives. In one way that's a good thing because we have seen that refined carbohydrates, which are the biggest constituent of most junk food, create stomach pain and uncomfortable dyspepsia, if and when those B vitamins are missing. Of course, people can just lose their appetites under quite normal circumstances too, and that appetite factor was central to the initial discovery of vitamins. Sir Robert McCarrison in his 1921 treatise found that adding brewer's yeast, naturally rich in B-complex vitamins did the trick[1213] – made people more hungry that is. He learned that loss of appetite was one of the most fundamental signs of vitamin deprivation and considered it as a kind of warning sign which indicated that there was a dietary problem.

Thomas Osborne and Lafayette Mendel found out at roughly the same time that if they had poor quality, nutrient deficient food, they could still get animals to eat it, as long as brewer's yeast (aka vitamin B) was added in sufficient quantities[1214]. They likened this to the problems sometimes encountered when feeding infants, because we are less hungry when fed nutrition-less food – unless it has been previously 'vitamized'. In an article questioning the entire role of food enrichment:

> *In other words, enriching refined foods—and "educating" people to eat those foods—tricks the body into craving a food that it would otherwise lose its appetite for… this is exactly what the American Bakers Association did to Americans. Enriching white flour enables people to eat refined junk food.* [1215]

We forget or simply don't know that the historical context for those early days of adding vitamins to food in the USA was very different from that found today. Many Americans, particularly young men, considered themselves to be scrawny, with bodybuilding advertisements becoming popular and 'ironized yeast' featured as the best way to promote weight gain as well as to stimulate your appetite. Steadily, people were learning that they could gain weight on a relatively poor diet, as long as the food was enriched, or you were taking the right blend of B vitamins.

Much more recently, Dr. Shi-Sheng Zhou et al. published six papers linking vitamin B food enrichment to the obesity epidemic and related metabolic diseases, including diabetes[1216,1217,1218,1219,1220,1221]. In 2014, Zhou wrote of the strong correlations between increases to enrichment levels and rising obesity trends in developed countries: "*We therefore hypothesize that excess vitamins may play a causal role in the increased prevalence of obesity.*" [1222] What he was also able to show was that developed countries who choose not to fortify food have much less obesity. In general, those include several European countries such as France and Denmark who traditionally forbid the fortification of carbohydrates. There is a lot of institutional pressure on this situation however and Denmark which used to ban the sale of all fortified Kellogg's products for this very reason, has recently started to make exceptions[1223].

Turning that correlation between food enrichment and obesity into a possible causation proved difficult and somewhat tenuous for Dr. Zhou and his team. Although he pursued the idea of a vitamin overload, the simpler explanation, that enrichments stimulate the appetite seems to us the most likely. Yet are there some countries where obesity is on the rise and yet B-vitamins are not being added? Zhou comments on this, saying that those countries where more meat is eaten also correlate with higher levels of obesity. Meat in general does contain particularly high natural levels of the B vitamins so perhaps a clearer statement would be that you can maintain your appetite as long as you are getting your B vitamins from somewhere. Meat is after all, more available than ever, thanks to modern, intensive farming.

The increasingly well-known case of William Banting provides us with an example of that relatively rare situation where someone could become obese on a diet of pure non-enriched carbohydrates[1224]. The corpulent Mr. Banting was a famous British undertaker living in mid-Victorian times. He buried everyone from King George III in 1820 to the Duke of Wellington upon his death in 1852 and Prince Albert himself in 1861. Today he is more famous for both getting very fat and losing a lot of weight, and in certain countries such as South Africa, his name has become synonymous with successful low-carb dietary approaches. He enjoyed the privileged position of being able to afford to eat lots of sugary foods (yes, they were expensive back then) and other unenriched carbohydrates, but he also enjoyed his beer. In doing so, he put on a considerable amount of weight. His doctor, William Harvey referred to this weight gain as happening when he ate "*low*", meaning lots of bread and potatoes, versus "*well*", when he ate mostly meat. On these so-called low days, he also consumed "*large quantities of beer, milk and sugar*" which were effectively giving him his B vitamins and stimulating his appetite for refined carbohydrates. If as in earlier centuries, he had been obtaining all those vitamins from whole plants and grains, he would have had to eat an immense quantity to get enough, and such foods are very filling. Banting's story was widely discussed, partly because obesity was something of a rarity in Victorian England, although beer was known to promote weight gain in sedentary people. Highly active brewery workers stayed slim, even those who drank similar quantities to shoemakers for example, who were famous for putting on the pounds.

It seems clear, whether you are a farm animal, a rodent, or a human, you need some source of B vitamins to maintain your appetite, and it doesn't matter from where the B vitamins come. The interesting hypothesis that arises in this connection is the following. If you were to remove all additives from U.S. cereal-based foods, bread, and flour, would the demand and the resulting consumption go down? Our conclusion is that it would, simply because we would all have to look elsewhere for our B-vitamins.

The avoidance of enrichments in many other developed countries has preserved the consumption of local, traditional foods, but cooking culture becomes less relevant and necessary when vitamins are in abundance. From an early age, Americans are more or less indoctrinated into believing that vitamins are essential additives, with messaging taking pride of place on cereal packages and milk cartons. However, **if flour fortification went away, sales of junk food would almost certainly decline.** William Banting, were he alive today, may well have become even more corpulent with access to so much vitamin enriched junk food, and yet had he been born in France, things may have worked out differently for him.

Let's be clear here, the effect of enrichment is quite 'subtle' because the process normalizes your appetite. If you were to eat truly pure, nutrition-less, refined carbohydrates and soda all day, you would over time, lose your appetite and as a result, become deficient and sick. **What the enrichments facilitate is your ability to eat a junk food diet, the direct cause of so much obesity today**. That is why Americans do not lose their appetites even when they remain sedentary and eat lots of refined foods. You would not be able to eat such food in sufficient quantities without getting enough B vitamins, and the current levels of enrichment are enough to do so. We have read that a single slice of enriched white bread contains as much appetite-stimulating B vitamins as a medium sweet potato and more riboflavin and niacin than a cup of beans. That's borderline irresponsible, particularly when you consider that the big push to add enrichments to the food supply did not come from the government, but rather from the American Bakers Association (ABA), who are effectively an industry lobby group. The ABA website portrays their most recent activities in this and other areas with pride, but it also presents a window into how the voice of industry may be having a larger impact on your daily food than you think.

Chapter 6 – Fats That Make You Fat, Fats That Make You Lean

Fat has the highest caloric content out of all the macronutrients. It has more than double the amount of calories per gram than protein or carbs (9 vs 4). That makes it easy to think that eating fat promotes weight gain. Cross-sectional studies do show that obese patients obtain a larger percentage of their calories from fat than individuals with a healthy BMI[1225]. However, **going into a calorie surplus by eating too many calories will inevitably make you gain weight regardless if the calories come from fat, carbohydrates or protein.** Sources of dietary fat are much smaller in volume; for example, 100 grams of butter is nearly half the volume as 100 grams of broccoli, yet it has up to 30x more calories (900 vs 30). Granted, most people are more likely to eat broccoli than just pure butter but **adding a lot of extra fats and oils to your food can unknowingly increase your total daily caloric intake quite significantly**. What's more, fat tends to make food more palatable and tastier. Regular broccoli isn't that appealing, and you get satiated quite fast eating it, but if you cook it in a lot of fat and oil it becomes a lot more hyperpalatable. In this form, broccoli could indeed make you gain weight because it has a lot more calories than it does in its natural form. Such tricks have been used for decades by the processed food industry by adding fats into their products to make them tastier.

However, the ratio of fat in the American diet hasn't increased over recent decades, it's actually decreased. NHANES data from 1971-2000 has discovered that the percentage of calories from fat has decreased from 36.9% to 32.8% in men and 36.1% to 32.8% in women[1226]. Calories from saturated fat has also dropped from 13.5% to 10.9% in men and 13.0% to 11% in women. However, this decrease is attributed to an increase in total calories consumed and absolute intake of fat in grams has increased[1227]. Thus, it's not that people are eating less fat, they're eating more calories from carbohydrates. During this same time frame, in men, the percentage of calories from carbohydrates have increased from 42.4% to 49.0% and in women from 45.4% to 51.6%. Protein contribution has also dropped from 16.5% to 15.5% in men and 16.9% to 15.1% in women.

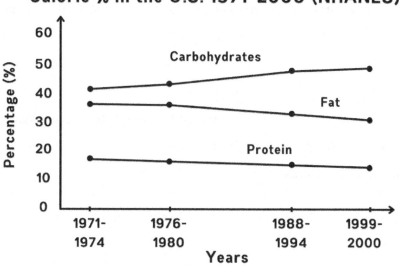

Redrawn From: CDC (2004)

Despite not eating a significantly higher amount of fat, obesity rates have been steadily increasing. Obviously, an excess of dietary fat can make you gain weight by putting you into an energy surplus. However, the data doesn't suggest that consuming more fat is to blame for the rise in calorie consumption or the obesity epidemic. Rather, the culprit may be the types of fat people have been consuming and in what forms they come. Different types of fat have different effects on your metabolic rate, energy expenditure, insulin sensitivity and metabolic health. In this chapter, we're going to look at the impact of dietary fats on weight loss and metabolic health.

Which Fats Make You Fat, Which Ones Make You Lean

Fat is an essential nutrient and humans have been eating fats throughout history. Populations consuming large amounts of fat from olive oil or fish show significantly lower rates of cardiovascular disease risk, meaning the quality of fat is just as important as the quantity[1228]. **Over the past 100 years we've started to consume a higher intake of omega-6 fat from seed oils, which can lead to inflammation and cardiovascular disease**. Nowadays, the average American diet consists of 20% energy from soybean oil, with over 7% of daily calories coming from the omega-6 fat linoleic acid[1229]. It's been noted that the rise in obesity, diabetes and asthma has paralleled an increase of omega-6 linoleic acid in adipose tissue of U.S adults[1230]. **In the U.S., soybean oil intake has increased by over 1,000-fold from 1909 to 1999**[1231]. On the flip side, saturated fat consumption has decreased[1232].

% Caloric Intake from Linoleic Acid in the United States[1233]

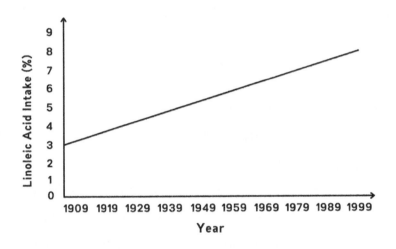

Redrawn From: Blasbalg et al (2011)

156

Linoleic Acid in Subcutaneous Adipose Tissue in the United States[1234]

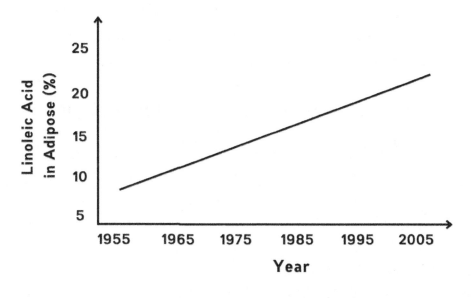

Redrawn From: Guyenet et al (2015)

In animals, a high omega-6 intake promotes fat deposition and decreases muscle insulin sensitivity, whereas omega-3 fats have the opposite effect[1235,1236,1237,1238,1239]. Rats fed fish oil have been seen to have lower visceral fat and less insulin resistance compared to rats fed corn oil or lard[1240]. Human clinical studies also affirm that oxidized omega-6 fats raise pro-inflammatory cytokines, whereas supplementing long chain omega-3 fatty acids like EPA and DHA lowers inflammation[1241]. EPA and DHA reduce inflammatory cytokines and interleukins[1242,1243,1244,1245,1246,1247,1248]. Thus, getting an excess of omega-6 fatty acids in your diet and not enough omega-3s makes it easier for you to develop metabolic syndrome, cardiovascular disease, and inflammatory fat gain[1249,1250,1251]. Hunter-gatherers are thought to have consumed an omega-6 to omega-3 a ratio of about 1:1 or up to 4:1[1252]. However, today the average American diet has an omega-6/3 ratio of 20-50:1, significantly favoring omega-6s[1253]. In other words, the omega-6/3 ratio has increased by about 30-fold compared to traditional intakes[1254]. Virtually all of that comes from the consumption of omega-6 seed oils (soybean, corn, canola, sunflower, safflower, rice bran, grapeseed, peanut, etc.) contained in processed packaged foods, such as frozen pizzas, cookies, donuts, salad dressings, etc. These oils are also used for cooking, which further creates oxidation products in the oil.

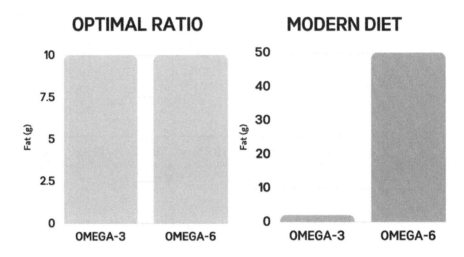

Not all omega-6 fats are bad, and they are essential fatty acids. The main omega-6 fats are linoleic acid (LA) and arachidonic acid (AA), which are involved in the body's inflammatory response to infections, by promoting swelling, inflammation, redness, heat and pain[1255]. In contrast, omega-3s eicosapentaenoic acid (EPA) and docosahexaenoic acid (DHA) have anti-inflammatory properties that help to resolve inflammation[1256,1257]. Thus, you do need both but in the right balance.

It's not even the excess consumption of omega-6 fats that's the most harmful thing about them but rather the fact that the omega-6 fats people do consume nowadays are oxidized. Polyunsaturated fats (PUFAs), which most refined oils are made of, become very easily oxidized when exposed to heat, oxygen, pressure, or light during the extraction process. This leads to lipid peroxidation (just a fancy term for oxidation) and aldehyde formation which causes DNA damage, mutagenesis, and carcinogenesis[1258]. The overconsumption of omega-6 seed oils can even increase the susceptibility of LDL to oxidation[1259,1260,1261,1262,1263], which is associated with heart disease[1264,1265,1266,1267]. Oxidized LDL causes direct damage and inflammation to cells, promoting atherosclerosis[1268]. Coronary heart disease patients have higher levels of oxidized LDL[1269,1270,1271]. The primary catalyst for the oxidation of LDL cholesterol is the oxidized linoleic acid inside LDL particles[1272]. After oxidation, LDL won't be recognized by LDL receptors on the liver anymore, promoting atherosclerosis and heart disease[1273,1274]. Linoleic acid rich HDL and VLDL can also become oxidized, which contributes to cardiovascular disease risk as well[1275]. What this means is that the more omega-6 fats you consume, the more gets into all your lipoproteins (LDL, VLDL and HDL), the higher the likelihood they become oxidized[1276]. Cholesterol bound to saturated fat is less susceptible to oxidation because of the higher heat-stability of saturated fats[1277]. Eating the right PUFAs from unoxidized fats like fish will also help to lower cholesterol because PUFAs increase LDL receptor activity, which lowers cholesterol[1278,1279]. A low intake of omega-3s also makes cholesterol levels go up in response to a high saturated fat intake, whereas this doesn't happen when you consume enough of omega-3s[1280]. The hypercholesterolemia and dyslipidemia that may occur when eating saturated fats is thought to be caused by low omega-3 fatty acid intake[1281].

How omega-6 seed oils cause inflammation

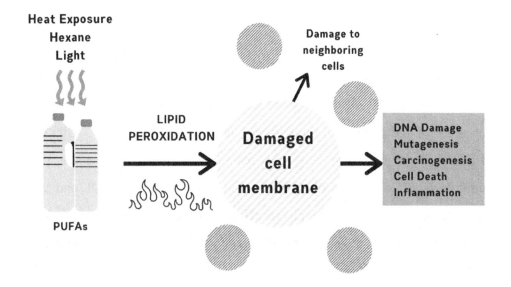

Lipid peroxidation is also damaging to the skin and promotes inflammatory acne[1282]. Exposure to sunlight can also trigger lipid peroxidation in your skin and promote the development of skin cancer if your fat tissue and cell membranes consist of a lot of heat sensitive omega-6 PUFAs[1283,1284,1285,1286,1287,1288,1289,1290,1291,1292,1293,1294,1295,1296,1297,1298,1299,1300,1301,1302]. Having a high amount of lipid peroxidation contributes to weight gain, insulin resistance, heart disease and the development of metabolic syndrome[1303,1304,1305,1306]. However, lipid peroxidation isn't a prerequisite for obesity and diabetes, meaning you can gain weight even without consuming oxidized fats[1307]. However, obese individuals have higher markers of lipid peroxides and weight loss decreases them[1308].

PUFAs include both omega-6 and omega-3 fats, such as linoleic acid (LA) and arachidonic acid (AA), which are omega-6 fats and alpha-linolenic acid (ALA), eicosapentaenoic acid (EPA) and docosahexaenoic acid (DHA), which are omega-3 fats. Arachidonic acid is present mostly in meat, eggs, and fish, whereas EPA/DHA is found in oily fish and marine oils. ALA and LA are predominantly in plants, although they are found in animal foods. Refined seed oils like canola oil, rapeseed oil, soybean oil, corn oil, sunflower oil, etc. have to go through intense amounts of heat during processing, which damages their fatty acid composition causing lipid peroxidation. If you process them even further by hydrogenizing them, you will get margarine and other solid vegetable oil spreads. Consumption of these trans fats is linked to obesity, metabolic syndrome, visceral fat gain, oxidative stress, heart disease, cancer, and Alzheimer's[1309,1310,1311,1312,1313,1314,1315]. Thus, for optimal metabolic health you should avoid these kind of refined fats, especially those that have been processed with heat or have sat on store shelves under bright lights for months. Some natural animal foods like milk, meat and butter also contain some trans fats but of the *cis* kind, which doesn't appear to cause the same negative side-effects[1316,1317]. A lot of fish oil supplements are also found to be rancid[1318]. Thus, make sure to obtain a certificate of analysis indicating low peroxidation values for your fish oil. All fats can become oxidized and rancid – they just have different thresholds at which it happens, depending on their structure.

How to protect against oxidation of lipids:

- Avoid the consumption of refined omega-6 seed oils and trans fats
- Do not cook with and reduce or eliminate the intake of omega-6 seed oils, such as corn, soybean, safflower, cottonseed, sunflower, canola, grapeseed, rice bran, peanut, etc.
- Extra virgin olive oil protects against lipid peroxidation thanks to its antioxidant and polyphenol content[1319]. Unfortunately, many olive oil products are mixed with canola oil and may be rancid. You should only consume olive oil that's been kept in air-tight dark glass bottles. If it tastes slightly peppery and spicy, then the olive oil has polyphenols.

- Get enough vitamin C and/or E from vegetables, fruits, fish and pastured eggs/meat[1320,1321]

- Get enough copper to bolster your antioxidant defense[1322]
  - Ideally this would come from liver or organ blends

- Don't overheat PUFAs[1323]

- Prevent iron accumulation by limiting the consumption of iron-fortified foods[1324]
  - Excess iron can be balanced with copper that also contributes to the body's antioxidant defense[1325]

- Consume carotenoids from colorful vegetables and grass-fed animal foods[1326,1327]

- Take 2-3 grams of spirulina with a meal that has heated fats[1328,1329]

- Eat crushed garlic with meals[1330]

- Add turmeric or curry to your fatty meals[1331,1332]

- Get enough magnesium (400-500 mg/d)[1333,1334,1335,1336]

- Consume olive oil, cacao, coffee, tea, spices, and other foods that contain a lot of polyphenolic compounds[1337,1338,1339,1340,1341,1342,1343,1344]

- Supplement glycine 3-6 grams/d[1345,1346]
  - Glycine can also lower the blood sugar response to glucose by >50%[1347]

Monounsaturated fats (MUFAs) are quite stable during cooking. Olive oil is about 73% MUFAs and 14% saturated fat[1348,1349]. In other words, 87% of the fats in olive oil are heat resistant. The polyphenols and vitamin E in olive oil also protect against lipid peroxidation, making it one of the best fats to cook with[1350,1351]. Consumption of MUFAs is linked to a reduced risk of diabetes, weight gain and heart disease[1352,1353]. MUFAs from olive oil, but not animal fats, is associated with a reduction in all-cause mortality, cardiovascular mortality, cardiovascular events, and stroke[1354,1355,1356]. In one study, people who ate bread with oleic acid that's found in olive oil in high amounts felt fuller and ate fewer calories over the following 24 hours compared to those who ate the bread with low oleic acid sunflower oil[1357]. A similar benefit has been shown with olive oil versus butter, with those consuming olive oil eating 23% less bread when at restaurants[1358]. High oleic acid sunflower oil with the bread also resulted in a significant reduction in energy intake, which indicates that the oleic acid content of a meal can help improve satiety.

Fatty Acid Composition of Certain Fats[1359]

Type of Fat or Oil	% Saturated	% Monounsaturated	% Polyunsaturated
Coconut Oil	91	6	3
Butter	66	30	4
Lamb Tallow	58	38	4
Palm Oil	51	40	9
Beef Tallow	49-54	42-48	3-4
Lard	44	45	11
Duck Fat	35	50	14
Chicken Fat (Schmaltz)	30-32	48-50	18-23
Cottonseed Oil	29	19	52
Peanut Oil	17	56	26
Olive Oil	16	73	11

Soybean Oil	15	23	62
Sesame Oil	15	41	43
Corn Oil	14	27	59
Sunflower Oil	13	18	69
Grapeseed Oil	11	16	73
Safflower Oil	9	11	80
Flaxseed Oil	9	17	74
High-Oleic Sunflower Oil	9	81	9
Canola Oil	7	65	28

BEST to WORST COOKING FATS

1. Coconut oil, pastured butter, ghee, tallow, and extra virgin olive oil (BEST)

2. Avocado oil

3. Argan oil

4. Macadmia nut/peanut oil (LIMIT)

DO NOT COOK WITH THE BELOW

5. Canola

6. Sunflower

7. Rice bran

8. Grapeseed (WORST)

The optimal dietary fat ratio between monounsaturated fatty acids (MUFAs) to polyunsaturated fatty acids (PUFAs) to saturated fatty acids (SFAs) should be 6:1:1, respectively[1360]. The ideal ratio of omega-6 and omega-3 PUFAs is 1:1 or 4:1 at the most. That can be achieved relatively easily if one eliminates the majority of added refined omega-6 seed oils from their diet and stops cooking with processed seed oils. Instead, you should cook with things like extra virgin olive oil, tallow, coconut oil, avocado oil, or butter. To manage the total calorie content, it's still recommended to try to get most of your dietary fat from whole foods, such as meat, eggs, fish, or nuts instead of butter or oil. The only exception would be extra virgin olive oil that has a long track record of improving risk factors of metabolic health and disease. Extra virgin olive oil that's high in polyphenols is excellent for both cooking and salad dressing but it docsn't mean you can't gain weight from consuming it. Overall, the effect of saturated fats on health appears to be not that significant based on meta-analyses and reviews[1361,1362]. The American Heart Association recommends that 5-6% of your daily calories should come from saturated fats[1363].

Estimated dietary fat composition during the Paleolithic versus the modern diet[1364]

Dietary Fat	Paleolithic Era	Current Day	Change
Linoleic Acid (Omega-6)	7.5–14 g[1365] (None from industrial seed oils)	11–22.5 g/day[1366] (Almost entirely industrial seed oils)	23% decrease up to 3-fold increase
Alpha-Linoleic Acid (Omega-3)	12–15 g (None from industrial seed oils)	1.4 g/day (Mostly from industrial seed oils)	8.5–10-fold decrease
EPA and DHA (Omega-3)	660–14,250mg	100–200 mg/day	3–142-fold decrease
Omega-6/3 Ratio	0.79	15–20[1367]	19–25-fold increase
Saturated Fat	32–39 g	22–55 g[1368,1369]	1.8-fold decrease up to 1.7-fold increase
Industrial Trans Fat	0 g	5.4 g[1370] (2.6% of calories)	Entirely introduced in the modern diet; completely void in the Paleolithic diet

Here's a list of the different oils and their fatty acid content

FOOD	OMEGA-6 (g)	OMEGA-3 (g)	RATIO 6:3
FISH			
Salmon (4 oz/113 g)	0.2	2.3	1:12
Mackerel (4 oz/113 g)	0.2	2.2	1:11
Swordfish (4 oz/113 g)	0.3.	1.7	1:6
Sardines (4 oz/113 g)	4.0	1.8	2.2:1
Canned Tuna (4 oz/113 g)	3.0	0.2	15:1
Lobster (4 oz/113 g)	0.006	0.12	1:20
Cod (4 oz/113 g)	0.1	0.6	1:6
VEGETABLES			
Spinach (1 cup/110 g)	30.6	166	1:5.4
Kale (1 cup/110 g)	0.1.	0.1	1:1
Collards (1 cup/110 g)	133	177	1:1.3
Chard (1 cup/110 g)	43.7	5.3	8.2:1
Sauerkraut (1 cup/110 g)	37	36	1:1
Brussels Sprouts (1 cup/110 g)	123	270	1:1.3
NUTS AND SEEDS			
Walnuts (1 oz/28 g)	10.8	2.6	4.2:1
Flaxseeds (1 oz/28 g)	1.6	6.3	1:4
Pecans (1 oz/28 g)	5.7	0.3	21:1
Poppy Seeds (1 oz/28 g)	7.9	0.1	104:1
Pumpkin Seeds (1 oz/28 g)	2.5	0.1	114:1
Sesame Seeds (1 oz/28 g)	6	0.1	57:1
Almonds (1 oz/28 g)	3.3	0.002	1987:1
Cashews (1 oz/28 g)	2.1	0.017	125:1
Chia Seeds (1 oz/28 g)	1.6	4.9	1:3
Pistachios (1 oz/28 g)	3.7	0.071	52:1
Sunflower Seeds (1 oz/28 g)	6.5	0.021	312:1
Lentils (1 oz/28 g)	0.0384	0.0104	3.7:1
OILS AND FATS			
Butter (1 Tbsp)	0.18	0.83	1:1.5
Lard (1 Tbsp)	1.0	0.1	10:1
Cod Liver Oil (1 Tbsp)	2.8	1.3	2.2:1
Grain-Fed Tallow (1 Tbsp)	3.35	0.2	16.8:1
Grass-Fed Tallow (1 Tbsp)	1.2	0.8	1.5:1

Peanut Oil (1 Tbsp)	4.95	Trace	1:0.0
Soybean Oil (1 Tbsp)	7.0	0.9	7.8:1
Canola Oil (1 Tbsp)	2.8	1.3	2.2:1
Walnut Oil (1 Tbsp)	7.2	1.4	5.1:1
Sunflower Oil (1 Tbsp)	6	0.0	6:1
Margarine (1 Tbsp)	2.4	0.04	6:1
Peanut Butter (1 Tbsp)	1.4	0.008	17:1
Almond Butter (1 Tbsp)	1.2	0.04	2.8:1
Flaxseed Oil (1 Tbsp)	2.0	6.9	1:3.5
Olive Oil (1 Tbsp)	1.1	0.1	11:1
MEAT			
Ground Pork (6 oz/170 g)	2.83	0.119	23.8:1
Chicken	2.2	0.16	13.8:1
Grain-Fed Beef	0.73	0.08	9:1
Grass-Fed Beef	0.72	0.15	4.9:1
Domestic Lamb	1.9	0.6	3.3:1
Grass-Fed Lamb	1.7	2.2	0.7:1
Farmed Salmon	1.7	4.5	0.39:1
Wild Salmon	0.3	3.6	0.08:1

Fatty acids are divided into short-chain fatty acids (SCFAs), medium-chain triglycerides (MCTs), long-chain fatty acids (LCFAs) and very long chain fatty acids (VLCFAs)[1371]. SCFAs consist of less than 6 carbon atoms, MCTs 6-12, LCFAs 13-21 and VLCFAs more than 22[1372]. SCFAs like butyrate, acetate and propionate are produced in the colon through fermentation of fiber or consumption of fats like butter[1373]. They regulate appetite and cardiometabolic health factors[1374,1375]. MCTs (C6, C8, C10 and C12) have a thermic effect, increasing fat oxidation and metabolic rate[1376,1377,1378]. Because MCTs are shorter than LCFAs, they provide faster energy by passively diffusing from the GI tract into the portal vein, skipping steps SCFAs and LCFAs go through. It's been found that MCTs decrease subsequent energy consumption without influencing appetite[1379][1380]. Thus, they may have a better weight loss effect compared to LCFAs. Animal milk consists of mostly LCFAs and about 10-20% of MCTs[1381].

How Much Fat Should You Eat?

Although fat has had a negative connotation in terms of weight loss for decades, it's still an essential nutrient needed for metabolic, cognitive, neurobehavioral, hormonal, and structural functions[1382][1383][1384][1385][1386]. You also need fat to absorb fat-soluble vitamins, such as vitamin A, D, E and K. Technically, you could produce fat inside the body from carbohydrates via the process of *de novo lipogenesis*, but this is quite an energy-wasteful process[1387]. This is how people in South-East Asia like Vietnam or Thailand have sustained themselves on diets comprising of only 6-7% fat in their diet[1388]. However, **it is suggested that one should get at least a minimum of 15% of their daily calories as dietary fat, which includes 2.5% as linoleic acid and 0.5% as alpha-linoleic acid**[1389]. Eating 20% of your calories as fat appears to result in lower testosterone levels than a 40% fat intake but there is no additional increase beyond the 40% mark[1390]. Thus, it is recommended to get over 20% of your daily calories from fat but more than 40% isn't inherently needed nor does it provide additional benefits.

Although the body can convert ALA into EPA and DHA, it's not a very efficient process. Most people are only able to convert 5% of ALA to EPA and 0.5% into DHA, with the exception of women in their reproductive age who may convert up to 21% of ALA into EPA and 9% into DHA[1391]. It's recommended to get at a minimum 250-500 mg of combined DHA and EPA per day[1392]. **Thus, consuming seafood and fish that contain preformed DHA/EPA is a more bioavailable and effective way to cover your omega-3 requirements**. Physically active individuals who exercise a lot may need to get more omega-3s to curb inflammation[1393]. Strenuous exercise promotes pro-inflammatory biomarkers, such as C-reactive protein (cRP) and tumor necrosis factor-alpha (TNF-alpha), which omega-3 supplementation can mitigate[1394,1395]. Omega-3 fatty acids also decrease muscle damage caused by exercise[1396,1397,1398,1399]. For those who perform strenuous exercise on a consistent basis, we recommend 3-4 grams of EPA/DHA per day.

Fish consumption has a long epidemiological history of decreased risk of cardiovascular disease (CVD), lower inflammation and better metabolic health[1400]. People who eat fish 1-2 times a week have a 50% reduced risk of CVD, 34% lower risk of dying to CVD and 50% less strokes compared to those who eat no fish[1401,1402]. The Diet and Reinfarction Trial (DART) found that telling patients who had a history of a heart attack to consume more fatty fish dropped all-cause mortality by 29% compared to those who didn't get this recommendation[1403]. Supplementing with omega-3s may reduce CVD mortality[1404]. Giving omega-3s with EPA/DHA reduces all-cause mortality by over 50% even in those without established heart disease[1405,1406]. In patients with heart failure, EPA/DHA supplementation has been found to significantly reduce non-fatal second heart attacks, stroke and all-cause mortality[1407,1408,1409].

Fish oil supplementation does decrease CVD risk factors but hasn't proven to definitively prevent it[1410]. However, oxidized and rancid fish oil would still promote lipid peroxidation and inflammation. Most commercial fish oil brands tend to be exposed to heat, sunlight and humidity, which determines the amount of spoilage[1411]. They should be stored in a dark glass bottle and inside a refrigerator or freezer, away from oxygen and sunlight. According to consumerlabs.com a lot but not all fish oil supplements are rancid[1412]. If your fish oil smells or tastes bad, then it's most likely oxidized. Krill oil has less EPA/DHA but has been found to have essentially the same metabolic benefits[1413]. The omega-3s in krill oil are bound to phospholipids, which increases their likelihood of crossing the blood-brain barrier instead of getting destroyed in the gut[1414].

Here is a table that compares the current AHA recommendations for fatty acids to evidence-based recommendations that we have outlined in this chapter[1415]

Current AHA Recommendations	Evidence-based Recommendations
Consume at least 5–10% of total daily calories as omega-6.	You need only 0.5-2% of total calories as linoleic acid to support essential bodily functions. The upper limit for linoleic acid is 3% to prevent enzymatic competition with ALA and to avoid inflammation. In any case, linoleic acid should come from only whole food sources.[1416]
Industrial vegetable oils and seed oils are considered heart healthy	Avoid industrial seed oils. Omega-6 should come from whole foods like nuts, seeds, fish, eggs, poultry, etc.
No advice given about the optimal omega-6/3 ratio	The ideal omega-6/3 ratio is 1:1 but 4:1 is also acceptable
500 mg EPA/DHA a day to prevent heart disease. Those who already have heart disease should consume 1000 mg EPA/DHA	Get about 2-4 grams of EPA/DHA a day for both primary and secondary prevention of heart disease. However, EPA/DHA consumption should be titrated to maintain an omega-3 index (EPA+DHA in red blood cells) of at least 8% or more[1417]

Low Fat vs High Fat Diet

A low-fat diet is characterized by less than 30% of your calories coming from fat[1418]. Reducing fat consumption, especially saturated fat and trans-fat, has been used as an effective way to lower serum cholesterol levels, making it widely recommended for managing cardiovascular disease[1419,1420,1421]. However, there are multiple potential issues with going on a low-fat diet, which inherently warrants a higher carbohydrate intake. For example, products labeled as low-fat may not always be healthier as the fat in them has been replaced with added sugar, high fructose corn syrup or refined carbohydrates. It's been found that replacing saturated fat with refined carbs and sugars doesn't lower rates of cardiovascular disease, whereas doing so with polyunsaturated fats or monounsaturated fats does[1422,1423,1424]. Consumption of too many refined carbohydrates lowers HDL cholesterol, which has cardioprotective effects, and raises triglycerides, which are risk factors for metabolic syndrome[1425,1426,1427,1428]. A low-fat diet can certainly work and result in long-term weight loss as South-East Asian populations consume significantly less fat than people in the Western countries. However, you would have to make sure that the calories you replace the low-fat intake with do not jeopardize your metabolic health. **Thus, we think a fat intake between 20-40% is probably the most optimal for the majority of people**. That's the approximate ratio of the Mediterranean Diet as well, which is associated with reduced heart disease risk and central obesity[1429,1430,1431,1432,1433]. The Mediterranean Diet rich in extra-virgin olive oil and nuts has also been found to reduce oxidized LDL particles[1434].

Dietary Fat Intake Ratios

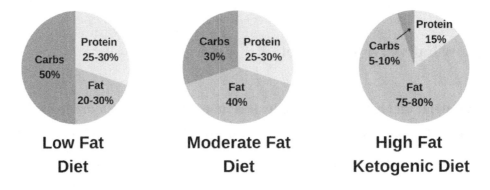

| Low Fat Diet | Moderate Fat Diet | High Fat Ketogenic Diet |

The standard ketogenic diet consists of up to 75-80% fat, 15% protein and 5-10% carbohydrates because you have to be very restrictive with carbs and protein to achieve ketosis[1435]. Ketone bodies do have anti-inflammatory, antioxidant, and neuroprotective effects[1436,1437,1438,1439,1440,1441]. They also have been found to suppress appetite, reduce the hunger hormone ghrelin and stabilize blood sugar levels[1442,1443,1444,1445]. It's said that a state of ketosis begins when your blood ketone concentrations are above 0.5 mmol[1446]. Ketogenic diets were originally created to manage epileptic seizures in children by mimicking the physiology of fasting in the 1920s[1447,1448,1449]. A 24-week study of a low-carb ketogenic diet (30 grams of carbs, 1 g/kg of protein and 20% of the fat as saturated fat and 80% as polyunsaturated) resulted in significant weight loss in obese patients, while improving metabolic health markers[1450]. Even in normal-weight men, a short-term ketogenic diet may improve the lipid profile[1451].

For optimal insulin sensitivity and glucose tolerance it's not recommended to be in ketosis all the time because it can cause a state of physiological insulin resistance. An 8-week study on mice on a ketogenic diet discovered that a high carbohydrate meal in ketosis does show decreased glucose control but these effects are quick to reverse after returning to a regular diet[1452]. Similar results have been seen in humans who follow a ketogenic diet in the long-term[1453,1454]. If you're restricting carbs and go into ketosis for a while, the muscles and liver become slightly insulin resistant as to preserve glucose for the brain. It's not actually characterized by any pathological symptoms, such as elevated fasting insulin, high fasting blood sugar or triglycerides. The only negative reaction occurs when you consume a large amount of carbohydrates in a state of ketosis wherein the muscle and liver cells aren't ready yet to pick up the glucose. As a result, your blood sugar may stay elevated for some time. A much more accurate term to describe this phenomenon would be 'decreased glucose demand' or 'glucose sparing' because that's what essentially causes this[1455]. Regardless, it's still probably not ideal to be in chronic ketosis because of this reason as well as the potential downregulation of thyroid hormones. That's why for optimal insulin sensitivity and metabolic health it's recommended to do ketosis cyclically.

In conclusion, the recommended amount of fat you should consume is somewhere between 20-40%, depending on your preference and adherence. More than that will not provide any additional benefits for fat loss or satiety because fat is still higher in calories than carbs or protein. The best sources of those fats should be from whole foods, such as fatty fish, eggs, meat, nuts, seeds, avocados, and olives. Olive oil is technically processed but it's done so minimally and without causing lipid peroxidation. Based on epidemiological studies, extra virgin olive oil is probably one of the healthiest fats to consume. Medium-chain triglyceride fats like MCT oil and coconut oil may increase thermogenesis and energy expenditure but only to a small degree. Too many added fats, even of the healthy kind, add to your total daily calorie intake, which will interfere with weight loss. Thus, if your goal is to lose fat you should be sparing with how much fat you add to your food in the form of salad dressing, cooking fat, etc. If you're doing a ketogenic diet, you naturally would end up eating more fat but that occurs at the expense of reduced carbohydrate intake, keeping total calorie intake at a balance. Eating too much fat, even when in ketosis, can result in weight gain.

Chapter 7 – Structuring a Diet for Sustainable Weight Loss

You often hear about people who struggle with weight loss who go on semi-starvation diets that consist of less than 1000 calories per day. Unfortunately, those diets are never sustainable and the individuals will eventually regain their weight. Some of them may even end up heavier than they started and their subsequent attempts to shed a few pounds become increasingly more difficult. The most striking example of this are participants of weight loss TV programs. A 2016 study on the Biggest Loser competitors 6 years post-show discovered that the participants had regained 70% of the weight they lost[1456]. The participants also lost 25 lbs of lean muscle during the show and only regained about half of that lean mass. Their metabolic rate also decreased and they experienced a drop in their resting energy expenditure.

Is there a way to avoid the fate of The Biggest Loser competitors who regained their weight, lost muscle, and dropped their metabolic rate? Clearly, there are millions of people on less restrictive and intense programs who've seen far better results. One of the biggest reasons the participants regained their weight has to do with losing motivation and not being able to maintain their extreme physical activity combined with severe calorie restriction. No one can maintain severe caloric restriction indefinitely and eventually they will break, leading to potential binge-eating and weight rebounding. However, **it's been found that a more modest calorie restriction of 20% and vigorous exercise 20 min/day is enough to maintain substantial weight loss[1457]. That's why most successful weight loss programs recommend only an energy deficit of no more than 20-33%.** A bigger calorie deficit makes you lose weight faster, but you'll also lose much more muscle, which decreases resting energy expenditure and makes it harder to sustain the weight loss[1458,1459]. Thus, the goal shouldn't be to eat as little as possible, thinking it's going to be beneficial for weight loss, but instead to eat as many calories as possible while gradually losing weight and maintaining muscle mass.

A successful diet program should make you lose as much fat as possible while keeping as much muscle as possible and maintaining those results for as long as possible. Our mission with this book is to give you a blueprint with commonalities of successful diets that enable you to maintain a healthy body composition for the long-term.

How to Not Crash Diet and Rebound

If you're trying to lose weight, there are three primary strategies, 1.) reduce caloric intake, 2.) increase calorie burning through physical activity and 3.) fix underlying hormonal abnormalities (#1 and #2 can help here but improving the overall quality of the diet is the best way to do this). Combining all 3 strategies will lead to faster and synergistic effects. Unfortunately, your body will eventually get used to a certain calorie intake, leading to a reduction in energy expenditure or in some cases increasing it – a term called metabolic adaptation[1460]. Most of the decrease in metabolic rate is the result of having less bodyweight or muscle, which lowers your basal metabolic rate[1461,1462,1463]. Such metabolic adaptations can persist even after dieting stops, making it progressively harder to keep losing weight or maintain the accomplished weight loss[1464,1465].

Your body adapts to a decreased calorie consumption primarily by adaptive thermogenesis and reducing metabolic rate[1466,1467,1468,1469], which makes you burn fewer calories and the activity you engage in is done more efficiently

with less calories burned. There is also a drop in non-exercise activity thermogenesis (NEAT) and deliberate exercise[1470,1471,1472,1473]. To make matters worse, your desire to eat increases through an elevation of hunger hormones, such as ghrelin and reduced leptin[1474]. Thyroid hormones down-regulate as well during long periods of calorie restriction, which results in lower total daily energy expenditure (TDEE)[1475]. This is inevitable to a certain degree as you do need to experience some form of energy deficit to lose weight, especially when reaching lower levels of body fat. However, there are ways to keep the negative effects of metabolic adaptation to a minimum and prevent them from undermining your future attempts to stay at an optimal bodyweight. These strategies include being more moderate with your calorie restriction, taking diet breaks, building muscle mass and optimizing your health and overall diet[1476,1477]. By raising leptin and thyroid hormones, you increase the body's metabolic rate, which prevents metabolic adaptation and helps to break weight loss plateaus. Carbohydrates have the largest effect on raising leptin and thyroid function[1478,1479]. Eating a bit more calories can also increase your non-exercise activity thermogenesis (NEAT) as well, making you burn more calories without you realizing it[1480].

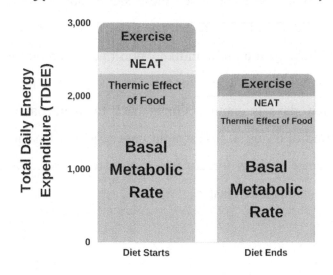

Hypothetical Scenario of Metabolic Adaptation

Chronic dieting and calorie restriction is less effective over the long-term than intermittent energy restriction. One 2018 study called MATADOR (Minimising Adaptive Thermogenesis And Deactivating Obesity Rebound) took 51 obese men and divided them randomly into 2 groups: (1) continuous energy restriction (CON) or (2) intermittent energy restriction (INT) for 16 weeks[1481]. The CON group consumed 67% of their calorie maintenance all throughout the time period, whereas the INT group ate 67% of their maintenance calories 2 weeks in a row, followed by eating 100% of their calorie balance for 2 weeks and swapping between these 2 cycles until the end of those 16 weeks. Importantly, the INT subjects saw more weight loss (14.1±5.6 vs 9.1±2.9 kg), more fat loss (12.3±4.8 vs 8.0±4.2 kg) and experienced less metabolic adaptation than the CON group. **The main idea behind MATADOR dieting is to eat at about 25-33% calorie deficit for 2 weeks and then return to maintenance calories for 1-2 weeks and repeating this cycle as many times as needed to hit your desired body weight.** This mitigates the downregulation of thyroid hormones and metabolism. You could even do MATADOR with 1 week on and 1 week off. However, to warrant the need for taking a diet break, you would need to be in a steeper calorie deficit of at least 30% as in the original study. At less of a deficit, such as 10-20%, you don't really see these significant metabolic adaptations affecting leptin and thyroid hormones. In most cases of a moderate calorie restriction of 25-33%, you more than likely don't need to return to maintenance calories for any longer than 1 week. For some people, even eating at maintenance calories for a few days is enough. Going back to maintenance calories may prolong the period of trying to lose weight unnecessarily. Essentially, if you go back to maintenance calories for 1 week, instead of 2 weeks, you can achieve your weight loss results much faster.

Here's an example block of a MATADOR diet for a moderately active 35-year-old 200 lb. man who is 30 pounds overweight:

Calories to maintain 200 pounds = ~ 2,800/day

Calories to maintain 170 pounds = ~ 2,600/day

- 4 weeks of consuming 2,800 calories/day to get you accustomed to eating an amount of food that does not lead to weight gain

- Week 1-2 at a 30% calorie deficit of around 2,000 calories

- Week 2-4 consume the number of calories that provides weight maintenance (~ 2,800 calories/day if you weigh 200 pounds). You can use this calculator to determine how many calories you should be consuming to maintain your body weight https://www.healthline.com/nutrition/how-many-calories-per-day#calculator

- Repeat until you've reached goal bodyweight

- Once you have reached your goal bodyweight (170 pounds in this case)

  o Maintain 2,600 calories consumed per day

These are just averages and caloric needs will increase depending on activity level

Here's an example block of a MATADOR diet for a moderately active 35-year-old 170 lb. woman who is 30 pounds overweight:

Calories to maintain 170 pounds = ~ 2,200/day

Calories to maintain 140 pounds = ~ 2,000/day

- 4 weeks of consuming 2,200 calories/day to get you accustomed to eating an amount of food that does not lead to weight gain

- Week 1-2 at a 30% calorie deficit of around 1,500 calories

- Week 2-4 at maintenance calories of around 2,200 calories (this will go down as you lose weight)

  - You can use this calculator to determine how many calories you should be consuming to maintain your body weight https://www.healthline.com/nutrition/how-many-calories-per-day#calculator

- Repeat until you've reached your goal bodyweight of 140 pounds

- Once you've achieved your goal bodyweight (in this case 140 pounds)

  - Maintain 2,000 calories consumed per day

These are just averages and caloric needs will increase depending on activity level

Another reason why people rebound after dieting has to do with their body not being used to their new body fat setpoint. Based on the body fat setpoint theory, your body tries to maintain a specific homeostatic weight range[1482]. Like a thermostat or an autopilot, feedback loops between the brain and food intake leads to weight maintenance withing a certain range[1483]. When you eat too many calories past your body fat setpoint, you'll experience countermeasures that include higher satiety, increased energy expenditure and less desire to eat. Going too low or below your body fat setpoint also leads to increasing hunger, cravings and decreasing energy expenditure.

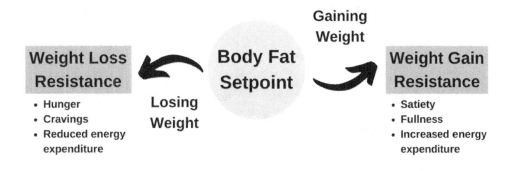

There are both genetic and epigenetic factors that affect your body fat setpoint, but the main idea is that everyone has a different homeostatic balance[1484]. Losing a significant amount of weight does disrupt that equilibrium, which is uncomfortable and hunger-inducing in the short term. However, after a certain amount of time, you will get used to that new setpoint, making the new bodyweight your new normal. That's the reason why extreme calorie restriction tends to result in weight rebounding and yo-yo dieting. Conversely, a more moderate calorie deficit of about 20-33%, with 1-2 week breaks in between, allows your body to accommodate to its new body fat setpoint preventing the countermeasures from occuring that are meant to stop the weight loss. Additionally, a more step-by-step reduction in calorie intake, where you drop your caloric intake by 25% slowly over the course of a week may improve compliance. As your bodyweight decreases, so does your total daily energy expenditure and because you weigh less, your body also needs fewer calories per day. A more stepwise reduction in caloric intake also gives your body more time to adjust to the lower calorie intake. When calorie restriction is done gradually it won't create a significant amount of resistance.

MATADOR Diet Period Example

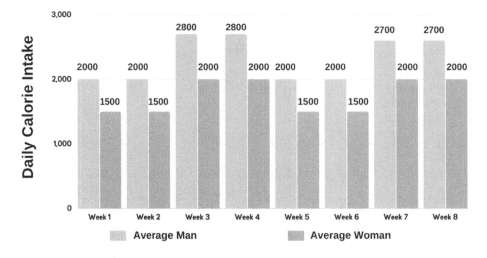

Gradual Intermittent Energy Restriction

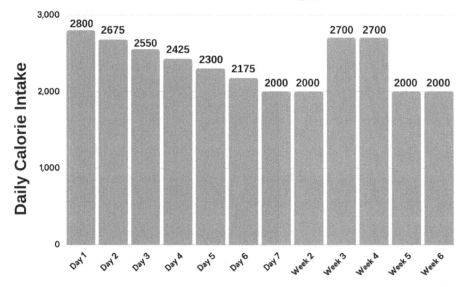

These type of dieting periods should be done until you reach your target goal weight. Of course, you could even apply intermittent energy restriction followed by refeeding even when you're not trying to lose weight. The reason being that weight loss or weight gain isn't only determined by your daily calorie balance but more so by your calorie balance over the course of weeks and months. If you eat 10% less calories for 5 days of the week but then consume 50% more calories on day 6 the weekly energy balance stays neutral and you're not really gaining or losing weight. However, if you're trying to lose weight, then this kind of intermittent energy restriction can help to keep you in a net negative calorie balance. If you've lost 2% of your body weight to dieting after 2 weeks, then your new calorie maintenance is also lower than it was before. Thus, to not end up in a calorie surplus you have to adapt your maintenance calories to your new bodyweight. Authors of the original MATADOR study did state that to discover your maintenance calories, it may be better to go through a few weeks of stabilization[1485]. If you have no clue how to start, first consume enough calories for weight maintenance for 4 weeks before trying MATADOR. After that, begin the weight loss phase by going into a 25-33% calorie deficit. **After you've reached your desired fat loss, you should try and maintain a caloric intake that will maintain your desired weight**. If you were previously completely sedentary and slightly overweight, then you can even build muscle in a calorie deficit[1486,1487]. Thus, you may find yourself in a situation where you need to be eating more calories to prevent losing too much weight due to an increased activity level. However, the average person who is maintaining a similar amount of activity as before should not need to increase their calorie intake. It's a natural urge to want to eat more food after weight loss but that's the body desiring to return to its previous bodyweight. The average amount of calories needed to maintain a healthy body weight for a moderately active 140-pound woman and a 170-pound man is 2,000 calories and 2,600 calories per day, respectively. However, if you are highly active this will increase to around 2,400 and 3,000 calories per day, respectively. Unfortunately, most adults in the United States are not very active and likely only need 2,000-2,600 calories/day for women and men, respectively. However, the average American consumes 3,600 calories per day[1488]. It's the consumption of highly processed foods that has led us to consume so many calories. Thus, the idea is to bring back whole nutritious foods so you can naturally drop your caloric intake. We are going to provide examples for moderately active adults for weight loss using the MATADOR method.

How to avoid weight regain after dieting:

- **MATADOR method** – First, we should note that in many instances simply improving the overall quality of your diet can automatically lead to your desired weight/fat loss, no calorie counting required. Focusing on eating high protein, moderate fat and moderate whole food carbohydrate intake will lead to effortless weight loss due to sustained satiety throughout the day. However, for those who are struggling to lose weight even when switching over to a whole food diet, then periods of calorie restriction may be required. Here is how we suggest this can be done in a manageable way. Reduce caloric intake by 25-33% for 1-2 weeks. You can take a step-wise approach and slowly reduce the caloric intake over 1-2 weeks. Then consume the amount of calories needed to maintain your desired weight for 1-2 weeks (using the healthline calculator mentioned previously). To count the calories in your diet you can use apps like MyFitnessPal, Lose It!, FatSecret, Cronometer and Noom. You can continue this cycle based on your goals. If you desire a greater degree of weight loss, then you can reduce the baseline calorie intake as desired to reach your goals.

After weight loss, your body is the most vulnerable to gaining fat as you're hungrier and you have a lower metabolic rate. To get used to your new body fat setpoint, you have to spend a bit of time at your newly reached bodyweight.

Here is how you can maintain a healthy bodyweight effortlessly

- **Eat an Abundance of Protein and Fiber** – Protein and fiber are the most satiating food compounds. Fiber fills you up faster than any other macronutrient and protein leads to sustained satiety. When you start to increase calorie intake again after caloric restriction, consuming more protein will help to mitigate unnecessary fat gain thanks to its higher thermic effect, which makes your body burn more calories to digest the protein. Thus, even after you've stopped dieting, a slightly higher protein intake will still help to keep the extra pounds off. The goal should be to consume around 1-1.25 grams of protein per pound of lean body weight per day (more on the higher end if you have more lean muscle mass). Having some whole food carbohydrates (in the range of ~ 60-150 grams depending on the person) is also advised to raise leptin and thyroid hormones.

- **Fat, protein and carbohydrate intake and options**

  o **Protein options** (~ 1-1.25 grams per pound of lean body weight) – grassfed meat, fish, pastured eggs, yogurt (Greek or Icelandic with low or no sugar added), cottage cheese, etc.

  o **Carbohydrate options** (~ 60-150 grams/day, which can be higher if activity is high) – organic potatoes, sweet potatoes, greenish bananas, berries (any kind), mango, pineapple, apples, oranges, clementines, etc. Apples are an exceptional fruit option as they are very filling and low sugar.

o **Fat options** ($\sim$ 80-120 grams of fat) – Fat should mostly come from pastured eggs, meat, fish, yogurt, cheese and a little from cooking fats (grass-fed animal fats, coconut oil or extra virgin olive oil), nut butters (almond butter) and full-fat milk (if tolerated).

- **Continue Exercising** – Physical activity after the Biggest Loser show is associated with less weight regain[1489]. By exercising you're burning more calories, building muscle and improving insulin sensitivity, which makes it easier to eat more calories without gaining weight[1490]. Try and maintain a similar amount of exercise while on a lower calorie intake as when you are eating more calories. The goal is to make sure you are exercising in a sustainable way. For optimal fat loss and muscle gain you should aim to exercise 5 times per week and including daily walking, especially after meals.

Here is what we recommend for exercise

o Resistance training (body weight exercises, resistance bands, weights, resistance machines, etc.) 3-6 times per week (work your way up to 6 days per week if you can). You can train more often by exercising a different muscle group the next time you work out. This gives the previous muscle groups that you worked out time to recover. By exercising almost every day your body will become used to the routine and you will actually crave exercise. If you are just starting out, you may only be able to exercise 2-3 days per week.

- View exercise just like you view brushing your teeth, eating, or going to the bathroom. Exercise should be part of your daily routine.

  o High intensity interval sprints 2-3 times per week (work your way up to hill sprints and even push ups, squats or jumping jacks at the bottom of the hill before running up it)

  o Daily walking of at least 10-12,000 steps per day (especially after a large meal)

- **Maintain Gut Health** – The microbiome has a huge impact on weight loss by making you crave certain foods, usually junk food, and even absorb more or less calories from food[1491]. Phenolic compounds found in dark berries, vegetables and fermented foods (pickles, sauerkraut, natto, kimchi, etc.) promote the proliferation of strains of bacteria, such as lactobacillus, bifidobacteria and akkermansia that are associated with losing weight and better metabolic health[1492].

- **Control Your Cravings** – Getting cravings for sugar or food in general is natural and part of being in an energy deficit. That's why you should be prepared for dealing with them in advance. Here are some strategies to help you fight food/sugar cravings.

  o Get enough protein and fiber, especially if you are someone who eats breakfast. This can help reduce cravings later in the day.

  o Eat a piece of dark chocolate with/without nuts.

  o Have Greek or Icelandic yogurt with berries, nuts, and a little raw honey.

  o Have a scoop of raw honey.

- o Have some pickle juice

- o Have some Redmond Real Salt®

- o Have a scoop of Redmond Re-Lyte® electrolyte mix

Sometimes restrictive diets like keto, carnivore, or no sugar makes it easier for you to stick to your goals. For others it's easier to eat whatever fits your daily calorie balance. Whatever it is, find out what works best for you and execute.

How to Lose Fat Not Muscle

It's estimated that one pound of fat loss requires a 3,500 calorie deficit[1493]. However, you can also lose muscle and lean tissue while keeping the fat when losing weight[1494,1495]. There's also a significant loss of water and glycogen with weight loss[1496,1497]. Thus, **focusing solely on weight loss may result in net negative effects on overall body composition and health as you'll end up with less lean muscle tissue after dieting, which often leads to weight rebounding**[1498,1499]. Losing muscle tissue is also detrimental to sustaining weight loss and keeping a healthy bodyweight as skeletal muscle contributes up to 15-17% of your resting metabolic rate[1500,1501,1502].

When dieting and being in a calorie deficit, you're inevitably going to lose some lean muscle tissue just by virtue of restricting energy intake. However, you can attenuate that effect a lot. The most effective way to do that is through exercise, especially resistance training, which has been shown to mitigate the loss of fat free mass during low calorie intakes[1503,1504,1505,1506,1507]. In fact, **it's more important to do resistance training in a calorie deficit than when not in a calorie deficit, at least in terms of maintaining lean body mass because it's** the biggest signal for the body to keep muscle and burn fat instead[1508,1509,1510,1511]. Doing only cardio without resistance training tells the body that there's no need for muscle and thus it becomes less of a priority to keep it around. As a result, you'll end up with less muscle and a lower basal metabolic rate at the end of a diet than you began with.

A study on subjects consuming 800 liquid calories a day found that those who did resistance training experienced no loss of lean body mass after 12 weeks, whereas those who did only aerobic exercise (cardio) saw a 3-5 kg drop in their lean body mass[1512]. To make matters worse, their metabolic rate was lower as well. Thus, you could consider lifting weights and doing any form of resistance training almost mandatory during dieting or low calorie intakes as to maintain more muscle. Chances are your strength and power will decrease due to the reduced calorie intake but you can compensate that by increasing overall volume with slightly lower intensities. Of course, cardio and engaging in more low intensity activities, such as hiking and walking, can still help to accelerate fat loss by increasing your daily energy expenditure. However, you don't want to do that exclusively in the absence of resistance training.

Resistance training helps with fat loss directly as well besides just increasing your basal metabolic rate. A 2021 study discovered that mechanical overload from lifting weights releases extracellular vesicles holding muscle-specific microRNA-1 that are favorably picked up by epidydimal white adipose tissue (eWAT)[1513]. When the microRNA enters the eWAT, it promotes fat breakdown and metabolic adaptations towards greater fat burning. Resistance training is also one of the top ways to improve insulin sensitivity and glucose disposal[1514,1515,1516,1517], directing the food you eat more towards glycogen storage instead of fat storage[1518,1519]. Obesity-induced insulin resistance predominantly decreases glucose disposal in skeletal muscle[1520]. Contracting muscles at near-maximal intensity, as you would during resistance training, activates glucose transporters, such as GLUT4, that directs glucose into the cells[1521]. Thus, resistance training gears your body to burn more fat at all times through many mechanisms. It's also one of the best methods for improving overall glucose control and insulin sensitivity. Virtually all of your biomarkers of metabolic health improve when you do regular resistance training. **Resistance training or high intensity interval training (HIIT), like interval sprints, combined with a higher protein intake (2.3 g/kg or 35% of total calories) has been found to be more effective in preserving lean mass and losing fat mass than a low protein diet (1 g/kg or 15% of total calories) at a 40% calorie deficit over the course of 2 weeks**[1522]. A high protein diet of 2.4 g/kg of body weight is more effective for fat loss than a diet of 1.2 g/kg when combined with high intensity exercise[1523]. Consuming whey protein versus the same caloric amount of sugar in people doing low-intensity movement, such as walking, during extreme calorie restriction of 320 calories per day for 1 week has been shown to preserve significantly more lean mass[1524]. **Thus, ensuring you get a high amount of protein of at least 2-2.4 g/kg of bodyweight or 25-35% of total calories and possibly supplementing essential amino acids during severe calorie deficits helps to attenuate the potential loss of lean tissue**. Exercising on top of that, especially resistance training, is also vital because exercised muscles are more sensitive to the effects of circulating amino acids and testosterone[1525,1526], while being more resistant towards the catabolic effects of cortisol and calorie restriction[1527,1528].

Recommended Protein Intakes

| Maintenance Calories | Moderate Calorie Restriction (10-30%) | Severe Calorie Restriction (>33%) |

Here are the things that make you lose more muscle than fat:

- Sleep deprivation or short sleep of less than 6 hours
- Low protein diet (< 0.8 g/kg per day)
- No resistance training
- Too much cardio without resistance training
- Very low calorie intake for too long
- Prolonged fasting for several days
- Prolonged periods of zero or low protein intake

Here's how to preserve more muscle when in a calorie deficit:

- Doing resistance training and strength training
- Higher protein intake (2-3.3 g/kg per day)
- HMB supplementation at 3 mg/day
- Taking EAAs 10-15 g/day or whey protein (20-40 g/day)
- Moderate calorie restriction of about 20-30%
- Intermittent energy restriction (MATADOR)
- Getting at least 7-8 hours of sleep per night
- Chromium picolinate supplementation 200-1000 mcg/day
- Inositol supplementation 1-2 grams twice daily (improves thyroid and insulin signaling)

Bodybuilders are known to supplement amino acids to help with muscle preservation, especially during dieting. **Branched chain amino acids (BCAAs) have evidence for reducing muscle soreness and accelerating recovery, but they don't improve exercise performance**[1529,1530,1531]. **BCAAs don't have an extra benefit on muscle growth if you're getting enough dietary protein**[1532]. For protein synthesis to occur, you need all 9 essential amino acids (EAAs) out of which 3 are BCAAs[1533,1534]. The primary amino acid for protein synthesis is leucine[1535,1536,1537,1538,1539]. Taking leucine alone hasn't been found to prevent or treat age-related muscle loss[1540]. **However, supplementing HMB at doses of 1.5-3 grams/day combined with training has been shown to promote muscle growth and strength in untrained people and the elderly**[1541,1542,1543,1544]. HMB or β-Hydroxy β-Methyl Butyrate is a by-product of leucine metabolism that reduces exercise-induced muscle catabolism[1545,1546,1547,1548,1549,1550]. In already trained individuals, HMB has less of an effect[1551,1552,1553,1554] and it's more beneficial for patients who experience sarcopenia, cachexia, or muscle wasting[1555,1556]. Regardless, HMB before exercise has been found to reduce protein breakdown even in resistance-trained men[1557]. Meaning, you could benefit from supplementing HMB or EAAs that contain leucine when you're either a beginner or during severe calorie restriction. The maximum effective dose for HMB appears to be 3 grams/day[1558] and 6 grams has no additional benefits in terms of suppressing muscle catabolism[1559]. To obtain 3 grams of HMB from whole food you would have to ingest up to 60 grams of leucine, which is equal to roughly 600 grams of protein[1560]. In humans, HMB is safe and may even decrease risk factors of cardiovascular disease[1561,1562,1563].

Chromium picolinate helps maintain lean tissue during a diet[1564,1565,1566]. The mechanisms for better nutrient partitioning and body composition include improved insulin sensitivity and glucose regulation[1567,1568,1569,1570,1571]. Chromium is needed for binding insulin to the surface of cells so it could exert its effects[1572]. A 2019 meta-analysis stated that doses of chromium at 200-1000 mcg/d for 9-24 weeks in obese subjects can lead to a 0.75 kg greater weight loss than the placebo[1573]. However, supplementing chromium appears to have less of a benefit in already health normo-glycemic non-obese people[1574,1575,1576].

In professional swimmers, 400 mcg/day of chromium picolinate for 24 weeks increased lean body mass by 3.5% and decreased fat mass by 4.5% compared to placebo[1577]. A double-blind study on 10 male college students saw that 200 mcg of chromium picolinate a day caused a 3.4 kg fat loss and 2.6 kg lean mass gain after 24 days of resistance training, whereas individuals in the placebo group only lost 1 kg of fat and gained only 1.8 kg of lean tissue[1578]. The authors of the study hypothesized that this was due to chromium's ability to help drive amino acids and nutrients into the muscle. Although chromium has little effect on muscle growth, many athletes can still be deficient in it[1579]. Exercise doubles the average urinary chromium to 0.2-0.4 mcg/d[1580]. To replace that 0.2-0.4 mcg of chromium lost during exercise, you would have to consume 8-100 mcg of chromium from dietary sources because the absorption rate of chromium from food is only 0.4-2.5%[1581]. Sweating causes an additional loss of chromium and 1 hour of exercise can lead to the excretion of up to 7.5 mcg of chromium, which would necessitate the consumption of 600-750 mcg of chromium from diet (as dietary bioavailability of chromium is only ~ 1%)[1582,1583,1584]. You get chromium from mussels, oysters, seafood, shrimp, some meat, broccoli, and oatmeal. However, if you sweat a lot through exercise or saunas, supplementing 200-1000 mcg/d can also be beneficial for improved blood sugar regulation, especially if you have impaired glucose tolerance or insulin resistance.

Low Carb vs Low Fat Diets

Very low-calorie diets (VLCD), composed of less than 800 calories a day can lead to weight loss, including fat loss, but it comes at a substantial cost on lean muscle tissue as well[1585]. **It's been found that very low-calorie diets cause about 75% fat loss and 25% lean body mass loss**[1586]. The loss of lean tissue occurs mostly to support endogenous glucose production[1587]. Your body is converting muscle into glucose to satisfy the brain's and other glucose-dependent tissues' glucose demands. To meet the brain's demand of 110-120 grams of glucose a day, you would need to break down 160-200 grams of protein because synthesizing 1 gram of glucose requires 1.6 grams of amino acids[1588,1589]. Granted, people on a VLCD still consume some glucose and they wouldn't burn that much protein to meet those requirements, but during extreme dieting you would still be losing muscle tissue. Fortunately, there are ways to mitigate and reduce that sacrifice of lean muscle tissue that occurs during energy restriction in many ways.

The brain can also use ketones for fuel and after keto-adaptation, you can meet ~ 50% of the brain's energy demands with ketone bodies[1590,1591]. These ketone bodies will be derived from either dietary fat or your already present adipose tissue. Glucose can also be created from glycerol – the backbone of triglycerides or fatty acid molecules – contributing up to 21.6% of glucose produced by the liver through gluconeogenesis[1592]. This decreases the conversion of protein into glucose even further, resulting in less muscle being used to meet the body's glucose demand. The brain can also use lactate, which is the byproduct of burning glycogen, for fuel[1593]. So, in a best-case scenario, you could cover up to 75% of your brain's glucose requirement with alternative fuel sources, which would greatly reduce the conversion of muscle protein into glucose. Ketone bodies also have additional anti-catabolic effects even during inflammation[1594,1595,1596]. Thus, some degree of nutritional ketosis would be beneficial when under severe calorie restriction of less than 800 calories/day.

Although a low carb ketogenic diet may provide additional anti-catabolic effects during extreme dieting, it's probably not superior during moderate calorie deficits of 500-1000 fewer calories per day. It's been found that both low-carb and low-fat diets result in a similar distribution of weight loss with 75% coming from fat and 25% from lean tissue[1597,1598]. However, ketogenic diets may result in slightly higher loss of visceral fat and less of a drop in energy expenditure[1599,1600,1601]. **The overall loss of body weight on a low carb diet is identical to a low-fat diet when calorie intakes are equal even when carbohydrate restriction causes a higher rate of fat oxidation**[1602]. Both low carb and low fat diets can improve risk factors of metabolic syndrome and reduce weight[1603,1604].

Claims that low carb diets are metabolically superior to low fat diets even without calorie restriction[1605,1606] are based on epidemiological findings, which are often inaccurate due to false self-reporting[1607,1608,1609]. Self-reported calorie intake can be underestimated by up to 14%[1610]. When people lose weight while restricting carbs without seemingly restricting calories, then it's most likely because of replacing carbohydrates with protein, which automatically creates increased energy expenditure through the higher thermic effect of protein, or by spontaneously eating less food thanks to protein's appetite suppressing effects[1611]. Studies that control for total calorie intake have consistently found that carbohydrate restriction isn't superior to high carbohydrate intake or when total calorie intake is the same[1612,1613,1614,1615]. However, to be fair, controlling for total calorie intake isn't what happens in the real world. If a lower carbohydrate intake, for example, is more satiating than a low fat diet but you control for the lower calories, then that is taking away one of the real world benefits of going on a low carbohydrate diet (i.e. a lower intake of calories). So nuance is important in these discussions.

On the flip side, being on a very low-carb high-fat ketogenic diet may prevent weight loss if the person ends up eating too many calories from added fats. **If you avoid many low calorie plant-based foods, such as fruits and vegetables, you may end up in a calorie surplus from higher calorie cheeses, fats and meats.** Even the slightly higher energy expenditure and lower insulin levels will not prevent you from gaining weight in that scenario. We do have a lot of evidence that fiber intake helps with weight loss and maintaining a lower bodyweight[1616,1617,1618]. Fiber also reduces the amount of fat you absorb during digestion by binding to fatty acids, which helps to establish an even greater calorie deficit, similar to protein[1619,1620]. A 2021 controlled-feeding trial on 20 adults showed that a low-fat higher carb diet led to a 500-700 lower spontaneous total calorie intake compared to the low-carb control group during 3 weeks of ad libitum feeding[1621]. That can be a significant benefit in the real world where people aren't measuring their calories – eating a lot of low calorie fibrous vegetables makes you fuller faster and you end up eating less calories. Thus, deliberately restricting fiber-rich foods does not appear to be beneficial in diet adherence and overall weight loss (if you tolerate those types of foods), especially when we know that being in ketosis or eating low carb doesn't necessarily provide any additional benefits for weight loss. Ultimately, in the real world, most people find that going on a low-carb diet is easier to maintain versus a low-fat diet but they typically make the mistake of consuming too many added fats (heavy cream butter) or dairy (full fat cheese, milk, etc.) and not enough foods that provide quick satiety (such as vegetables, potatoes, greenish bananas, etc.) and sustained satiety (meat). With a high protein and high fiber intake, you will more than likely feel very satiated and that is enough to cause a spontaneous decrease in calorie intake. However, at the end of the day you need to know which diet and macronutrient ratio works best for you. You need to experiment whether you do better on a low, moderate or high carb diet. Just know that the studies find generally no difference when total calorie and protein intake is matched. However, selecting the correct diet for you, one that leads to sustained satiety and an optimal body weight, is ultimately going to be the best diet for you.

Many people suffer from what's called the "keto flu" when they start a low carbohydrate diet. This is due to the salt loss that occurs due to drops in insulin. Here are the below sodium losses that occur when starting a low-carbohydrate diet. You can use this information to supplement back the necessary amount of sodium that is lost.

Sodium losses on a low-carb diet

- **On a 2,000 calorie carbohydrate free diet the average losses of sodium out the urine per day are as follows[1622]:**

  o   Day 1: 3 grams of sodium/day

  o   Day 2: 1.3 grams of sodium/day

  o   Day 3: 437 mg of sodium/day

- **On a 1,500 calorie carbohydrate-free diet the average losses of sodium out the urine per day are as follows[1623]:**

  o   Day 1: 2.4 grams of sodium/day

  o   Day 2: 2.2 grams of sodium/day

  o   Day 3: 1 gram of sodium/day

Sodium losses on a very low calorie, low-carb diet

- On a very low calorie diet (420 calories) consisting of only 105 grams of carbohydrates, the average sodium losses out the urine per day are as follows[1624]:

  - Day 1-2: 1.38 grams of sodium/day

  - Day 3-4: 0.68 grams of sodium/day

  - Day 5-6: 0.60 grams of sodium/day

  - Day 7-8: 0.45 grams of sodium/day

  - Day 9-10: 0.33 grams of sodium/day

Intermittent Fasting

Another popular method for weight loss is intermittent fasting (IF). Instead of eating 3-6 meals a day as many people do, you confine your daily eating window to a certain timeframe. Most commonly, people who do IF eat 1-3 meals a day over the course of 2-8 hours. Time restricted eating (TRE) is the more scientifically acquainted term for describing intermittent fasting but they're basically the same thing. Alternate day fasting (ADF) is another form of IF where you eat normally for one day and the following day you eat around 500 calories. **Studies show that time restricted eating or intermittent fasting improves aspects of metabolic syndrome, diabetes, insulin resistance, cardiovascular disease, and hypertension**[1625,1626,1627,1628,1629,1630,1631,1632,1633,1634]. ADF has been found to decrease risk factors for diabetes, heart disease and high blood pressure similar to calorie restriction[1635,1636].

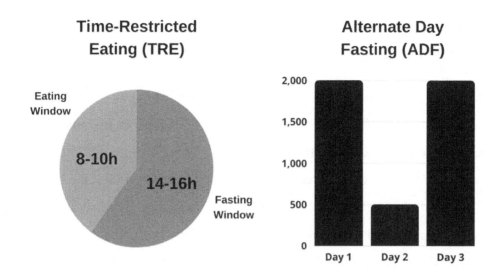

Time-Restricted Eating (TRE)

Eating Window

8-10h

14-16h

Fasting Window

Alternate Day Fasting (ADF)

2,000
1,500
1,000
500
0

Day 1   Day 2   Day 3

For weight loss, intermittent fasting helps with adhering to a diet and controlling daily calorie intake. Some people may find eating larger-sized meals more satiating even when they get to eat less often compared to small frequently eaten meals. Research does find that time restricted eating (TRE) in humans can result in weight loss and fat loss[1637,1638,1639]. It also reduces triglycerides, inflammatory biomarkers, blood pressure and atherogenic lipids[1640,1641,1642]. Granted, these studies are based on self-reported calorie intake not done in metabolic wards.

It's been found that when calorie intakes are equal, TRE isn't more effective for weight loss than eating throughout the day[1643,1644]. However, free living individuals who practice TRE will likely end up reducing their spontaneous food consumption and thus lose weight through an energy deficit. The average American consumes their food over the course of 15 hours[1645], which essentially means they have their first bite of food right after waking up, eat several times throughout the day, snack frequently and have their last calories before bed. That increases their likelihood of consuming more calories by the end of the day, whereas imposing some self-defined time restrictions, such as skipping a single meal or avoiding deliberate snacking, creates a calorie deficit with little effort.

ADF isn't superior to daily calorie restriction either[1646,1647]. **However, one advantage of ADF may be the mitigation of adaptive thermogenesis over long periods of energy restriction.** Calorie restriction can result in a 4.5% drop in metabolic rate, but fortunately ADF has been found to do so only by 1.8% after 23 weeks[1648]. ADF doesn't appear to increase hunger exponentially either as people report less hunger when doing it[1649]. Many individuals claim that after 2 weeks of ADF their overall hunger decreases[1650]. That may be due to increased keto adaptation and fat oxidation that keeps the body tapped into its adipose stores. **Alternate day fasting, wherein you consume 500 calories a day on low calorie days, is found to be more tolerable and adherable by regular people compared to complete fasting with zero calorie intake**[1651]. Such very low calorie intake resembles a lot of the physiological effects of complete fasting[1652]. Unfortunately, a 2021 randomized controlled trial on ADF saw that it wasn't superior to daily calorie restriction in terms of losing fat and actually resulted in slightly higher loss of lean mass[1653]. Thus, **ADF is not recommended for very physically active individuals and for them a daily reduction in calories and time restricted eating is better.**

In 2015, a study tested how eating an entire day's caloric intake within a 10–12-hour window before 8 PM affected overweight individuals[1654]**. They lost about 4% body weight in 16 weeks and retained it for up to a year. This was accompanied by a spontaneous 20% reduction in calories**. The participants also reported improved sleep and higher alertness during daytime. Thus, if you are dieting and your calorie intake is limited, you may find it more convenient and sustainable to eat less often and limit snacking as to ensure you do maintain a calorie deficit. This is especially effective if you're not counting and weighing all your food for their calories. **By just skipping a meal you will automatically cut down on a large proportion of calories you would've otherwise eaten.** You just have to make sure you're not going to binge after you stop fasting. There are several ways to prevent that from happening as well, such as consuming salted water to not develop refeeding syndrome that occurs in the absence of sodium[1655,1656]. Additionally, during fasting salt is continuously lost out in the urine. Here are the below amounts of sodium that are lost when fasting.

Sodium losses when fasting

- **During fasting the average losses of sodium out the urine per day are as follows[1657]:**

    o Day 1: 2.32 grams of sodium/day

    o Day 2: 1.84 grams of sodium/day

    o Day 3: 1.77 grams of sodium/day

    o Day 4: 1.98 grams of sodium/day

    o Day 5: 1.95 grams of sodium/day

    o Day 6: 1.98 grams of sodium/day

    o Day 7: 1.87 grams of sodium/day

    o Day 8: 1.78 grams of sodium/day

    o Day 9: 1.67 grams of sodium/day

    o Day 10: 1.56 grams of sodium/day

- Other fasting studies show that the average sodium loss per day for the first 4 days of a fast is ~ 1.38 grams of sodium, dropping to a 1 gram sodium loss per day by day 5, 600 mg of sodium by day 6, 500 mg by day 7 and then around 230 mg of sodium loss per day from day 8-10[1658,1659].

- On average around 1.38-2 grams of sodium is lost our the urine every day for a 4 day fast.

  - That means for every day that you fast you should eventually replace 1.38-2 grams of sodium. You will also need to calculate how much sodium was lost through sweat and add that to the 1.38-2 grams of sodium lost out the urine per day to get the total amount of sodium needed to be consumed upon rehydration.

- On a normal diet, most people feel best consuming 3,000-5,000 mg of sodium per day. When fasting, that means most people will feel best consuming ~ 4,380-7,000 mg of sodium per day.

- Sweating and coffee/caffeine will also increase sodium losses and also need to be taken into account when considering salt intake for the day.

  - If you consume 2 cups of coffee, you lose ~ 600 mg of sodium. So if you do that twice daily that means you would need another 1,200 mg of sodium to replace the losses.

- The body becomes mildly acidic after 2 days of a fast. This can be counteracted by consuming sodium citrate or bicarbonate mineral waters like Gerolsteiner or Magnesia water.

Ghrelin, the hunger hormone, does have a circadian rhythm, peaking in the evening and reaching its bottom in the morning[1660]. This was confirmed by a 2013 study that found that the subjects weren't that hungry in the morning after an overnight's fast and their hunger peaked at 8 PM instead of 8 AM when it was at its trough[1661]. Your body adapts to your habitual mealtime and starts optimizing digestion around those time periods. Meaning, if you're used to eating breakfast at 8 AM, you'll start getting hungry around that time. Likewise, if you're used to skipping breakfast and eating your first meal at 11 AM, then you'll get hungry then, etc. Another 2015 study confirmed this as well – that the negative side-effects of skipping breakfast, such as increased hunger, decreased satiety and higher insulin and free fatty acid responses to eating lunch after skipping breakfast, occurred only in those individuals who were regularly eating breakfast[1662]. Others who were used to skipping it didn't see those adverse ramifications. That also explains why some people are more likely to overeat and binge in the following meal if they skip a habitual meal. Nevertheless, intermittent fasting may not be a viable eating strategy for a lot of people who tend to experience the negative side-effects more often, including bingeing.

Some epidemiological studies do suggest that skipping breakfast increases the risk of developing type-2 diabetes and obesity[1663]. However, that is almost always caused by overcompensating the higher levels of hunger with overeating calories. In studies where the subjects don't eat very late and don't overeat calories, there is no causal link between skipping breakfast and weight gain or poorer metabolic health[1664,1665,1666]. **Regardless, it is more likely that early time restricted eating (eTRE), meaning eating early in the day, is more suitable for the human physiology and optimal metabolic health.** Your body's insulin sensitivity and glucose tolerance are by default higher earlier in the day[1667,1668,1669]. A 2019 study published by Jamshed et al in May showed that eTRE, between 8 AM and 2 PM, improves 24-hour blood glucose levels, lipid metabolism and circadian clock gene expression[1670]. However, that was compared to a non-TRE group eating between 8 AM and 8 PM. Another 2019 study published by Hutchinson et al 2 months earlier in April didn't see a difference in glucose homeostasis, glycemic control, bodyweight, or hunger responses between eTRE from 8 AM to 5 PM and late-TRE from 12 PM to 9 PM[1671]. In athletes doing resistance training, late TRE (12-8 PM) decreases fat mass without changes in fat-free mass[1672].

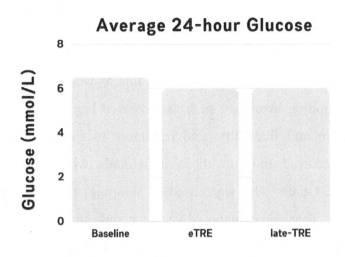

Average 24-hour Glucose

Redrawn From: Hutchinson et al (2019)

A 2022 study discovered that a single meal per day in the evening reduces more body weight, increases fat oxidation and results in lower 24-hour blood glucose levels than 3 meals a day with the same amount of calories among 30-year-old lean individuals[1673]. The individuals consuming one meal a day lost more bodyweight (-1.4 ± 0.3 kg) than those consuming 3 meals a day (−0.5 ± 0.3 kg). Among that weight loss, the one meal a day group lost 0.7 kg as fat and 0.7 kg as lean mass, whereas the 3 meals a day one lost 0.1 kg as fat and 0.4 kg as lean mass. Thus, a larger fasting window and a smaller eating window may make you lose more weight, but it can also predispose you to greater muscle loss. There are ways to mitigate that effect as well as discussed earlier. However, if you're very physically active, eating once a day is probably not ideal for your goals. Fortunately, fasting for only 16 hours and eating within 8 hours among resistance-trained men has been found to be equally effective for muscle and strength growth as a 12-hour eating window[1674].

Multiple studies have shown that eating your entire days' protein requirements in a smaller eating window has no negative effect on muscle preservation as long as the protein intake is sufficiently high[1675,1676,1677,1678].

Women eating their daily protein goal of 79 grams in either 4 meals or a single meal made no difference in their protein absorption[1679]. In fact, a 1999 study on elderly women found that pulse feeding 80% of their daily protein in one meal vs 4 meals spread out resulted in a bigger positive nitrogen balance, protein synthesis and protein turnover[1680]. Of course, this was done on non-athletes, and they didn't build more muscle, but it does challenge the commonly held idea that you need to be eating frequently to preserve muscle. Muslim bodybuilders who train during Ramadan and dry fast don't show decreases in muscle either[1681].

Overall, time-restricted eating has little to no superior effect over regular calorie restriction except the important fact that it's easier to be compliant with time-restricted eating vs. regular calorie restriction. To lose weight with TRE, you still need to be in a calorie deficit. It's just that skipping certain meals and confining your calories in a specific timeframe can improve diet adherence and satiety. Which meal you end up removing is also not that impactful if your daily calorie intake is the same. On paper, early time restricted eating appears to be healthier for the human physiology and circadian rhythm. However, in the real world it also depends on the individual, how many calories they are eating, and what's their current metabolic health like. Whatever the case may be, eating immediately before bed is most likely not beneficial for your biomarkers the following day and it also can decrease sleep quality and increase acid reflux. Your body does go through its maintenance and repair during sleep and one of the main antioxidants for that is NADPH. Fat storage and creation of new fat cells is one of the biggest consumers of NADPH[1682], meaning that if your body is storing calories while you're sleeping it has less resources for healing. This can leave you vulnerable to inflammation and oxidative stress. Melatonin, the sleep hormone, also inhibits insulin production by the pancreas, impairing your ability to regulate your blood sugar levels before bed[1683]. Thus, **it's recommended to have an early**

dinner instead of a late one and stop calorie consumption at least a few hours before bed.

How Not to Wreck Your Metabolism with Excessive Fasting

As said many times, losing weight will potentially decrease your overall metabolic rate through adaptive thermogenesis and reduced bodyweight. However, some of those negative adaptations can occur with excessive fasting and prolonged calorie restriction as well. **Fasting for 72+ hours has been found to lower serum T3 by 30% and TSH by 70% in healthy men due to downregulation of leptin**[1684,1685]. This is a completely normal physiological response to food scarcity as to preserve energy[1686]. Having a lower metabolic rate will also mitigate some muscle loss by making you burn less calories[1687]. Fortunately, T3 and reverse T3 will return to normal after the fasting stops and you refeed[1688]. These negative changes have not been found to occur on daily time restricted eating in the absence of severe calorie restriction. It's been even found that Ramadan fasting (approximately 12-14 hours of dry fasting during the day) doesn't affect thyroid hormones significantly and they stay within normal ranges[1689,1690].

Eating a lower calorie intake of 1500 calories a day for 5 days after a 10-day fast wasn't enough to restore T3 levels in obese subjects[1691]. However, refeeding with carbohydrates can reverse fasting-induced changes in T3 and reverse T3 even when being in an energy deficit[1692]. Carbohydrates are the primary fuel source for thyroid hormones and leptin. Insulin is also required to convert T4 into T3 and raise metabolism. Thus, consuming carbohydrates after prolonged fasting or severe calorie restriction can be a powerful way to break some aspects of metabolic adaptation, mainly adaptive thermogenesis, even while being hypocaloric. This makes it ideal during a reverse diet scenario wherein you shouldn't be eating a surplus of calories immediately. Making the main calories you re-introduce carbohydrates would enable you to raise your metabolism without reaching an energy surplus.

Protein Sparing Modified Fast (PSMF)

Another way to lose weight rapidly while preserving muscle is to practice what's called a Protein Sparing Modified Fast (PSMF)[1693]. Essentially, you eat virtually no carbohydrates with some fiber being allowed, as close to zero fat as possible and primarily lean protein at a severe calorie deficit. In a typical PSMF you consume only 800-1000 calories a day with nearly all of those calories coming from protein. PSMF originates from the 1970s as a method to treat obese patients or type-2 diabetics[1694]. It's also commonly used by bodybuilders and fitness competitors to lose a lot of body fat before stepping on stage. Because you are still eating a significant amount of protein, you're going to mitigate a lot of the muscle loss that would occur during complete fasting. In addition to weight loss, PSMF can also lower blood glucose, blood pressure, hemoglobin A1C and improve insulin resistance[1695,1696]. However, the PSMF can also have some dangerous side-effects if practiced for too long and if the calorie restriction is too severe, such as death due to unexpected heart issues[1697]. That's why we caution you to consult with your physician before trying anything like this as to assess your health condition beforehand. Generally, these harsh consequences occur in obese individuals who are doing the PSMF (again at only around 800 calories a day) for several weeks and months. Among fitness competitors, the PSMF phases last only for a few weeks.

Here's an example Protein Sparing Modified Fast (PSMF):

- ~ 800-1,000 calories a day

- ~ 2 grams of protein/kg of body weight

- Breakfast

    o 5 oz. of steak at breakfast (400 calories, 35 g protein)

    o 3 oz. cooked spinach (for potassium and magnesium)

- Lunch

    o 30-40 grams of whey protein

- Dinner

    o 5 oz. of 100% grass burger blend (75% muscle meat/25% heart and liver) for dinner (400 calories)

    o 3 oz. of spinach or berries

- 45 minutes prior to bedtime

    o 30 grams of casein protein (slower but longer acting protein)

Doing a PSMF tends to make you lose weight quite rapidly because you're eating only about 30-40% of your total daily energy expenditure. **People doing the PSMF appear to lose more weight initially compared to regular low-calorie dieting (minus 12.4% vs 2.6%)**[1698]. A study on 15 overweight individuals eating 500 calories a day with PSMF saw that they lost on average 32.4 lbs. (14.7 kg) of fat over the course of 6 weeks with virtually no muscle loss[1699]. Obese subjects experience weight loss plateaus only after several weeks or even months of such dieting, wherein you have to introduce refeeds[1700]. During refeeding you would eat some complex carbohydrates that would raise leptin and thyroid hormones. Generally, refeed days on the PSMF are done once after every few weeks or whenever needed. Leaner and already physically active people would see a drop in thyroid function much faster than obese individuals, which is why they may need to have refeeds more often. After you stop doing the PSMF diet, you start to increase your total calorie intake by introducing more carbohydrates and fats. The reason being the potential of regaining weight, as most obese PSMF patients tend to gain back nearly 50% of the weight they lost 2-3 years after the fact[1701].

Ultimately, to keep the weight off, you have to change your relationship with food, eat better quality food and develop better eating habits. **Most people aren't going to count every calorie they consume. Thus, the key to weight loss and optimal body composition is moderation in eating (portion out your meals) and the quality of the food that you eat.** This includes predominantly opting for foods that promote satiety, fullness and good health. There are many ways to reach that goal and you have to find what works for you. Certain dietary adjustments or extreme dieting can work in the short term and you can even be successful in maintaining those results. However, if you want to stay at a healthy bodyweight then you'll also have to structure your diet in a way that's sustainable for you.

Summary for the best strategies to lose weight

1.) Eat whole nutritious foods (cook at home most of the time)

2.) Avoid or limit junk food, fast food, pre-packaged foods and restaurant food

3.) Portion out your meals (so as not to overconsume food)

4.) Try skipping one meal (especially on non-exercise days) or eating an early dinner

    a. Consider skipping a meal that is easiest for you to skip. If you are someone who usually eats breakfast, then you may want to skip lunch or dinner. However, if time-restricted eating doesn't suit you, or you tend to overcompensate for it with overeating afterwards, then consuming 3 meals a day is still appropriate.

        i. If you ensure that your breakfast has a high amount of protein (~ 50 grams of protein give or take) this will make it easier to skip lunch and eat an early dinner.

5.) Try the MATADOR method – 25-33% calorie restriction for 1-2 weeks followed by a maintenance caloric intake for 1-2 weeks. You can take a step-wise approach to both the calorie reduction phase and maintenance phase.

6.) Try a protein sparing modified fast, but only at a 25-33% calorie restriction, for 1-2 weeks followed by a maintenance caloric intake for 1-2 weeks.

7.) For weight loss under doctor supervision - try a protein sparing modified fast (1,000 calories per day mostly from protein)

Chapter 8 – The Obesity Fix Diet

The goal of this book is to give you sustainable guidelines for maintaining an optimal body composition. To that end, there are certain characteristics commonly shared by all successful diets and eating routines. They all help you to stay satiated and satisfied without going into cycles of overeating while providing you with optimal amounts of macro- and micronutrients. In this chapter, we're going to outline the main take-aways of this book and give additional principles for losing weight and keeping it off for good.

What Kind of Macronutrients to Eat?

The U.S. Dietary Guidelines in 2015-2020 recommended that the average woman needs around 1,600-2,400 calories per day and the average man 2,000-3,000[1702]. Those numbers might not be suitable for someone who has a very low level of energy expenditure or who has a significant amount of fat to lose. If you're not exercising at all and are trying to lose weight, then you will probably have to consume a bit less than that to create a calorie deficit. Granted, an overweight person might have a higher basal metabolic rate due to being heavier but you obviously don't want to sustain the fat mass. Instead, you should create a negative energy balance based on the calorie intake that makes you lose weight.

However, **calories alone aren't enough to pay attention to as the macronutrient ratios of your diet will dramatically affect your energy balance and body composition**. For example, diets higher in protein tend to do better in weight loss studies even when you consume the same amount of calories, mostly because of the higher thermic effect of protein (you burn more calories breaking down protein than carbs or fat) but in the real world higher protein also translates to sustained satiety[1703]. People in industrialized societies consume 12-17% of their total calories as protein, whereas hunter-gatherers get up to 35%[1704]. Protein also has 4 calories per gram, the same as carbohydrates, compared to 9 calories with fat. Thus, protein is the most important macro for fat loss and maintaining muscle.

The Recommended Daily Allowance (RDA) for protein is only 0.36 g/lb or 0.8 g/kg of bodyweight[1705]. However, this is based on only covering essential structural requirements[1706]. Many nutritionists and experts consider the current RDA to be inadequate[1707], especially among the elderly who can't sustain their muscle mass with the RDA[1708]. For muscle growth, the optimal protein intake has been found to be 0.8 g/lb or 1.6 g/kg of lean bodyweight with no additional benefits beyond that[1709]. However, when you're in a calorie deficit, increasing your protein intake to 2.2-3.3 g/kg can help with more muscle preservation[1710,1711,1712,1713,1714]. To make it easier to remember, for protein, **aim for 1 g/lb or 2.2 g/kg of lean bodyweight**[1715]. Those with higher muscle mass may even benefit from consuming 1.25 grams of protein per pound of lean body weight. You could consume less than that and get 20-25% of calories as protein but because of the beneficial effects of high protein intakes on fat loss it's not advisable to get less than 20%.

You've probably heard that protein is bad for your kidneys, which is why you shouldn't eat a high protein diet. Fortunately, there's no evidence that would show that eating more protein would be harmful to the kidneys of healthy people[1716]. Kidney damage from too much protein has been seen to happen only in people with pre-existing kidney disease[1717]. Eating too much protein doesn't spike your blood sugar the same way as carbohydrates or sugar does either. Diabetics who eat a meal with 2 grams of protein per kilogram don't see a significant rise in their blood sugar after eating[1718]. However, eating 1 g/kg of carbohydrates does raise blood sugar significantly.

Here are the recommended macronutrient ratios for weight loss:

- **Protein 25-35%** - meat, fish, eggs, organ meat, poultry, cottage cheese, curd, Greek yogurt, beans, legumes, lentils, protein powder. Animal protein is more bioavailable and should comprise the majority of your protein calories.

- **Fat 25-40%** - fat from meat, eggs, fish, cod liver oil, olive oil, avocados, nuts, seeds, MCT oil; fats you cook with: olive oil, coconut oil, avocado oil, butter, tallow, lard.

- **Carbohydrates 10-25%** - potatoes, sweet potatoes, carrots, zucchini, asparagus, broccoli, peppers, buckwheat, Ezekiel bread (tastes better when toasted), beetroot, apples, bananas, pineapple, mangos, grapefruit, oranges, clementines, kiwis, blueberries, cranberries, strawberries, grapes, currants. Rice can be consumed but it should be minimized as it is high in carbohydrates and low in micronutrients.

The Obesity Fix
Recommended Fat Loss Macros

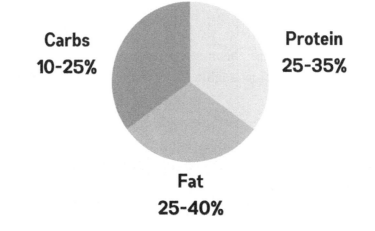

Carbs
10-25%

Protein
25-35%

Fat
25-40%

Alcohol cannot be used as a nutrient by the body but it does provide 7 calories per gram of ethanol[1719]. Because it's recognized as a toxin, the body starts to metabolize alcohol first and puts the oxidation of other macros on the backburner and overconsumption of alcohol can lead to insulin resistance[1720]. This is the reason drinking alcohol makes it easier to store fat and gain weight, especially if you eat calories alongside it[1721,1722]. On top of that, alcohol promotes visceral fat gain and reduces testosterone by raising estrogen[1723,1724,1725].

Protein and carbs have the second highest oxidative priority after alcohol and fat has the lowest. You can only store a limited amount of protein as amino acids and glucose as glycogen, whereas the storage capacity for fat in the adipose tissue is essentially unlimited. Thus, fat is the easiest macro to store and also burns the least number of calories to digest.

	Alcohol	Protein	Carbohydrates	Fat
Oxidative Priority	1	2	3	4
Calories Per Gram	7	4	4	9
Thermic Effect	15%	20-30%	7-15%	2-4%

The Obesity Fix Diet Tips

Here are some top tips for eating:

1. Dial up the protein (1-1.25 g/lb or 2.2-2.3 g/kg of lean bodyweight).
   a. For someone who weighs 150 pounds this would be ~150-180 grams of protein per day spread across 2-4 meals per day.
2. Dial down the carbs (10-25% of calories from carbohydrates vs. 55% in the Standard American Diet). This equates to around 65-165 grams of carbohydrates for a male adult weighing 170 pounds. Those who are less active should stick to the lower end of the range, whereas those who are more active should consume closer to the higher end of this range. Consuming at least 100 grams of carbohydrates from whole foods per day is beneficial for energy levels, hormone function, and vitality. While certain periods of very low carbohydrate intakes can be beneficial for weight loss (< 60 grams/day), especially in those who are sedentary, a moderate carbohydrate intake (~ 65-165 grams) is more sustainable and optimal for those who are moderately to highly active.
   a. Eliminate refined carbohydrates and sugars in your diet
   b. Stick to consuming whole food carbohydrates
3. Try to get your fat from whole foods instead of added oils or other fats
   a. Reduce the consumption of heavy cream or butter in coffee
4. Eat more foods that have fiber
   a. A little fiber goes a long way. You don't have to eat loads of fiber, however having one food item that contains fiber can help provide quick satiety.
5. Replace most of your high carb foods (pizza, cakes, cookies, chips, etc.) with low calorie fruits and vegetables

6. Avoid the consumption of refined sugars, especially sugary beverages

    a. Fruit juices should be limited

7. Limit or avoid the consumption of omega-6 seed oils (soybean oil, sunflower oil, safflower oil, cottonseed oil, canola oil, corn oil, grapeseed oil, rice bran oil, peanut oil, sesame oil, etc.)

8. Limit the consumption of fast food and ultra-processed foods (cake, pizza, subs, chips, cookies, etc.)

9. Try to avoid snacking and spontaneous food consumption in between meals.

    a. However, if you feel you need a snack, for example perhaps you worked out hard or didn't consume enough calories in your previous meal we have provided a list of snack options later in this chapter.

10. Be careful with the foods you eat in restaurants because they tend to have significantly more calories than home-made foods

The Obesity Fix Food Pyramid

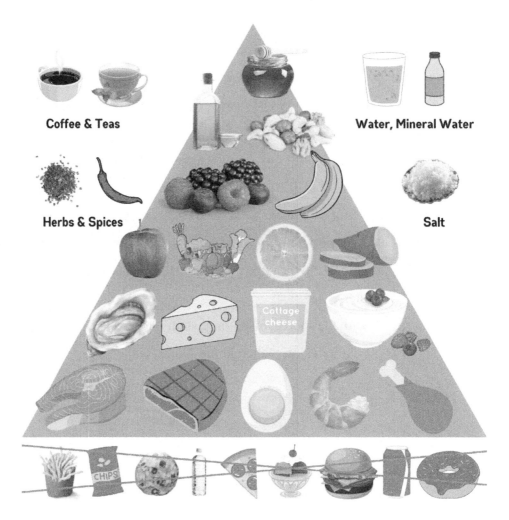

You should get the majority of your food in volume as protein and fibrous vegetables. However, the calories would be coming predominantly from animal foods given that vegetables are quite voluminous and large in size with relatively low weight. For example, to get 100 calories from meat, you'd only have to eat 2-3 ounces, depending on the amount of fat in it. To get 100 calories from broccoli you'd have to eat around 10 oz. That's why it's going to be quite difficult to eat 1000 calories of broccoli, whereas it's much easier to reach that with meat.

Average Plate Serving Size

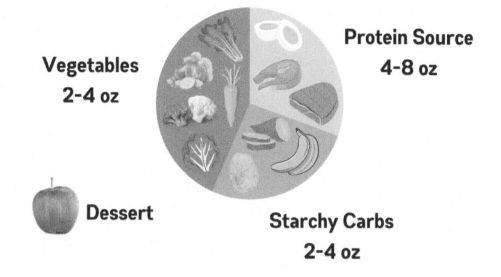

Vegetables
2-4 oz

Protein Source
4-8 oz

Dessert

Starchy Carbs
2-4 oz

The majority of your calories should be coming from animal sources, however, because vegetables are so low in calories, the actual proportion on your plate may take up more space than your animal foods. Importantly, if you do not tolerate vegetables, then you can replace those calories with fruit or more animal protein. Because of their filling effect, you'll end up consuming fewer calories per plate, enabling you to maintain a normal calorie intake. The more vegetables and greens you have, the less room there will be for calorie-dense fats, oils, and sugars from various sources. Although protein sources burn a lot of calories for digestion, they still have significantly more calories than low calorie vegetables. Starchy carbohydrates and olive oil as dressing should be complimentary parts of the dish not the star. **To reduce glucose spikes, eat protein, fat and vegetables before fruit and starchy carbs.**

Limit or Avoid	Consume to Satiety
Cereal	Greek Yogurt
Juice	Cottage Cheese
Muffins	Pastured Eggs
Waffles	Grass-Fed- Meat, Chicken, Beef, etc.
Bagels	Organic Bacon, Sausages
Donuts	Steel Cut Oats
Toast	Ezekiel Bread with Almond Butter, Bananas, and Cinnamon (snack)
Croissants	Fruit and Berries
McMuffins	Fish, Sardines, Salmon
Sausage Biscuits	Omelette
McGriddles	Cheddar Cheese Stick
Pancakes	Nuts (if tolerated)
Hotcakes	Nut Butters (consume in moderation, ensure there's no seed oils added)
Hash Browns	Celery, Peanut Butter, Raisins (snack)
Hot Dogs or Cheese Dogs	Cheddar Cheese Stick
Cheesecake	Pickles, Olives

Macaroni Salad or Potato Salad	Grass-Fed Jerky (Beef, venison, bison, etc.)

Healthy cooking oils

- Extra virgin olive oil
- Butter
- Ghee
- Tallow
- Coconut oil

Cooking oils to avoid

- Soybean oil
- Sunflower oil
- Safflower oil
- Cottonseed oil
- Canola oil (rapeseed)
- Corn oil
- Grapeseed oil
- Rice bran oil
- Peanut oil
- Sesame oil

Healthy eating isn't about eliminating all your favorite foods but more about eating healthy 80-90% of the time and finding versions of your favorite meals that contain healthier ingredients.

Replace or Limit This	Eat This Instead
Yellow Banana	Greenish Banana (more fiber)
Wheat Bread	Ezekiel Bread
Ice Cream	Yogurt or Cottage Cheese with Berries
Big Mac	Steak or Bun-less Burger Wrapped in Lettuce
French Fries	Organic Potatoes/Sweet Potatoes
Pizza	Cauliflower Crust Pizza
Sugary Cereal	Greek Yogurt with Nuts and Seeds
American Cheese	Raw Grass-fed Cheese
Salad Dressing	Extra Virgin Olive Oil
Butter and Margarine	Grass-Fed Butter
Eggs	Pastured Eggs
Grain-Fed Meat	Grass-Fed Meat
Milk Chocolate	70%+ Dark Chocolate
Fake Juices	Citrus Fruit (clementine, orange, etc.) or small amounts of 100% fruit juice
Peanut Butter	Almond Butter (small amounts of peanut butter on occasion is fine)
Potato Chips	Nuts with salt or pickles

The Obesity Fix Meal Plans

Here are meal plans for breakfast, lunch, and dinner that you can incorporate into your meal plan.

Breakfast Options

1. Ham and cheese omelet with grilled onions and peppers (you can add other vegetables if you like)
2. Steak, over easy or scrambled pastured eggs, greenish banana, or berries
3. Scrambled eggs with mushrooms, spring onion and cauliflower
4. Over easy pastured eggs with organic bacon and/or ham, fruit
5. Greek or Icelandic yogurt, nuts (pecans, walnuts, etc.), fruit
6. Cottage cheese with berries
7. Soft boiled eggs with half of an avocado and 2 raw carrots
8. Soft boiled eggs with steamed broccoli and milk
9. Frittata with tomatoes, mushrooms, and broccoli
10. Steel cut oats with cottage cheese and cinnamon
11. Steel cut oats with protein powder and berries
12. Pastured eggs, toasted Ezekiel bread and Greek or Icelandic yogurt
13. Toasted Ezekiel bread with nut butter, slices of banana, cinnamon, wild honey, and yogurt
14. Beef burger (can add tomato in a lettuce wrap if tolerated)
15. Beef burger with cooked asparagus and pickles
16. Casserole with turkey meat, spinach, onion, and eggs
17. Shredded cabbage slaw with minced meat, shredded carrot, and olive oil mayonnaise
18. Mashed cauliflower with liver sausage and pickles

19. Mashed cauliflower with scrambled eggs and meat

20. Roasted Bok Choy with minced beef, bell peppers and cheddar cheese

21. Chia pudding with coconut milk, berries, and chia seeds

22. Smoked salmon with asparagus and cherry tomatoes

23. Salted salmon with steamed vegetables and cucumber

24. Homemade cereal with nuts, coconut flakes, berries, and grass-fed milk

Lunch Options

1. Turkey Taco Salad - Organic ground turkey with roasted potatoes

2. Organic Chicken and roasted potatoes or wild rice or mushrooms

3. Pulled pork, roasted potatoes, green beans

4. Bacon burger, salad, sweet potatoes, side of fruit

5. Tacos (beef, chicken, steak) sour cream, cheese

6. Brisket, sweet potatoes, asparagus

7. Meat in roasted red peppers (with or without cheese or cream cheese)

8. Chicken wraps in lettuce with peppers and onions

9. Stuffed bell peppers with minced mead and tomatoes

10. Cooked salmon with asparagus and olive oil mayonnaise

11. Zucchini noodle pasta with scallops, herbs, and snow peas

12. Black bean wraps with tomatoes, onions, and peppers

13. Fried beef and broccoli with a potato

14. Air fried chicken drumsticks with cauliflower

15. Caesar salad with chicken, romaine lettuce, pumpkin seeds, and olive oil

16. Boiled chicken, shredded purple cabbage, celery and carrot wrapped in Bok Choy

17. Mediterranean grilled chicken salad with tomatoes, feta cheese, beans, and herbs

18. Chickpea salad with cucumber, tomatoes, red onions, and Romaine lettuce

19. Salted salmon sushi wrapped in zucchini slices and mustard

20. Strawberry spinach salad with feta cheese, wild shrimp, and red onions

21. Sweet potato with pork tenderloin and pickles

22. Roasted potatoes with beef brisket

23. Steak fajita bowl with black beans, tomatoes, onions, sour cream

24. Spinach salad with fried eggs and olive oil

25. Fried cod with steamed vegetables and rice

Dinner Options

1. Grass-fed beef, asparagus, green beans, or roasted potatoes or zucchini

2. Stuffed zucchini with minced meat, onion, and cooked vegetables

3. Stuffed bell peppers with steak, vegetables and topped with cheese

4. Zucchini noodles with cherry tomatoes, salmon, and herbs

5. Cabbage rolls with chicken, peppers, and onion

6. Chicken casserole with Brussel sprouts, carrots, and eggs

7. Roasted chicken with broccoli and cauliflower

8. Baked salmon with asparagus and rice

9. Chicken breast with sweet potato and asparagus

10. Cauliflower crust pizza with minced meat and tomato sauce topping

11. Chili con carne with beef, black beans, and cauliflower

12. Chicken Thai curry with squash and rice noodles

13. Ground turkey, squash borscht soup

14. Roasted pork with sauerkraut, buckwheat, and a slice of rye bread

15. Pho soup (Vietnamese soup with rice noodles and beef)

16. Cottage cheese with salted nuts and black beans

17. Beef steak with roasted potatoes, carrots, and rosemary

18. Cauliflower rice with shrimp, mushrooms, and romaine lettuce

19. Fried liver with onions, broccoli, and pineapple slices

20. Fried beef heart with green beans, potatoes, and carrots

21. Grilled shrimp skewers with bell peppers and zucchini

22. Ground turkey Bolognese with whole wheat pasta

23. Zucchini lamb meat balls with tomato sauce

24. Sugar free jelly with cottage cheese and berries

25. Egg frittata with mozzarella, beans, and broccoli

26. Organ blend cheeseburger (Northstar Bison) and mixed vegetables

Snack Options

1. Almond butter

2. Apples

3. Oranges, clementines, mandarin orange

4. Mango, peach, nectarine

5. Piece of 70-80% high cacao dark chocolate

6. Handful of nuts and seeds

7. Greek/Icelandic yogurt, nuts, raw wild honey

8. Beef jerky

9. Boiled egg

10. Meat sticks

11. Celery sticks

12. Raw carrot

13. Protein bar

14. Protein shake

15. Sugar-free jelly

16. Surimi sticks

17. Cottage cheese and berries

18. Wakame chips

19. Cucumber slices with hummus

20. Cherry tomatoes

21. Chia pudding

22. Baby carrots

23. Half an avocado

24. Roasted chickpeas

25. Cantaloupe slices

10 Meal Plans

Examples of 3 Meals per Day

Here are some examples of 3 meals per day meal plans. The below meal plans are simply a guide and will change depending on an individual's caloric needs.

3-Meal per Day Example 1

- **Breakfast:** 8 oz. grass-fed steak, 2 pastured eggs, 1 medium sized greenish banana.

- **Lunch:** 6 oz. wild salmon, 2-4 oz. asparagus, 4 oz. roasted potatoes.

- **Dinner:** 6 oz. ground beef (50% organ blend, 50% ground meat), which can be made into burgers or taco meat, 4 oz. mixed vegetables, 1 slice toasted Ezekiel bread dipped in organic extra virgin olive oil and salt, 2-4 pieces of organ dark chocolate (75% cacao).

3-Meal per Day Example 2

- **Breakfast:** 3 whole eggs, 2 raw carrots, 1 small persimmons, 2 tbsp peanut butter, 10g of dark chocolate.

- **Post workout meal:** 1 protein bar, 1 small banana

- **Lunch:** 3 eggs, 2 oz oatmeal, a handful of nuts

- **Dinner:** about 7 oz roasted lean pork, sauerkraut, 4 oz rye bread, 1 cup of buckwheat.

3-Meal per Day Example 3

- **Breakfast:** 1 whey protein shake, 1 oz dark chocolate, 1 raw carrot.

- **Snack:** 2 oz jerky beef, 2 Brazil nuts, cashews, walnuts, almonds, 1 carrot, 1 greenish banana, 2 tbsp peanut butter

- **Late Lunch (2pm):** 1 cup borscht soup no cream, 4 small Turkey breakfast sausage, 4 oz sautéed kale.

- **Dinner:** 10 oz chicken Thai curry, ½ cup squash, some rice noodles, one square of dark chocolate

3-Meal per Day Example 4

- **Breakfast:** 2 eggs, 1 big raw carrot, 1 nut bar, 3 Brazil nuts, 1 oz dark chocolate

- **Lunch:** 1 healthy pancake (10 oz egg whites, 4 oz sweet potato purée, 4 oz oatmeal, cinnamon, ginger, flax seeds), 1 small avocado, 1 small banana with 1.5 tbsp peanut butter.

- **Dinner:** 2 cups of pho (Vietnamese soup with rice noodles and beef)

3-Meal per Day Example 5

- **First Meal:** 3 fried eggs in 1 tbsp butter, 1 cup of spinach, 1 oz of cheese

- **Second Meal:** 8 oz/200 g ground beef in 1 tbsp butter, 1 oz/28 g cheese

- 2-4 cups of steamed broccoli, ½ avocado

- **Third Meal:** 1/2 cup of Greek yogurt, 1 tablespoon of coconut flakes, a handful of berries

3-Meal per Day Example 6

- **Breakfast:** 1 protein bar, one small apple, 3 almonds

- **Snack**: 1 small meat stick

- **Lunch:** 2 duck eggs, 2 chicken eggs, 1 avocado, sautéed cabbage, 1 tbsp extra virgin olive oil, 1 tbsp coconut milk (full fat), 3 Brazil nuts, 2 pecans, 2 cashews.

- **Dinner:** 6 oz ground Turkey, 9 oz of squash/pumpkin, borscht soup (no sour cream), 1 tbsp extra virgin olive oil.

Examples of 2 Meals per Day

Here are some examples of 2 meals per day meal plans.

Low Carb Day Example 1

- **First Meal:** 2-4 eggs, 8 oz. grass-fed meat, 2 cups of veggies, 1 cup of sauerkraut or kimchi, 1-2 raw carrots, 1-2 Brazil nuts

- **Snack:** If you do want a snack, raw carrots are good or a bit of beef jerky/meat sticks

- **Second Meal:** 10 oz. wild salmon or other wild fish, 1 oz liver (can get as organ blends), 2-4 cups of oven baked cauliflower or cabbage next to the fish, ½ cup of rice, ½ cup of beans

Low Carb Day Example 2

- **First Meal:** 2-4 eggs, 100 g cottage cheese, 2 cups of veggies, 1-2 raw carrots, 1-2 Brazil nuts

- **Snack:** If you do want to snack something, then some raw carrots are good or a bit of beef jerky/meat sticks

- **Second Meal:** 12 oz of any meat, 1.5 oz of liver (can get as organ blends), ½ cup of rice, ½ cup of beans, 2-4 cups of oven baked cauliflower or cabbage next to the fish

High Carb Day Example 1

- **First Meal:** 12 oz ground grass-fed beef or other meat, 2-4 cups of steamed broccoli, ½ cup of rice, ½ cup of beans, 1-2 raw carrots, 1-2 Brazil nuts

- **Second Meal:** 12 oz cod or other white fish, 7 oz cooked potatoes, 7 oz cooked beetroot or carrots, 1 kiwifruit, 2 cups of berries/strawberries etc., 3 oz cottage cheese, 200-1000 mcg of chromium with the meal is recommended

High Carb Example 2

- **First Meal:** 6 slices of bacon, 2 egg yolks or 3 oz fatty fish, 1 cup of veggies cooked, 2 oz of liver (can get as organ blends)

- **Second Meal:** 15 oz steak or other red meat, 1/3 cup of beans, 2-4 cups of oven baked potatoes

How to Combat Sugar Cravings

Many times, sugar cravings are your body craving carbohydrates for fuel. Here are some things to consume that can help stop a sugar craving in its tracks!

- Fruit - citrus, berries, grapes, mango, apple, etc.
- Redmond Real Salt
- Redmond Re-Lyte
- Pickle juice
- Pickles
- Cherry tomatoes and cucumber
- Piece of 70% or higher cacao dark chocolate
- Handful of nuts and seeds
- Beef jerky
- Toasted Ezekiel bread with nut butter
- Greenish banana
- Inositol powder dissolved in the mouth
- Small amount of dried fruit, e.g., raisins, cranberries, etc.

Sometimes, you get cravings in between meals because you didn't consume enough calories during your actual meals. This can be improved by consuming enough protein and fiber.

Consume to satiety during meals:

- Grass-fed meat
- Pastured eggs
- Wild salmon
- Greek yogurt
- Cottage cheese
- Fruit (citrus, berries, grapes, etc.)
- Potatoes
- Greenish bananas
- Raw grass-fed cheese
- Mushrooms
- Vegetables and salad

How to Read Food Labels:

As a rule, avoid or limit foods that have over 5 grams of added sugar per serving or more.

Ingredients that are fine:

- Salt
- Whole foods (meat, fruits, vegetables, dairy)

Ingredients to limit:

- Added sugars (see chapter 4 on all their different names)
- Flour (wheat flour, white flour, corn flour, etc.)
- Seed oils (soybean oil, sunflower oil, safflower oil, cottonseed oil, canola oil, corn oil, grapeseed oil, rice bran oil, peanut oil, sesame oil, etc.)
- Phosphates
- Nitrates/nitrites
- Artificial colors - red/yellow/blue dyes
- Artificial sweeteners - aspartame, saccharin, sucralose

Fiber and carbs

Subtract the fiber from the total carbohydrate to get the net carbohydrates. The higher the fiber content the lower the net carbohydrates.

Healthy labels to look for

- Organic
- Non-GMO (Non-genetically modified organisms)

Easy Guide for Workouts

For overall health and fat loss, it's recommended to do both cardio and resistance training.

- Perform 3 to 5, 30-60-minute weight training sessions per week
- Focus on 2-3 different exercises for each muscle group
- 3-4 sets per exercise, go close to failure or failure each time
- Cycle between push, pull and leg days.
    - Day 1: chest, triceps, and shoulders
    - Day 2: back, biceps and arms
    - Day 3: quads, hamstrings, glutes, and calves
    - Abs can be integrated into either one of the above days or performed on a separate day
- Aim for about 2-3 low intensity cardio sessions per week
- Go for long walks every day, several times a day if possible

How heavy to lift?

Where you get close to failure after you complete ~5-12 reps with weights but this can also be done to failure or close to failure with bodyweight exercises.

What types of exercises?

Resistance training

If starting out

- Focus on pull ups, push-ups, dips, and squats. You can add weight as body weight becomes easier. Go close to failure or failure each time.

- Try alternating bodyweight exercises: 20 squats, 1 push up, 19 squats, 2 push-ups, keep going until you get to 1 squat and 20 push-ups.

Exercise selection for muscle groups:

- Chest
  - Pushups, bench press, incline bench, decline bench, dumbbell press, chest flies
- Shoulders
  - Overhead press, military press, lateral raises, rear delt flies, handstand pushups
- Back
  - Deadlifts, barbell row, pullups, 1 hand dumbbell row, lat pulldown, lower back bench exercises
- Biceps
  - Barbell curls, hammer curls, z-bar curls
- Triceps
  - Dips, triceps pushdown, skull crushers, seated tricep press, diamond pushups, tiger pushups
- Forearms
  - Farmer's carries, deadlifts, forearm curls
- Legs
  - Barbell squats, split squats, walking lunges, leg press, leg curls, hamstring curls, Nordic curls, calf raises, stiff legged deadlifts, sumo deadlifts

Cardio

- Hill work outs
  - Squats
  - Sprint up a hill
  - Walk down the hill
  - Push-ups or jumping jacks
  - Sprint up a hill
  - Walk down
  - Repeat as many times as you can
- Run, jog, bike, or swim at low intensity for 30-45 minutes
- Interval sprints
  - 30 second sprint, 30 second rest
  - Repeat for as many times as you can

Concluding Remarks

We hope that you will take the information in this book to help you with your weight loss and muscle building goals. As a final summary, we are providing you with 21 final key takeaways when it comes to weight loss and good metabolic health.

The 21 Keys to Weight Loss and Optimal Health

1. **Eat real food**
   a. As close to nature as possible, for example, this means 100% grass-fed meat (not grain-finished meat), pastured eggs (not conventional eggs), etc.

2. **Build muscle**
   a. Lift weights, resistance/body weight workouts, etc. 3-6 X per week.

3. **Target protein**
   a. Consume 1-1.25 grams of protein per pound of lean body weight, those who lift more weights or perform more full body workouts should target the higher end of intake.

4. **Eliminate highly refined foods**
   a. Remove the refined carbohydrates, refined sugar, and seed oils

5. **Optimize sleep**
   a. 8-9 hours of sleep

6. **Conquer your mindset/stress**
   a. Eliminate negative thoughts, come up with strategies to handle stress

7. **Avoid a high omega-6/3 ratio**
   a. Avoid excessive consumption of foods high in omega-6 (still okay to consume eggs, chicken, and walnuts for example but you want to make sure you are consuming enough omega-3s to balance it out)

    b.   Consume omega-3s (wild salmon, sardines, high quality omega-3 supplements). Aim for 2-3 grams of EPA/DHA per day.

8. Reduce artificial sweetener intake

    a.   Particularly aspartame, sucralose and erythritol.

    b.   Stevia/monk fruit are better but still should not be overconsumed.

9. Avoid light at night

    a.   Turn off lights at night in the home

    b.   Turn down the light settings on your phone

    c.   Use blue light blocking glasses, especially if working on a computer at night

10. Avoid eating refined carbohydrates and fat bombs together

    a.   Eating refined carbs plus fats is one of the quickest ways to gain weight, this would include things like bagel with cream cheese, cereal with full-fat milk, milk chocolate, peanut butter and jelly sandwich, pizza, donuts, pasta with cheese, etc.

11. Keep fat bombs to a minimum

    a.   Keep butter/cream intake to a minimum

12. Eat healthy carbs that you tolerate

    a.   Ezekiel bread, organic spinach, berries, lightly cooked white/sweet/purple potatoes, onions, garlic, peppers, etc.

13. Drink mineral water or spring water

    a.   Gerolsteiner, Magnesia, San Pellegrino, Mountain Valley Spring Water

14. Eat real salt

    a.   Redmond Real Salt or Redmond Re-Lyte plus fluid should be used for boosting energy, powering workouts, and reducing sugar cravings

    b.   Pickle juice is also a great way to quickly provide salt and fluid and to help reduce sugar cravings

15. Balance acid-base status

    a.   Bicarbonate-mineral waters, sodium/potassium citrate, fruits/vegetables help balance the acid load from animal foods/grains.

16. Consume collagen

a. Skin on chicken/fish, grass-fed hydrolyzed collagen proteins, bone broth made from collagenous meats (where a lot of gelatin forms in the refrigerator), glycine supplements, etc.

17. Eat nuts for minerals

a. Walnuts, almonds, pecans, etc. can provide a nice mineral boost. Walnuts are high in omega-6 so don't overconsume.

18. Eat high cacao dark chocolate

a. 70-90% high cacao dark chocolate.

b. A few pieces will do for a sugar fix (especially if nuts are added). However, don't overconsume as there can still be fair amounts of sugar/fat.

19. Healthy snacks (if needed)

a. Venison, Bison, Grass-fed Beef jerky

    i. These can help reduce sugar cravings at night

20. Get appropriate sunlight, fresh air and get out in nature

a. Start enjoying the life outdoors!

21. Practice portion control

a. Portion out your meals and only eat until you are 80% full (not hungry but not stuffed)

The Obesity Fix Plan is relatively simple – you simply portion out your meals, eat whole nutritious foods, eat until you're 80% full, target the protein/carb/fat ratios presented in this book and incorporate daily movement while adding resistance training and certain forms of cardio that fits into your lifestyle. The goal is to eat healthy nutritious foods 80-90% of the time so that you can enjoy some of your favorite desserts every now and then. Ultimately, only you have the power to change your health for the better. This book gives you information about how to lose weight and build muscle, but at the end of the day it's going to be you who will have to put in the work. Losing weight doesn't have to be an extremely complex problem. With the guidance written in this book, we believe you're well on your way towards a leaner, healthier and happier version of yourself. We wish you all the best on your weight loss journey!

References

[1] WHO Obesity and Overweight [Online]. World Health Organization (2019). Available online at: https://www.who.int/news-room/fact-sheets/detail/obesity-and-overweight (accessed September 18, 2020).

[2] CDC (2020) 'Adult Obesity Facts', Overweight & Obesity, Accessed Online: https://www.cdc.gov/obesity/data/adult.html

[3] Moore, J. X., Chaudhary, N., & Akinyemiju, T. (2017). Metabolic Syndrome Prevalence by Race/Ethnicity and Sex in the United States, National Health and Nutrition Examination Survey, 1988–2012. Preventing Chronic Disease, 14. doi:10.5888/pcd14.160287

[4] WHO (2021) 'Obesity and overweight', Accessed Online March 5 2022: https://www.who.int/en/news-room/fact-sheets/detail/obesity-and-overweight

[5] Caballero B. (2007). The global epidemic of obesity: an overview. Epidemiologic reviews, 29, 1–5. https://doi.org/10.1093/epirev/mxm012

[6] Caballero B. (2007). The global epidemic of obesity: an overview. Epidemiologic reviews, 29, 1–5. https://doi.org/10.1093/epirev/mxm012

[7] Ng, M., Fleming, T., Robinson, M., Thomson, B., Graetz, N., Margono, C., Mullany, E. C., Biryukov, S., Abbafati, C., Abera, S. F., Abraham, J. P., Abu-Rmeileh, N. M., Achoki, T., AlBuhairan, F. S., Alemu, Z. A., Alfonso, R., Ali, M. K., Ali, R., Guzman, N. A., Ammar, W., … Gakidou, E. (2014). Global, regional, and national prevalence of overweight and obesity in children and adults during 1980-2013: a systematic analysis for the Global Burden of Disease Study 2013. Lancet (London, England), 384(9945), 766–781. https://doi.org/10.1016/S0140-6736(14)60460-8

[8] Peter G. Kopelman; Ian D. Caterson; Michael J. Stock; William H. Dietz (2005). Clinical obesity in adults and children: In Adults and Children. Blackwell Publishing. p. 493. ISBN 978-1-4051-1672-5.

[9] Flegal, K. M., Ogden, C. L., & Carroll, M. D. (2004). Prevalence and trends in overweight in Mexican-american adults and children. Nutrition reviews, 62(7 Pt 2), S144–S148. https://doi.org/10.1111/j.1753-4887.2004.tb00085.x

[10] Ogden, C. L., Carroll, M. D., Curtin, L. R., McDowell, M. A., Tabak, C. J., & Flegal, K. M. (2006). Prevalence of overweight and obesity in the United States, 1999-2004. JAMA, 295(13), 1549–1555. https://doi.org/10.1001/jama.295.13.1549

[11] Ogden, C. L., Yanovski, S. Z., Carroll, M. D., & Flegal, K. M. (2007). The epidemiology of obesity. Gastroenterology, 132(6), 2087–2102. https://doi.org/10.1053/j.gastro.2007.03.052

[12] Ogden, C. L., Troiano, R. P., Briefel, R. R., Kuczmarski, R. J., Flegal, K. M., & Johnson, C. L. (1997). Prevalence of overweight among preschool children in the United States, 1971 through 1994. Pediatrics, 99(4), E1. https://doi.org/10.1542/peds.99.4.e1

[13] Eurostat Statistics Explained (2019) 'Overweight and obesity - BMI statistics', Accessed Online March 5 2022: https://ec.europa.eu/eurostat/statistics-explained/index.php?title=Overweight_and_obesity_-_BMI_statistics

[14] Berrington de Gonzalez, A., Hartge, P., Cerhan, J. R., Flint, A. J., Hannan, L., MacInnis, R. J., Moore, S. C., Tobias, G. S., Anton-Culver, H., Freeman, L. B., Beeson, W. L., Clipp, S. L., English, D. R., Folsom, A. R., Freedman, D. M., Giles, G., Hakansson, N., Henderson, K. D., Hoffman-Bolton, J., Hoppin, J. A., … Thun, M. J. (2010). Body-mass index and mortality among 1.46 million white adults. The New England journal of medicine, 363(23), 2211–2219. https://doi.org/10.1056/NEJMoa1000367

[15] Flegal, K. M., Kit, B. K., Orpana, H., & Graubard, B. I. (2013). Association of all-cause mortality with overweight and obesity using standard body mass index categories: a systematic review and meta-analysis. JAMA, 309(1), 71–82. https://doi.org/10.1001/jama.2012.113905

[16] Xu et al (2018) 'Association of Obesity With Mortality Over 24 Years of Weight History: Findings From the Framingham Heart Study', JAMA Netw Open. 2018;1(7):e184587. doi:10.1001/jamanetworkopen.2018.4587

[17] Abdelaal, M., le Roux, C. W., & Docherty, N. G. (2017). Morbidity and mortality associated with obesity. Annals of translational medicine, 5(7), 161. https://doi.org/10.21037/atm.2017.03.107

[18] Nomura, D. K., Long, J. Z., Niessen, S., Hoover, H. S., Ng, S. W., & Cravatt, B. F. (2010). Monoacylglycerol lipase regulates a fatty acid network that promotes cancer pathogenesis. Cell, 140(1), 49–61. https://doi.org/10.1016/j.cell.2009.11.027

[19] Nakamura, K., Fuster, J. J., & Walsh, K. (2014). Adipokines: a link between obesity and cardiovascular disease. Journal of cardiology, 63(4), 250–259. https://doi.org/10.1016/j.jjcc.2013.11.006

[20] Riobó Serván P. (2013). Obesity and diabetes. Nutricion hospitalaria, 28 Suppl 5, 138–143. https://doi.org/10.3305/nh.2013.28.sup5.6929

[21] Kotchen, T. A., Grim, C. E., Kotchen, J. M., Krishnaswami, S., Yang, H., Hoffmann, R. G., & McGinley, E. L. (2008). Altered relationship of blood pressure to adiposity in hypertension. American journal of hypertension, 21(3), 284–289. https://doi.org/10.1038/ajh.2007.48

[22] Sjöström, L., Narbro, K., Sjöström, C. D., Karason, K., Larsson, B., Wedel, H., Lystig, T., Sullivan, M., Bouchard, C., Carlsson, B., Bengtsson, C., Dahlgren, S., Gummesson, A., Jacobson, P., Karlsson, J., Lindroos, A. K., Lönroth, H., Näslund, I., Olbers, T., Stenlöf, K., … Swedish Obese Subjects Study (2007). Effects of bariatric surgery on mortality in Swedish obese subjects. The New England journal of medicine, 357(8), 741–752. https://doi.org/10.1056/NEJMoa066254

[23] Adams, T. D., Gress, R. E., Smith, S. C., Halverson, R. C., Simper, S. C., Rosamond, W. D., Lamonte, M. J., Stroup, A. M., & Hunt, S. C. (2007). Long-term mortality after gastric bypass surgery. The New England journal of medicine, 357(8), 753–761. https://doi.org/10.1056/NEJMoa066603

[24] Christou, N. V., Sampalis, J. S., Liberman, M., Look, D., Auger, S., McLean, A. P., & MacLean, L. D. (2004). Surgery decreases long-term mortality, morbidity, and health care use in morbidly obese patients. Annals of surgery, 240(3), 416–424. https://doi.org/10.1097/01.sla.0000137343.63376.19

[25] Xiao, C., Giacca, A., & Lewis, G. F. (2008). Oral taurine but not N-acetylcysteine ameliorates NEFA-induced impairment in insulin sensitivity and beta cell function in obese and overweight, non-diabetic men. Diabetologia, 51(1), 139–146. https://doi.org/10.1007/s00125-007-0859-x

[26] Gordon, S. Alternative activation of macrophages. Nat Rev Immunol 3, 23–35 (2003). https://doi.org/10.1038/nri978

[27] Johnson, A. R., Justin Milner, J., & Makowski, L. (2012). The inflammation highway: metabolism accelerates inflammatory traffic in obesity. Immunological Reviews, 249(1), 218–238. doi:10.1111/j.1600-065x.2012.01151.x

[28] Soysal, P., Arik, F., Smith, L., Jackson, S. E., & Isik, A. T. (2020). Inflammation, Frailty and Cardiovascular Disease. Frailty and Cardiovascular Diseases, 55–64. doi:10.1007/978-3-030-33330-0_7

[29] Donath, M. Y., & Shoelson, S. E. (2011). Type 2 diabetes as an inflammatory disease. Nature Reviews Immunology, 11(2), 98–107. https://doi.org/10.1038/nri2925

[30] Willerson, J. T. (2004). Inflammation as a Cardiovascular Risk Factor. Circulation, 109(21_suppl_1), II-2–II-10. doi:10.1161/01.cir.0000129535.04194.38

31 Colotta, F., Allavena, P., Sica, A., Garlanda, C., & Mantovani, A. (2009). Cancer-related inflammation, the seventh hallmark of cancer: links to genetic instability. Carcinogenesis, 30(7), 1073–1081. doi:10.1093/carcin/bgp127

32 Grivennikov, S. I., Greten, F. R., & Karin, M. (2010). Immunity, Inflammation, and Cancer. Cell, 140(6), 883–899. doi:10.1016/j.cell.2010.01.025

[33] Pase, M. P., Himali, J. J., Beiser, A. S., DeCarli, C., McGrath, E. R., Satizabal, C. L., … Bis, J. C. (2019). Association of CD14 with incident dementia and markers of brain aging and injury. Neurology, 94(3), e254–e266. doi:10.1212/wnl.0000000000008682

[34] D. Trachootham, W. Lu, M. A. Ogasawara, N. R.-D. Valle, and P. Huang, "Redox regulation of cell survival," *Antioxidants & Redox Signaling*, vol. 10, no. 8, pp. 1343–1374, 2008.

[35] Hedström, A. K., Lima Bomfim, I., Hillert, J., Olsson, T., & Alfredsson, L. (2014). Obesity interacts with infectious mononucleosis in risk of multiple sclerosis. European Journal of Neurology, 22(3), 578–e38. doi:10.1111/ene.12620

[36] Nikoopour, E., Schwartz, J. A., & Singh, B. (2008). Therapeutic benefits of regulating inflammation in autoimmunity. Inflammation & allergy drug targets, 7(3), 203–210. https://doi.org/10.2174/187152808785748155

[37] Borrello, M. G., Degl'Innocenti, D., & Pierotti, M. A. (2008). Inflammation and cancer: the oncogene-driven connection. Cancer letters, 267(2), 262–270. https://doi.org/10.1016/j.canlet.2008.03.060

[38] Grivennikov, S. I., Greten, F. R., & Karin, M. (2010). Immunity, Inflammation, and Cancer. Cell, 140(6), 883–899. doi:10.1016/j.cell.2010.01.025

[39] Miller, A. H., Maletic, V., & Raison, C. L. (2009). Inflammation and Its Discontents: The Role of Cytokines in the Pathophysiology of Major Depression. Biological Psychiatry, 65(9), 732–741. doi:10.1016/j.biopsych.2008.11.029

[40] Colotta, F., Allavena, P., Sica, A., Garlanda, C., & Mantovani, A. (2009). Cancer-related inflammation, the seventh hallmark of cancer: links to genetic instability. Carcinogenesis, 30(7), 1073–1081. doi:10.1093/carcin/bgp127

41 Barbé-Tuana, F., Funchal, G., Schmitz, C.R.R. et al. The interplay between immunosenescence and age-related diseases. Semin Immunopathol (2020). https://doi.org/10.1007/s00281-020-00806-z

[42] Esposito, K., Pontillo, A., Di Palo, C., Giugliano, G., Masella, M., Marfella, R., & Giugliano, D. (2003). Effect of weight loss and lifestyle changes on vascular inflammatory markers in obese women: a randomized trial. JAMA, 289(14), 1799–1804. https://doi.org/10.1001/jama.289.14.1799

[43] Sun, Y., Wang, Q., Yang, G., Lin, C., Zhang, Y., & Yang, P. (2016). Weight and prognosis for influenza A(H1N1)pdm09 infection during the pandemic period between 2009 and 2011: a systematic review of observational studies with meta-analysis. Infectious Diseases, 48(11-12), 813–822. doi:10.1080/23744235.2016.1201721

[44] Van Kerkhove, M. D., Vandemaele, K. A. H., Shinde, V., Jaramillo-Gutierrez, G., Koukounari, A., … Donnelly, C. A. (2011). Risk Factors for Severe Outcomes following 2009 Influenza A (H1N1) Infection: A Global Pooled Analysis. PLoS Medicine, 8(7), e1001053. doi:10.1371/journal.pmed.1001053

[45] Drucker, D. J. (2021). Diabetes, obesity, metabolism, and SARS-CoV-2 infection: the end of the beginning. Cell Metabolism, 33(3), 479–498. https://doi.org/10.1016/j.cmet.2021.01.016

[46] Paich, H. A., Sheridan, P. A., Handy, J., Karlsson, E. A., Schultz-Cherry, S., Hudgens, M. G., … Beck, M. A. (2013). Overweight and obese adult humans have a defective cellular immune response to pandemic H1N1 Influenza a virus. Obesity, 21(11), 2377–2386. doi:10.1002/oby.20383

[47] Smith, A. G., Sheridan, P. A., Harp, J. B., & Beck, M. A. (2007). Diet-Induced Obese Mice Have Increased Mortality and Altered Immune Responses When Infected with Influenza Virus. The Journal of Nutrition, 137(5), 1236–1243. doi:10.1093/jn/137.5.1236

[48] Rebeles, J., Green, W. D., Alwarawrah, Y., Nichols, A. G., Eisner, W., Danzaki, K., … Beck, M. A. (2018). Obesity-Induced Changes in T-Cell Metabolism Are Associated With Impaired Memory T-Cell Response to Influenza and Are Not Reversed With Weight Loss. The Journal of Infectious Diseases, 219(10), 1652–1661. doi:10.1093/infdis/jiy700

[49] O'Brien, K. B., Vogel, P., Duan, S., Govorkova, E. A., Webby, R. J., McCullers, J. A., & Schultz-Cherry, S. (2012). Impaired wound healing predisposes obese mice to severe influenza virus infection. The Journal of infectious diseases, 205(2), 252–261. https://doi.org/10.1093/infdis/jir729

[50] Nakajima, N., Hata, S., Sato, Y., Tobiume, M., Katano, H., Kaneko, K., Nagata, N., Kataoka, M., Ainai, A., Hasegawa, H., Tashiro, M., Kuroda, M., Odai, T., Urasawa, N., Ogino, T., Hanaoka, H., Watanabe, M., & Sata, T. (2010). The first autopsy case of pandemic influenza (A/H1N1pdm) virus infection in Japan: detection of a high copy number of the virus in type II alveolar epithelial cells by pathological and virological examination. Japanese journal of infectious diseases, 63(1), 67–71.

[51] Gerberding, J. L., Morgan, J. G., Shepard, J. A., & Kradin, R. L. (2004). Case records of the Massachusetts General Hospital. Weekly clinicopathological exercises. Case 9-2004. An 18-year-old man with respiratory symptoms and shock. The New England journal of medicine, 350(12), 1236–1247. https://doi.org/10.1056/NEJMcpc049006

[52] Fleury, H., Burrel, S., Balick Weber, C., Hadrien, R., Blanco, P., Cazanave, C., & Dupon, M. (2009). Prolonged shedding of influenza A(H1N1)v virus: two case reports from France 2009. Euro surveillance : bulletin Europeen sur les maladies transmissibles = European communicable disease bulletin, 14(49), 19434.

[53] American Society for Microbiology. (2020, July 15). Obesity and metabolic syndrome are risk factors for severe influenza, COVID-19. ScienceDaily. Retrieved August 30, 2020 from www.sciencedaily.com/releases/2020/07/200715131234.htm

[54] Neidich, S. D., Green, W. D., Rebeles, J., Karlsson, E. A., Schultz-Cherry, S., Noah, T. L., … Beck, M. A. (2017). Increased risk of influenza among vaccinated adults who are obese. International Journal of Obesity, 41(9), 1324–1330. doi:10.1038/ijo.2017.131

[55] Sheridan, P. A., Paich, H. A., Handy, J., Karlsson, E. A., Hudgens, M. G., Sammon, A. B., … Beck, M. A. (2011). Obesity is associated with impaired immune response to influenza vaccination in humans. International Journal of Obesity, 36(8), 1072–1077. doi:10.1038/ijo.2011.208

[56] Honce, R., Karlsson, E. A., Wohlgemuth, N., Estrada, L. D., Meliopoulos, V. A., Yao, J., & Schultz-Cherry, S. (2020). Obesity-Related Microenvironment Promotes Emergence of Virulent Influenza Virus Strains. mBio, 11(2). doi:10.1128/mbio.03341-19

[57] Painter, S. D., Ovsyannikova, I. G., & Poland, G. A. (2015). The weight of obesity on the human immune response to vaccination. Vaccine, 33(36), 4422–4429. https://doi.org/10.1016/j.vaccine.2015.06.101

[58] Khunti, K., Singh, A. K., Pareek, M., & Hanif, W. (2020). Is ethnicity linked to incidence or outcomes of covid-19? BMJ, m1548. doi:10.1136/bmj.m1548

[59] Rochlani, Y., Pothineni, N. V., Kovelamudi, S., & Mehta, J. L. (2017). Metabolic syndrome: pathophysiology, management, and modulation by natural compounds. Therapeutic Advances in Cardiovascular Disease, 11(8), 215–225. doi:10.1177/1753944717711379

[60] Grundy, S. M., Hansen, B., Smith, S. C., Cleeman, J. I., & Kahn, R. A. (2004). Clinical Management of Metabolic Syndrome. Arteriosclerosis, Thrombosis, and Vascular Biology, 24(2). doi:10.1161/01.atv.0000112379.88385.67

[61] Mottillo, S., Filion, K. B., Genest, J., Joseph, L., Pilote, L., Poirier, P., ... Eisenberg, M. J. (2010). The Metabolic Syndrome and Cardiovascular Risk. Journal of the American College of Cardiology, 56(14), 1113–1132. doi:10.1016/j.jacc.2010.05.034

[62] Wang, Z., Du, Z., & Zhu, F. (2020). Glycosylated hemoglobin is associated with systemic inflammation, hypercoagulability, and prognosis of COVID-19 patients. Diabetes Research and Clinical Practice, 164, 108214. doi:10.1016/j.diabres.2020.108214

[63] Cooper, I. D., Crofts, C. A. P., DiNicolantonio, J. J., Malhotra, A., Elliott, B., Kyriakidou, Y., & Brookler, K. H. (2020). Relationships between hyperinsulinaemia, magnesium, vitamin D, thrombosis and COVID-19: rationale for clinical management. Open Heart, 7(2), e001356. https://doi.org/10.1136/openhrt-2020-001356

[64] Popkin, B. M., Du, S., Green, W. D., Beck, M. A., Algaith, T., Herbst, C. H., ... Shekar, M. (2020). Individuals with obesity and COVID-19: A global perspective on the epidemiology and biological relationships. Obesity Reviews. doi:10.1111/obr.13128

[65] Xie, J., Zu, Y., Alkhatib, A., Pham, T. T., Gill, F., Jang, A., ... Denson, J. L. (2020). Metabolic Syndrome and COVID-19 Mortality Among Adult Black Patients in New Orleans. Diabetes Care, dc201714. doi:10.2337/dc20-1714

[66] World Health Organization (2008), 'Waist Circumference and Waist–Hip Ratio: Report of a WHO Expert Consultation', Geneva, 8–11 December 2008

[67] Price et al (August 2006). "Weight, shape, and mortality risk in older persons: elevated waist-hip ratio, not high body mass index, is associated with a greater risk of death". *Am. J. Clin. Nutr.* 84 (2): 449–60.

[68] Price et al (August 2006). "Weight, shape, and mortality risk in older persons: elevated waist-hip ratio, not high body mass index, is associated with a greater risk of death". Am. J. Clin. Nutr. 84 (2): 449–60.

[69] Ancel Keys et al (1972) 'Indices of relative weight and obesity', Vol 25(6-7), p 329-343.

[70] Hedley, A. A., Ogden, C. L., Johnson, C. L., Carroll, M. D., Curtin, L. R., & Flegal, K. M. (2004). Prevalence of overweight and obesity among US children, adolescents, and adults, 1999-2002. JAMA, 291(23), 2847–2850. https://doi.org/10.1001/jama.291.23.2847

[71] Obesity: preventing and managing the global epidemic. Report of a WHO consultation. (2000). World Health Organization technical report series, 894, i–253.

[72] Prospective Studies Collaboration, Whitlock, G., Lewington, S., Sherliker, P., Clarke, R., Emberson, J., Halsey, J., Qizilbash, N., Collins, R., & Peto, R. (2009). Body-mass index and cause-specific mortality in 900 000 adults: collaborative analyses of 57 prospective studies. Lancet (London, England), 373(9669), 1083–1096. https://doi.org/10.1016/S0140-6736(09)60318-4

[73] Tobias and Hu (2018) 'The association between BMI and mortality: implications for obesity prevention', The Lancet, VOLUME 6, ISSUE 12, P916-917, DECEMBER 01, 2018.

[74] Meisinger, C., Döring, A., Thorand, B., Heier, M., & Löwel, H. (2006). Body fat distribution and risk of type 2 diabetes in the general population: are there differences between men and women? The MONICA/KORA Augsburg cohort study. The American journal of clinical nutrition, 84(3), 483–489. https://doi.org/10.1093/ajcn/84.3.483

[75] Isoyama et al (2014) 'Comparative Associations of Muscle Mass and Muscle Strength with Mortality in Dialysis Patients', CJASN October 2014, 9 (10) 1720-1728; DOI: https://doi.org/10.2215/CJN.10261013

76 Kraschnewski, JL. et al (2016) 'Is strength training associated with mortality benefits? A 15year cohort study of US older adults', Prev Med, Vol 87, p 121-127.

[77] Volaklis, KA. et al (2015) 'Muscular strength as a strong predictor of mortality: A narrative review', European Journal of Internal Medicine, Vol 26(5), p 303-310.

[78] Barry, VW. et al (2014) 'Fitness vs. fatness on all-cause mortality: a meta-analysis', Prog Cardiovasc Dis, Vol 56(4), p 382-390.

[79] Taylor, R., & Holman, R. R. (2015). Normal weight individuals who develop type 2 diabetes: the personal fat threshold. Clinical science (London, England : 1979), 128(7), 405–410. https://doi.org/10.1042/CS20140553

[80] Virtue, S., & Vidal-Puig, A. (2010). Adipose tissue expandability, lipotoxicity and the Metabolic Syndrome--an allostatic perspective. Biochimica et biophysica acta, 1801(3), 338–349. https://doi.org/10.1016/j.bbalip.2009.12.006

[81] Virtue, S., & Vidal-Puig, A. (2010). Adipose tissue expandability, lipotoxicity and the Metabolic Syndrome — An allostatic perspective. Biochimica et Biophysica Acta (BBA) - Molecular and Cell Biology of Lipids, 1801(3), 338–349. doi:10.1016/j.bbalip.2009.12.006

[82] Taylor, R., & Holman, R. R. (2014). Normal weight individuals who develop Type 2 diabetes: the personal fat threshold. Clinical Science, 128(7), 405–410. doi:10.1042/cs20140553

[83] Matsuzawa, Y., Funahashi, T., & Nakamura, T. (2011). The Concept of Metabolic Syndrome: Contribution of Visceral Fat Accumulation and Its Molecular Mechanism. Journal of Atherosclerosis and Thrombosis, 18(8), 629–639. doi:10.5551/jat.7922

[84] Laforest, S., Labrecque, J., Michaud, A., Cianflone, K., & Tchernof, A. (2015). Adipocyte size as a determinant of metabolic disease and adipose tissue dysfunction. Critical Reviews in Clinical Laboratory Sciences, 52(6), 301–313. doi:10.3109/10408363.2015.1041582

[85] Bergman, R. N., Kim, S. P., Catalano, K. J., Hsu, I. R., Chiu, J. D., Kabir, M. , Hucking, K. and Ader, M. (2006), Why Visceral Fat is Bad: Mechanisms of the Metabolic Syndrome. Obesity, 14: 16S-19S.

[86] Price et al (August 2006). "Weight, shape, and mortality risk in older persons: elevated waist-hip ratio, not high body mass index, is associated with a greater risk of death". Am. J. Clin. Nutr. 84 (2): 449–60.

[87] Haslam D. (2007). Obesity: a medical history. Obesity reviews : an official journal of the International Association for the Study of Obesity, 8 Suppl 1, 31–36. https://doi.org/10.1111/j.1467-789X.2007.00314.x

[88] Theodore Mazzone; Giamila Fantuzzi (2006). Adipose Tissue And Adipokines in Health And Disease (Nutrition and Health). Totowa, NJ: Humana Press. p. 222.

[89] Speakman, J. Thrifty genes for obesity, an attractive but flawed idea, and an alternative perspective: the 'drifty gene' hypothesis. Int J Obes 32, 1611–1617 (2008). https://doi.org/10.1038/ijo.2008.161

[90] Hippocrates 400BC De Priscina Medicina.

[91] Hyde E. Edward Hyde: Life of Edward, 1st Earl of Clarendon, by himself. Clarendon, Oxford: Oxford, 1759.

[92] Brillante, C., & Laffi, G. C. (1982). Profilo storico-sintetico della malattia diabetica (dal papiro di Ebers a Banting e Best) [Historically assembled profile of diabetic disease (from Ebers' papyrus to Banting and Best)]. Minerva medica, 73(17), 1087–1106.

[93] Osler W. Lectures on Angina Pectoris and Allied States. D. Appleton: New York, 1897.

[94] Hippocrates ~400BC De Flatibus

[95] Siculus 90BC–20BC Bibliotheca historica

[96] Herodotus ~440BC. Euterpe, section 77.

[97] Plato 360BC Republic

[98] Laertius, Diogenes 3rd century Life of Pythagoras. segm 9. Menag (ed.).

[99] R. W. Fogel, 1997. "The Global Struggle to Escape from Chronic Malnutrition since 1700," CPE working papers 0006, University of Chicago - Centre for Population Economics.

[100] Henderson, R. M. (2005). The bigger the healthier: Are the limits of BMI risk changing over time? Economics & Human Biology, 3(3), 339–366. https://doi.org/10.1016/j.ehb.2005.08.001

[101] Komlos, J., & Brabec, M. (2011). The trend of BMI values of US adults by deciles, birth cohorts 1882-1986 stratified by gender and ethnicity. Economics and human biology, 9(3), 234–250. https://doi.org/10.1016/j.ehb.2011.03.005

[102] Carson, S. A. (2009). Racial differences in body mass indices of men imprisoned in 19th Century Texas. Economics & Human Biology, 7(1), 121–127. https://doi.org/10.1016/j.ehb.2009.01.005

[103] CDC (2020) 'Adult Obesity Facts', Overweight & Obesity, Accessed Online: https://www.cdc.gov/obesity/data/adult.html

[104] Carson, S. A. (2013). Body mass, wealth, and inequality in the 19th century: joining the debate surrounding equality and health. Economics and human biology, 11(1), 90–94. https://doi.org/10.1016/j.ehb.2012.05.004

[105] Wilkinson, R. G., & Pickett, K. E. (2006). Income inequality and population health: a review and explanation of the evidence. Social science & medicine (1982), 62(7), 1768–1784. https://doi.org/10.1016/j.socscimed.2005.08.036

[106] Subramanian, S. V. (2004). Income Inequality and Health: What Have We Learned So Far? Epidemiologic Reviews, 26(1), 78–91. https://doi.org/10.1093/epirev/mxh003

[107] Poston, W. S., 2nd, & Foreyt, J. P. (1999). Obesity is an environmental issue. Atherosclerosis, 146(2), 201–209. https://doi.org/10.1016/s0021-9150(99)00258-0

[108] Popkin, B., Gordon-Larsen, P. The nutrition transition: worldwide obesity dynamics and their determinants. Int J Obes 28, S2–S9 (2004). https://doi.org/10.1038/sj.ijo.0802804

[109] McLaren (2007) 'Socioeconomic Status and Obesity', Epidemiologic Reviews, Volume 29, Issue 1, 2007, Pages 29–48, https://doi.org/10.1093/epirev/mxm001

[110] Goodman, E., Adler, N. E., Daniels, S. R., Morrison, J. A., Slap, G. B., & Dolan, L. M. (2003). Impact of objective and subjective social status on obesity in a biracial cohort of adolescents. Obesity research, 11(8), 1018–1026. https://doi.org/10.1038/oby.2003.140

[111] Björntorp P. (2001). Do stress reactions cause abdominal obesity and comorbidities?. Obesity reviews : an official journal of the International Association for the Study of Obesity, 2(2), 73–86. https://doi.org/10.1046/j.1467-789x.2001.00027.x

[112] Mozaffarian, D., Hao, T., Rimm, E. B., Willett, W. C., & Hu, F. B. (2011). Changes in Diet and Lifestyle and Long-Term Weight Gain in Women and Men. New England Journal of Medicine, 364(25), 2392–2404. https://doi.org/10.1056/nejmoa1014296

[113] Schwartz, M. W., Seeley, R. J., Zeltser, L. M., Drewnowski, A., Ravussin, E., Redman, L. M., & Leibel, R. L. (2017). Obesity Pathogenesis: An Endocrine Society Scientific Statement. Endocrine Reviews, 38(4), 267–296. https://doi.org/10.1210/er.2017-00111

[114] Centers for Disease Control and Prevention (CDC) (2004). Trends in intake of energy and macronutrients--United States, 1971-2000. MMWR. Morbidity and mortality weekly report, 53(4), 80–82.

[115] Rosenheck, R. (2008). Fast food consumption and increased caloric intake: a systematic review of a trajectory towards weight gain and obesity risk. Obesity Reviews, 9(6), 535–547. https://doi.org/10.1111/j.1467-789x.2008.00477.x

[116] Nielsen, S. J., Siega-Riz, A. M., & Popkin, B. M. (2002). Trends in energy intake in U.S. between 1977 and 1996: similar shifts seen across age groups. Obesity research, 10(5), 370–378. https://doi.org/10.1038/oby.2002.51

[117] Striegel-Moore, R. H., Thompson, D., Affenito, S. G., Franko, D. L., Obarzanek, E., Barton, B. A., Schreiber, G. B., Daniels, S. R., Schmidt, M., & Crawford, P. B. (2006). Correlates of beverage intake in adolescent girls: the National Heart, Lung, and Blood Institute Growth and Health Study. The Journal of pediatrics, 148(2), 183–187. https://doi.org/10.1016/j.jpeds.2005.11.025

[118] Rajeshwari, R., Yang, S.-J., Nicklas, T. A., & Berenson, G. S. (2005). Secular trends in children's sweetened-beverage consumption (1973 to 1994): The Bogalusa Heart Study. Journal of the American Dietetic Association, 105(2), 208–214. https://doi.org/10.1016/j.jada.2004.11.026

[119] Malik, V. S., Schulze, M. B., & Hu, F. B. (2006). Intake of sugar-sweetened beverages and weight gain: a systematic review. The American journal of clinical nutrition, 84(2), 274–288. https://doi.org/10.1093/ajcn/84.1.274

[120] Olsen, N. J., & Heitmann, B. L. (2009). Intake of calorically sweetened beverages and obesity. Obesity reviews : an official journal of the International Association for the Study of Obesity, 10(1), 68–75. https://doi.org/10.1111/j.1467-789X.2008.00523.x

[121] FAO (2002) 'World agriculture: towards 2015/2030', Rome, Italy: Food and Agriculture Organization of the United Nations, 2002.

[122] Hiza, HAB and Bente L (2007) 'Nutrient Content of the U.S. Food Supply, 1909-2004, A Summary Report', Center for Nutrition Policy and Promotion, Home Economics Research Report No. 57.

[123] Drewnowski, A., & Specter, S. (2004). Poverty and obesity: the role of energy density and energy costs. The American Journal of Clinical Nutrition, 79(1), 6–16. https://doi.org/10.1093/ajcn/79.1.6

[124] Drewnowski, A., & Specter, S. E. (2004). Poverty and obesity: the role of energy density and energy costs. The American journal of clinical nutrition, 79(1), 6–16. https://doi.org/10.1093/ajcn/79.1.6

[125] Levine, J. A. (2011). Poverty and Obesity in the U.S. Diabetes, 60(11), 2667–2668. https://doi.org/10.2337/db11-1118

[126] Bojanowska, E., & Ciosek, J. (2016). Can We Selectively Reduce Appetite for Energy-Dense Foods? An Overview of Pharmacological Strategies for Modification of Food Preference Behavior. Current Neuropharmacology, 14(2), 118–142. https://doi.org/10.2174/1570159x14666151109103147

[127] Hall, K. D., Ayuketah, A., Brychta, R., Cai, H., Cassimatis, T., Chen, K. Y., Chung, S. T., Costa, E., Courville, A., Darcey, V., Fletcher, L. A., Forde, C. G., Gharib, A. M., Guo, J., Howard, R., Joseph, P. V., McGehee, S., Ouwerkerk, R., Raisinger, K., Rozga, I., … Zhou, M. (2019). Ultra-Processed Diets Cause Excess Calorie Intake and Weight Gain: An Inpatient Randomized Controlled Trial of Ad Libitum Food Intake. Cell metabolism, 30(1), 67–77.e3. https://doi.org/10.1016/j.cmet.2019.05.008

[128] Monteiro, C. A., Cannon, G., Moubarac, J. C., Levy, R. B., Louzada, M., & Jaime, P. C. (2018). The UN Decade of Nutrition, the NOVA food classification and the trouble with ultra-processing. Public health nutrition, 21(1), 5–17. https://doi.org/10.1017/S1368980017000234

[129] Katz, D. L., & Meller, S. (2014). Can we say what diet is best for health?. Annual review of public health, 35, 83–103. https://doi.org/10.1146/annurev-publhealth-032013-182351

[130] Schatzker M (2015). The dorito effect: The surprising new truth about food and flavor. (New York, NY: Simon & Schuster;).

[131] Moss M (2013). Salt, sugar, fat: how the food giants hooked us. (New York: Random House;).

132 Poti, J. M., Mendez, M. A., Ng, S. W., & Popkin, B. M. (2015). Is the degree of food processing and convenience linked with the nutritional quality of foods purchased by US households?. The American journal of clinical nutrition, 101(6), 1251–1262. https://doi.org/10.3945/ajcn.114.100925

133 Weaver, C. M., Dwyer, J., Fulgoni, V. L., 3rd, King, J. C., Leveille, G. A., MacDonald, R. S., Ordovas, J., & Schnakenberg, D. (2014). Processed foods: contributions to nutrition. The American journal of clinical nutrition, 99(6), 1525–1542. https://doi.org/10.3945/ajcn.114.089284

134 Brownson, R. C., Boehmer, T. K., & Luke, D. A. (2005). DECLINING RATES OF PHYSICAL ACTIVITY IN THE UNITED STATES: What Are the Contributors? Annual Review of Public Health, 26(1), 421–443. https://doi.org/10.1146/annurev.publhealth.26.021304.144437

135 WHO (2022) 'More physical activity', Accessed Online March 11 2022: https://www.who.int/teams/health-promotion/physical-activity

136 Ness-Abramof, R., & Apovian, C. M. (2006). Diet modification for treatment and prevention of obesity. Endocrine, 29(1), 5–9. https://doi.org/10.1385/endo:29:1:5

137 Centers for Disease Control and Prevention (CDC) (2003). Prevalence of physical activity, including lifestyle activities among adults-- United States, 2000-2001. MMWR. Morbidity and mortality weekly report, 52(32), 764–769.

138 Borodulin et al (2008) 'Thirty-year trends of physical activity in relation to age, calendar time and birth cohort in Finnish adults', European Journal of Public Health, Volume 18, Issue 3, June 2008, Pages 339–344, https://doi.org/10.1093/eurpub/ckm092

139 McDonald N. C. (2007). Active transportation to school: trends among U.S. schoolchildren, 1969-2001. American journal of preventive medicine, 32(6), 509–516. https://doi.org/10.1016/j.amepre.2007.02.022

140 CDC (2009) 'Youth Physical Activity: The Role of Schools', Division of Adolescent and School Health, Accessed Online March 10 2022: https://www.cdc.gov/healthyschools/physicalactivity/toolkit/factsheet_pa_guidelines_schools.pdf

141 Centers for Disease Control and Prevention. Youth Risk Behavior Surveillance—United States, 2007. MMWR. 2008;57(No. SS-4):1-131.

142 Andersen, R. E., Crespo, C. J., Bartlett, S. J., Cheskin, L. J., & Pratt, M. (1998). Relationship of physical activity and television watching with body weight and level of fatness among children: results from the Third National Health and Nutrition Examination Survey. JAMA, 279(12), 938–942. https://doi.org/10.1001/jama.279.12.938

143 Vioque, J., Torres, A., & Quiles, J. (2000). Time spent watching television, sleep duration and obesity in adults living in Valencia, Spain. International Journal of Obesity, 24(12), 1683–1688. https://doi.org/10.1038/sj.ijo.0801434

144 Tucker, L. A., & Bagwell, M. (1991). Television viewing and obesity in adult females. American journal of public health, 81(7), 908–911. https://doi.org/10.2105/ajph.81.7.908

145 Gortmaker, S. L., Must, A., Sobol, A. M., Peterson, K., Colditz, G. A., & Dietz, W. H. (1996). Television viewing as a cause of increasing obesity among children in the United States, 1986-1990. Archives of pediatrics & adolescent medicine, 150(4), 356–362. https://doi.org/10.1001/archpedi.1996.02170290022003

146 Emanuel EJ (2008). "Media + Child and Adolescent Health: A Systematic Review" (PDF). Common Sense Media. Accessed Online March 11 2022: https://ipsdweb.ipsd.org/uploads/IPPC/CSM%20Media%20Health%20Report.pdf

147 Schmidt, M., Affenito, S. G., Striegel-Moore, R., Khoury, P. R., Barton, B., Crawford, P., Kronsberg, S., Schreiber, G., Obarzanek, E., & Daniels, S. (2005). Fast-food intake and diet quality in black and white girls: the National Heart, Lung, and Blood Institute Growth and Health Study. Archives of pediatrics & adolescent medicine, 159(7), 626–631. https://doi.org/10.1001/archpedi.159.7.626

148 Boynton-Jarrett, R., Thomas, T. N., Peterson, K. E., Wiecha, J., Sobol, A. M., & Gortmaker, S. L. (2003). Impact of television viewing patterns on fruit and vegetable consumption among adolescents. Pediatrics, 112(6 Pt 1), 1321–1326. https://doi.org/10.1542/peds.112.6.1321

149 Keith, S. W., Redden, D. T., Katzmarzyk, P. T., Boggiano, M. M., Hanlon, E. C., Benca, R. M., Ruden, D., Pietrobelli, A., Barger, J. L., Fontaine, K. R., Wang, C., Aronne, L. J., Wright, S. M., Baskin, M., Dhurandhar, N. V., Lijoi, M. C., Grilo, C. M., DeLuca, M., Westfall, A. O., & Allison, D. B. (2006). Putative contributors to the secular increase in obesity: exploring the roads less traveled. International Journal of Obesity, 30(11), 1585–1594. https://doi.org/10.1038/sj.ijo.0803326

150 Cappuccio, F. P., Taggart, F. M., Kandala, N. B., Currie, A., Peile, E., Stranges, S., & Miller, M. A. (2008). Meta-analysis of short sleep duration and obesity in children and adults. Sleep, 31(5), 619–626. https://doi.org/10.1093/sleep/31.5.619

151 Miller, M. A., Kruisbrink, M., Wallace, J., Ji, C., & Cappuccio, F. P. (2018). Sleep duration and incidence of obesity in infants, children, and adolescents: a systematic review and meta-analysis of prospective studies. Sleep, 41(4). https://doi.org/10.1093/sleep/zsy018

152 Flegal, K. M., Troiano, R. P., Pamuk, E. R., Kuczmarski, R. J., & Campbell, S. M. (1995). The influence of smoking cessation on the prevalence of overweight in the United States. The New England journal of medicine, 333(18), 1165–1170. https://doi.org/10.1056/NEJM199511023331801

153 Gerlach, G., Herpertz, S., & Loeber, S. (2015). Personality traits and obesity: a systematic review. Obesity reviews : an official journal of the International Association for the Study of Obesity, 16(1), 32–63. https://doi.org/10.1111/obr.12235

154 Jokela, M., Hintsanen, M., Hakulinen, C., Batty, G. D., Nabi, H., Singh-Manoux, A., & Kivimäki, M. (2013). Association of personality with the development and persistence of obesity: a meta-analysis based on individual-participant data. Obesity reviews : an official journal of the International Association for the Study of Obesity, 14(4), 315–323. https://doi.org/10.1111/obr.12007

155 Lauder, W., Mummery, K., Jones, M., & Caperchione, C. (2006). A comparison of health behaviours in lonely and non-lonely populations. Psychology, health & medicine, 11(2), 233–245. https://doi.org/10.1080/13548500500266607

156 Albuquerque et al (2017) 'The contribution of genetics and environment to obesity', British Medical Bulletin, Volume 123, Issue 1, September 2017, Pages 159–173, https://doi.org/10.1093/bmb/ldx022

157 Loos, R. J., & Bouchard, C. (2008). FTO: the first gene contributing to common forms of human obesity. Obesity reviews : an official journal of the International Association for the Study of Obesity, 9(3), 246–250. https://doi.org/10.1111/j.1467-789X.2008.00481.x

158 Walley, A. J., Asher, J. E., & Froguel, P. (2009). The genetic contribution to non-syndromic human obesity. Nature reviews. Genetics, 10(7), 431–442. https://doi.org/10.1038/nrg2594

159 Roseboom, T. J., van der Meulen, J. H., Ravelli, A. C., Osmond, C., Barker, D. J., & Bleker, O. P. (2001). Effects of prenatal exposure to the Dutch famine on adult disease in later life: an overview. Molecular and cellular endocrinology, 185(1-2), 93–98. https://doi.org/10.1016/s0303-7207(01)00721-3

160 Ravelli, A. C., van Der Meulen, J. H., Osmond, C., Barker, D. J., & Bleker, O. P. (1999). Obesity at the age of 50 y in men and women exposed to famine prenatally. The American journal of clinical nutrition, 70(5), 811–816. https://doi.org/10.1093/ajcn/70.5.811

161 Jones, A. P., Simson, E. L., & Friedman, M. I. (1984). Gestational undernutrition and the development of obesity in rats. The Journal of nutrition, 114(8), 1484–1492. https://doi.org/10.1093/jn/114.8.1484

[162] Jones, A. P., & Friedman, M. I. (1982). Obesity and adipocyte abnormalities in offspring of rats undernourished during pregnancy. Science (New York, N.Y.), 215(4539), 1518–1519. https://doi.org/10.1126/science.7063860

[163] Adair, L. S., & Prentice, A. M. (2004). A critical evaluation of the fetal origins hypothesis and its implications for developing countries. The Journal of nutrition, 134(1), 191–193. https://doi.org/10.1093/jn/134.1.191

[164] Valdez, R., Athens, M. A., Thompson, G. H., Bradshaw, B. S., & Stern, M. P. (1994). Birthweight and adult health outcomes in a biethnic population in the USA. Diabetologia, 37(6), 624–631. https://doi.org/10.1007/BF00403383

[165] Caballero B (March 2001). "Introduction. Symposium: Obesity in developing countries: biological and ecological factors". The Journal of Nutrition (Review). 131 (3): 866S–870S.

[166] James, W.P. (2008). The fundamental drivers of the obesity epidemic. Obesity Reviews, 9.

[167] Nestle, M., & Jacobson, M. F. (2000). Halting the obesity epidemic: a public health policy approach. Public health reports (Washington, D.C. : 1974), 115(1), 12–24. https://doi.org/10.1093/phr/115.1.12

[168] Lau, D. C., Douketis, J. D., Morrison, K. M., Hramiak, I. M., Sharma, A. M., Ur, E., & Obesity Canada Clinical Practice Guidelines Expert Panel (2007). 2006 Canadian clinical practice guidelines on the management and prevention of obesity in adults and children [summary]. CMAJ : Canadian Medical Association journal = journal de l'Association medicale canadienne, 176(8), S1–S13. https://doi.org/10.1503/cmaj.061409

[169] Bleich, S., Cutler, D., Murray, C., & Adams, A. (2008). Why is the developed world obese?. Annual review of public health, 29, 273–295. https://doi.org/10.1146/annurev.publhealth.29.020907.090954

[170] Yach, D., Stuckler, D., & Brownell, K. D. (2006). Epidemiologic and economic consequences of the global epidemics of obesity and diabetes. Nature medicine, 12(1), 62–66. https://doi.org/10.1038/nm0106-62

[171] DiNicolantonio, J. J., & Lucan, S. C. (2014). The wrong white crystals: not salt but sugar as aetiological in hypertension and cardiometabolic disease. Open heart, 1(1), e000167. https://doi.org/10.1136/openhrt-2014-000167

[172] DiNicolantonio, J. J., Lucan, S. C., & O'Keefe, J. H. (2016). The Evidence for Saturated Fat and for Sugar Related to Coronary Heart Disease. Progress in cardiovascular diseases, 58(5), 464–472. https://doi.org/10.1016/j.pcad.2015.11.006

[173] DiNicolantonio, J. J., Mehta, V., Onkaramurthy, N., & O'Keefe, J. H. (2018). Fructose-induced inflammation and increased cortisol: A new mechanism for how sugar induces visceral adiposity. Progress in cardiovascular diseases, 61(1), 3–9. https://doi.org/10.1016/j.pcad.2017.12.001

[174] DiNicolantonio, J. J., & OKeefe, J. H. (2017). Added sugars drive coronary heart disease via insulin resistance and hyperinsulinaemia: a new paradigm. Open heart, 4(2), e000729. https://doi.org/10.1136/openhrt-2017-000729

[175] DiNicolantonio, J. J., Subramonian, A. M., & O'Keefe, J. H. (2017). Added fructose as a principal driver of non-alcoholic fatty liver disease: a public health crisis. Open heart, 4(2), e000631. https://doi.org/10.1136/openhrt-2017-000631

[176] DiNicolantonio, J. J., & Berger, A. (2016). Added sugars drive nutrient and energy deficit in obesity: a new paradigm. Open heart, 3(2), e000469. https://doi.org/10.1136/openhrt-2016-000469

[177] DiNicolantonio, J. J., & O'Keefe, J. H. (2016). Hypertension Due to Toxic White Crystals in the Diet: Should We Blame Salt or Sugar?. Progress in cardiovascular diseases, 59(3), 219–225. https://doi.org/10.1016/j.pcad.2016.07.004

[178] DiNicolantonio, J. J., & Lucan, S. C. (2015). Is fructose malabsorption a cause of irritable bowel syndrome?. Medical hypotheses, 85(3), 295–297. https://doi.org/10.1016/j.mehy.2015.05.019

[179] DiNicolantonio, J. J., Mehta, V., Zaman, S. B., & O'Keefe, J. H. (2018). Not Salt But Sugar As Aetiological In Osteoporosis: A Review. Missouri medicine, 115(3), 247–252.

[180] DiNicolantonio, J. J. (2016). Increase in the intake of refined carbohydrates and sugar may have led to the health decline of the Greenland Eskimos. Open heart, 3(2), e000444. https://doi.org/10.1136/openhrt-2016-000444

[181] DiNicolantonio, J. J., & O'Keefe, J. (2017). Markedly increased intake of refined carbohydrates and sugar is associated with the rise of coronary heart disease and diabetes among the Alaskan Inuit. Open heart, 4(2), e000673. https://doi.org/10.1136/openhrt-2017-000673

[182] Marriott, B. P., Olsho, L., Hadden, L., & Connor, P. (2010). Intake of Added Sugars and Selected Nutrients in the United States, National Health and Nutrition Examination Survey (NHANES) 2003—2006. Critical Reviews in Food Science and Nutrition, 50(3), 228–258. https://doi.org/10.1080/10408391003626223

[183] DiNicolantonio, J. J., & Lucan, S. C. (2014). The wrong white crystals: not salt but sugar as aetiological in hypertension and cardiometabolic disease. Open heart, 1(1), e000167. https://doi.org/10.1136/openhrt-2014-000167

[184] Johnson et al (2007) 'Potential role of sugar (fructose) in the epidemic of hypertension, obesity and the metabolic syndrome, diabetes, kidney disease, and cardiovascular disease', The American Journal of Clinical Nutrition, Volume 86, Issue 4, October 2007, Pages 899–906, https://doi.org/10.1093/ajcn/86.4.899

[185] Strom (2012) 'U.S. Cuts Estimate of Sugar Intake', NY Times, 27th October 2012, Accessed Online March 3rd 2022: https://www.nytimes.com/2012/10/27/business/us-cuts-estimate-of-sugar-intake-of-typical-american.html

[186] Cordain, L., Eades, M. R., & Eades, M. D. (2003). Hyperinsulinemic diseases of civilization: more than just Syndrome X. Comparative biochemistry and physiology. Part A, Molecular & integrative physiology, 136(1), 95–112. https://doi.org/10.1016/s1095-6433(03)00011-4

[187] Yudkin (2012) 'Pure, white and deadly', Penguin Books

[188] Yudkin (2012) 'Pure, white and deadly', Penguin Books

[189] Johnson et al (2007), 'Potential role of sugar (fructose) in the epidemic of hypertension, obesity and the metabolic syndrome, diabetes, kidney disease, and cardiovascular disease', The American Journal of Clinical Nutrition, Volume 86, Issue 4, October 2007, Pages 899–906, https://doi.org/10.1093/ajcn/86.4.899

[190] Johnson et al (2007), 'Potential role of sugar (fructose) in the epidemic of hypertension, obesity and the metabolic syndrome, diabetes, kidney disease, and cardiovascular disease', The American Journal of Clinical Nutrition, Volume 86, Issue 4, October 2007, Pages 899–906, https://doi.org/10.1093/ajcn/86.4.899

[191] Cordain, L., Eades, M. R., & Eades, M. D. (2003). Hyperinsulinemic diseases of civilization: more than just Syndrome X. Comparative biochemistry and physiology. Part A, Molecular & integrative physiology, 136(1), 95–112. https://doi.org/10.1016/s1095-6433(03)00011-4

[192] Gross, L. S., Li, L., Ford, E. S., & Liu, S. (2004). Increased consumption of refined carbohydrates and the epidemic of type 2 diabetes in the United States: an ecologic assessment. The American journal of clinical nutrition, 79(5), 774–779. https://doi.org/10.1093/ajcn/79.5.774

[193] Tordoff, M. G., & Alleva, A. M. (1990). Effect of drinking soda sweetened with aspartame or high-fructose corn syrup on food intake and body weight. The American journal of clinical nutrition, 51(6), 963–969. https://doi.org/10.1093/ajcn/51.6.963

[194] Mattes, R. D. (1996). Dietary Compensation by Humans for Supplemental Energy Provided as Ethanol or Carbohydrate in Fluids. Physiology & Behavior, 59(1), 179–187. https://doi.org/10.1016/0031-9384(95)02007-1

[195] Raben, A., Vasilaras, T. H., Møller, A. C., & Astrup, A. (2002). Sucrose compared with artificial sweeteners: different effects on ad libitum food intake and body weight after 10 wk of supplementation in overweight subjects. The American journal of clinical nutrition, 76(4), 721–729. https://doi.org/10.1093/ajcn/76.4.721

[196] DiMeglio, D., & Mattes, R. (2000). Liquid versus solid carbohydrate: effects on food intake and body weight. International Journal of Obesity, 24(6), 794–800. https://doi.org/10.1038/sj.ijo.0801229

[197] Johnson et al (2007) 'Potential role of sugar (fructose) in the epidemic of hypertension, obesity and the metabolic syndrome, diabetes, kidney disease, and cardiovascular disease', The American Journal of Clinical Nutrition, Volume 86, Issue 4, October 2007, Pages 899–906, https://doi.org/10.1093/ajcn/86.4.899

[198] DiNicolantonio, J. J., O'Keefe, J. H., & Wilson, W. L. (2018). Sugar addiction: is it real? A narrative review. British journal of sports medicine, 52(14), 910–913. https://doi.org/10.1136/bjsports-2017-097971

[199] DiNicolantonio, J. J., O'Keefe, J. H., & Wilson, W. L. (2018). Sugar addiction: is it real? A narrative review. British journal of sports medicine, 52(14), 910–913. https://doi.org/10.1136/bjsports-2017-097971

[200] Bray and Popkin (2014) 'Dietary Sugar and Body Weight: Have We Reached a Crisis in the Epidemic of Obesity and Diabetes?: Health Be Damned! Pour on the Sugar', Diabetes Care 2014;37(4):950–956

[201] Trust for America's Health (2018) 'The State of Obesity 2018: Better Policies for a Healthier America', Accessed Online March 14th 2022: https://www.tfah.org/report-details/the-state-of-obesity-2018/

[202] Putnam and Allshouse (1999), 'Food Consumption, Prices and Expenditures, 1970–1997'. Washington, DC: Economic Research Service, US Dept of Agriculture.

[203] Duffey, K. J., & Popkin, B. M. (2007). Shifts in patterns and consumption of beverages between 1965 and 2002. Obesity (Silver Spring, Md.), 15(11), 2739–2747. https://doi.org/10.1038/oby.2007.326

[204] Flegal, K. M. (2002). Prevalence and Trends in Obesity Among US Adults, 1999-2000. JAMA, 288(14), 1723. https://doi.org/10.1001/jama.288.14.1723

[205] Duffey, K. J., & Popkin, B. M. (2007). Shifts in patterns and consumption of beverages between 1965 and 2002. Obesity (Silver Spring, Md.), 15(11), 2739–2747. https://doi.org/10.1038/oby.2007.326

[206] Lucan, S. C., & DiNicolantonio, J. J. (2015). How calorie-focused thinking about obesity and related diseases may mislead and harm public health. An alternative. Public health nutrition, 18(4), 571–581. https://doi.org/10.1017/S1368980014002559

[207] DiNicolantonio, J. J., O'Keefe, J. H., & Lucan, S. C. (2015). Added fructose: a principal driver of type 2 diabetes mellitus and its consequences. Mayo Clinic proceedings, 90(3), 372–381. https://doi.org/10.1016/j.mayocp.2014.12.019

[208] Trust for America's Health (2018) 'The State of Obesity 2018: Better Policies for a Healthier America', Accessed Online March 14th 2022: https://www.tfah.org/report-details/the-state-of-obesity-2018/

[209] Bray and Popkin (2014) 'Dietary Sugar and Body Weight: Have We Reached a Crisis in the Epidemic of Obesity and Diabetes?: Health Be Damned! Pour on the Sugar ', Diabetes Care 2014;37(4):950–956

[210] Ludwig, D. S., Peterson, K. E., & Gortmaker, S. L. (2001). Relation between consumption of sugar-sweetened drinks and childhood obesity: a prospective, observational analysis. Lancet (London, England), 357(9255), 505–508. https://doi.org/10.1016/S0140-6736(00)04041-1

[211] Tordoff, M. G., & Alleva, A. M. (1990). Effect of drinking soda sweetened with aspartame or high-fructose corn syrup on food intake and body weight. The American journal of clinical nutrition, 51(6), 963–969. https://doi.org/10.1093/ajcn/51.6.963

[212] Raben, A., Vasilaras, T. H., Møller, A. C., & Astrup, A. (2002). Sucrose compared with artificial sweeteners: different effects on ad libitum food intake and body weight after 10 wk of supplementation in overweight subjects. The American journal of clinical nutrition, 76(4), 721–729. https://doi.org/10.1093/ajcn/76.4.721

[213] Vartanian, L. R., Schwartz, M. B., & Brownell, K. D. (2007). Effects of soft drink consumption on nutrition and health: a systematic review and meta-analysis. American journal of public health, 97(4), 667–675. https://doi.org/10.2105/AJPH.2005.083782

[214] Bes-Rastrollo, M., Schulze, M. B., Ruiz-Canela, M., & Martinez-Gonzalez, M. A. (2013). Financial conflicts of interest and reporting bias regarding the association between sugar-sweetened beverages and weight gain: a systematic review of systematic reviews. PLoS medicine, 10(12), e1001578. https://doi.org/10.1371/journal.pmed.1001578

[215] Berry (2019) '68 different names for sugar', Accessed Online 11th March 2022: https://www.garciaweightloss.com/blog/68-different-names-for-sugar/

[216] Campos (2020) '70 Names Used For Just One Sugar', Accessed Online 11th March 2022: https://www.whatsugar.com/post/sucrose-one-sugar-70-names

[217] Brillat-Savarin, Jean Anthelme (1970). The Physiology of Taste. trans. Anne Drayton. Penguin Books. pp. 208–209.

[218] Sir William, O (1920) 'The principles and practice of medicine', New York, London, D. Appleton and company, Accessed: https://archive.org/details/principlesandpr00mccrgoog/page/n6

[219] Edwards, C. H., Grundy, M. M., Grassby, T., Vasilopoulou, D., Frost, G. S., Butterworth, P. J., Berry, S. E., Sanderson, J., & Ellis, P. R. (2015). Manipulation of starch bioaccessibility in wheat endosperm to regulate starch digestion, postprandial glycemia, insulinemia, and gut hormone responses: a randomized controlled trial in healthy ileostomy participants. The American Journal of Clinical Nutrition, 102(4), 791–800. https://doi.org/10.3945/ajcn.114.106203

[220] The Diabetes Control And Complications Trial Research Group, (2001) 'Influence of Intensive Diabetes Treatment on Body Weight and Composition of Adults With Type 1 Diabetes in the Diabetes Control and Complications Trial', Diabetes Care. 2001 Oct; 24(10): 1711–1721.

[221] Henry, RR et al (1993) 'Intensive Conventional Insulin Therapy for Type II Diabetes: Metabolic effects during a 6-mo outpatient trial', Diabetes Care 1993 Jan; 16(1): 21-31.

[222] Putnam et al (2001) 'U. S. Per Capita Food Supply Trends: More Calories, Refined Carbohydrates, and Fats', Food Review/ National Food Review, Vol 25, Issue 3, Page 2-15.

[223] Storlien et al (1988) 'Effects of sucrose vs starch diets on in vivo insulin action, thermogenesis, and obesity in rats', The American Journal of Clinical Nutrition, Volume 47, Issue 3, March 1988, Pages 420–427, https://doi.org/10.1093/ajcn/47.3.420

[224] Hulman, S., & Falkner, B. (1994). The effect of excess dietary sucrose on growth, blood pressure, and metabolism in developing Sprague-Dawley rats. Pediatric research, 36(1 Pt 1), 95–101. https://doi.org/10.1203/00006450-199407001-00017

[225] Pagliassotti, M. J., Shahrokhi, K. A., & Moscarello, M. (1994). Involvement of liver and skeletal muscle in sucrose-induced insulin resistance: dose-response studies. American Journal of Physiology-Regulatory, Integrative and Comparative Physiology, 266(5), R1637–R1644. https://doi.org/10.1152/ajpregu.1994.266.5.r1637

[226] Pugazhenthi, S., Angel, J. F., & Khandelwal, R. L. (1993). Effects of high sucrose diet on insulin-like effects of vanadate in diabetic rats. Molecular and cellular biochemistry, 122(1), 77–84. https://doi.org/10.1007/BF00925740

[227] Gutman et al (1987) 'Long-term hypertriglyceridemia and glucose intolerance in rats fed chronically an isocaloric sucrose-rich diet.', Metabolism: Clinical and Experimental, 01 Nov 1987, 36(11):1013-1020

[228] Wright, D. W., Hansen, R. I., Mondon, C. E., & Reaven, G. M. (1983). Sucrose-induced insulin resistance in the rat: modulation by exercise and diet. The American Journal of Clinical Nutrition, 38(6), 879–883. https://doi.org/10.1093/ajcn/38.6.879

[229] Reiser, S., & Hallfrisch, J. (1977). Insulin sensitivity and adipose tissue weight of rats fed starch or sucrose diets ad libitum or in meals. The Journal of nutrition, 107(1), 147–155. https://doi.org/10.1093/jn/107.1.147

[230] Reiser, S., Handler, H. B., Gardner, L. B., Hallfrisch, J. G., Michaelis, O. E., 4th, & Prather, E. S. (1979). Isocaloric exchange of dietary starch and sucrose in humans. II. Effect on fasting blood insulin, glucose, and glucagon and on insulin and glucose response to a sucrose load. The American journal of clinical nutrition, 32(11), 2206–2216. https://doi.org/10.1093/ajcn/32.11.2206

[231] Beck-Nielsen et al (1980) 'Impaired cellular insulin binding and insulin sensitivity induced by high-fructose feeding in normal subjects', The American Journal of Clinical Nutrition, Volume 33, Issue 2, February 1980, Pages 273–278, https://doi.org/10.1093/ajcn/33.2.273

[232] Stanhope, K. L., Schwarz, J. M., Keim, N. L., Griffen, S. C., Bremer, A. A., Graham, J. L., Hatcher, B., Cox, C. L., Dyachenko, A., Zhang, W., McGahan, J. P., Seibert, A., Krauss, R. M., Chiu, S., Schaefer, E. J., Ai, M., Otokozawa, S., Nakajima, K., Nakano, T., Beysen, C., … Havel, P. J. (2009). Consuming fructose-sweetened, not glucose-sweetened, beverages increases visceral adiposity and lipids and decreases insulin sensitivity in overweight/obese humans. The Journal of clinical investigation, 119(5), 1322–1334. https://doi.org/10.1172/JCI37385

[233] Reiser, S., Handler, H. B., Gardner, L. B., Hallfrisch, J. G., Michaelis, O. E., 4th, & Prather, E. S. (1979). Isocaloric exchange of dietary starch and sucrose in humans. II. Effect on fasting blood insulin, glucose, and glucagon and on insulin and glucose response to a sucrose load. The American journal of clinical nutrition, 32(11), 2206–2216. https://doi.org/10.1093/ajcn/32.11.2206

[234] Reiser, S., Bohn, E., Hallfrisch, J., Michaelis, O. E., 4th, Keeney, M., & Prather, E. S. (1981). Serum insulin and glucose in hyperinsulinemic subjects fed three different levels of sucrose. The American journal of clinical nutrition, 34(11), 2348–2358. https://doi.org/10.1093/ajcn/34.11.2348

[235] Gross, L. S., Li, L., Ford, E. S., & Liu, S. (2004). Increased consumption of refined carbohydrates and the epidemic of type 2 diabetes in the United States: an ecologic assessment. The American journal of clinical nutrition, 79(5), 774–779. https://doi.org/10.1093/ajcn/79.5.774

[236] PM Kris-Etherton, Denise Shaffer Taylor, Shaomei Yu-Poth, Peter Huth, Kristin Moriarty, Valerie Fishell, Rebecca L Hargrove, Guixiang Zhao, Terry D Etherton; Polyunsaturated fatty acids in the food chain in the United States, The American Journal of Clinical Nutrition, Volume 71, Issue 1, 1 January 2000, Pages 179S–188S.

[237] Simopoulos, A. P., & DiNicolantonio, J. J. (2016). The importance of a balanced ω-6 to ω-3 ratio in the prevention and management of obesity. Open Heart, 3(2), e000385. https://doi.org/10.1136/openhrt-2015-000385

[238] Russo GL (2009) 'Dietary n-6 and n-3 polyunsaturated fatty acids: from biochemistry to clinical implications in cardiovascular prevention', Biochem Pharmacol. 2009 Mar 15;77(6):937-46.

[239] Leaf A and Weber PC (1988) 'Cardiovascular effects of n-3 fatty acids', AGRIS, Accessed: http://agris.fao.org/agris-search/search.do?recordID=US8845581.

[240] Blasbalg, T. L., Hibbeln, J. R., Ramsden, C. E., Majchrzak, S. F., & Rawlings, R. R. (2011). Changes in consumption of omega-3 and omega-6 fatty acids in the United States during the 20th century. The American Journal of Clinical Nutrition, 93(5), 950–962. https://doi.org/10.3945/ajcn.110.006643

[241] Guyenet, S. J., & Carlson, S. E. (2015). Increase in adipose tissue linoleic acid of US adults in the last half century. Advances in nutrition (Bethesda, Md.), 6(6), 660–664. https://doi.org/10.3945/an.115.009944

[242] Guyenet and Carlson (2015) 'Increase in Adipose Tissue Linoleic Acid of US Adults in the Last Half Century', Advances in Nutrition, Volume 6, Issue 6, November 2015, Pages 660–664, https://doi.org/10.3945/an.115.009944

[243] Simopoulos, A. P., & DiNicolantonio, J. J. (2016). The importance of a balanced ω-6 to ω-3 ratio in the prevention and management of obesity. Open Heart, 3(2), e000385. https://doi.org/10.1136/openhrt-2015-000385

[244] Alvheim, A. R., Torstensen, B. E., Lin, Y. H., Lillefosse, H. H., Lock, E. J., Madsen, L., Frøyland, L., Hibbeln, J. R., & Malde, M. K. (2014). Dietary linoleic acid elevates the endocannabinoids 2-AG and anandamide and promotes weight gain in mice fed a low fat diet. Lipids, 49(1), 59–69. https://doi.org/10.1007/s11745-013-3842-y

[245] Best, K. P., Gold, M., Kennedy, D., Martin, J., & Makrides, M. (2016). Omega-3 long-chain PUFA intake during pregnancy and allergic disease outcomes in the offspring: a systematic review and meta-analysis of observational studies and randomized controlled trials. The American Journal of Clinical Nutrition, 103(1), 128–143. doi:10.3945/ajcn.115.111104

[246] Guyenet, S. J., & Carlson, S. E. (2015). Increase in Adipose Tissue Linoleic Acid of US Adults in the Last Half Century. Advances in Nutrition, 6(6), 660–664. doi:10.3945/an.115.009944

[247] Flachs, P., Rossmeisl, M., Kuda, O., & Kopecky, J. (2013). Stimulation of mitochondrial oxidative capacity in white fat independent of UCP1: A key to lean phenotype. Biochimica et Biophysica Acta (BBA) - Molecular and Cell Biology of Lipids, 1831(5), 986–1003. doi:10.1016/j.bbalip.2013.02.003

[248] Flachs, P., Mohamed-Ali, V., Horakova, O., Rossmeisl, M., Hosseinzadeh-Attar, M. J., Hensler, M., … Kopecky, J. (2006). Polyunsaturated fatty acids of marine origin induce adiponectin in mice fed a high-fat diet. Diabetologia, 49(2), 394–397. doi:10.1007/s00125-005-0053-y

[249] Hensler, M., Bardova, K., Jilkova, Z. M., Wahli, W., Meztger, D., Chambon, P., Kopecky, J., & Flachs, P. (2011). The inhibition of fat cell proliferation by n-3 fatty acids in dietary obese mice. Lipids in health and disease, 10, 128. https://doi.org/10.1186/1476-511X-10-128

[250] Ruzickova, J., Rossmeisl, M., Prazak, T., Flachs, P., Sponarova, J., Veck, M., Tvrzicka, E., Bryhn, M., & Kopecky, J. (2004). Omega-3 PUFA of marine origin limit diet-induced obesity in mice by reducing cellularity of adipose tissue. Lipids, 39(12), 1177–1185. https://doi.org/10.1007/s11745-004-1345-9

[251] Hill JO, Peters JC, Lin D, et al. Lipid accumulation and body fat distribution is influenced by type of dietary fat fed to rats. Int J Obes Relat Metab Disord. 1993 Apr;17(4):223-36.

[252] Hiza, HAB and Bente L (2007) 'Nutrient Content of the U.S. Food Supply, 1909-2004, A Summary Report', Center for Nutrition Policy and Promotion, Home Economics Research Report No. 57.

[253] Blasbalg, T. L., Hibbeln, J. R., Ramsden, C. E., Majchrzak, S. F., & Rawlings, R. R. (2011). Changes in consumption of omega-3 and omega-6 fatty acids in the United States during the 20th century. The American Journal of Clinical Nutrition, 93(5), 950–962. https://doi.org/10.3945/ajcn.110.006643

[254] Guyenet, S. J., & Carlson, S. E. (2015). Increase in Adipose Tissue Linoleic Acid of US Adults in the Last Half Century. Advances in Nutrition, 6(6), 660–664. https://doi.org/10.3945/an.115.009944

[255] Rupp (2014) 'The Butter Wars: When Margarine Was Pink', National Geographic, Accessed Online March 14th 2022: https://web.archive.org/web/20180801063420/https://www.nationalgeographic.com/people-and-culture/food/the-plate/2014/08/13/the-butter-wars-when-margarine-was-pink/

[256] AHA (2018) 'History of the American Heart Association', Accessed Online March 14th 2022: https://www.heart.org/-/media/Files/About-Us/History/History-of-the-American-Heart-Association.pdf

[257] Braun (2014) 'Turning Bacon Into Bombs: The American Fat Salvage Committee', The Atlantic, Accessed Online March 14th 2022: https://www.theatlantic.com/health/archive/2014/04/reluctantly-turning-bacon-into-bombs-during-world-war-ii/360298/

[258] Barnard N et al (2014) 'Saturated and trans fats and dementia: a systematic review', Neurobiology of Aging, Volume 35, Supplement 2, September 2014, Pages S65-S73.

[259] Pase CS et al (2013) 'Influence of perinatal trans fat on behavioral responses and brain oxidative status of adolescent rats acutely exposed to stress', Neuroscience. 2013 Sep 5;247:242-52.

[260] *Nutrition Week* Mar 22, 1991 21:12:2-3

[261] US FDA, Trans Fat, Accessed 2018: https://www.fda.gov/food/ucm292278.htm

[262] Putnam et al (2002) 'U.S. Per Capita Food Supply Trends: More Calories, Refined Carbohydrates, and Fats', Food Review/ National Food Review, Vol 25, Issue 3, P 2-15.

[263] Putnam et al (2002) 'U.S. Per Capita Food Supply Trends: More Calories, Refined Carbohydrates, and Fats', Food Review/ National Food Review, Vol 25, Issue 3, P 2-15.

[264] Putnam et al (2002) 'U.S. Per Capita Food Supply Trends: More Calories, Refined Carbohydrates, and Fats', Food Review/ National Food Review, Vol 25, Issue 3, P 2-15.

265 Wanders, A. J., van den Borne, J. J., de Graaf, C., Hulshof, T., Jonathan, M. C., Kristensen, M., Mars, M., Schols, H. A., & Feskens, E. J. (2011). Effects of dietary fibre on subjective appetite, energy intake and body weight: a systematic review of randomized controlled trials. Obesity reviews : an official journal of the International Association for the Study of Obesity, 12(9), 724–739. https://doi.org/10.1111/j.1467-789X.2011.00895.x

266 Clark, M. J., & Slavin, J. L. (2013). The effect of fiber on satiety and food intake: a systematic review. Journal of the American College of Nutrition, 32(3), 200–211. https://doi.org/10.1080/07315724.2013.791194

267 Burton-Freeman B. (2000). Dietary fiber and energy regulation. The Journal of nutrition, 130(2S Suppl), 272S–275S. https://doi.org/10.1093/jn/130.2.272S

268 Kristensen, M., Jensen, M. G., Aarestrup, J., Petersen, K. E., Søndergaard, L., Mikkelsen, M. S., & Astrup, A. (2012). Flaxseed dietary fibers lower cholesterol and increase fecal fat excretion, but magnitude of effect depend on food type. Nutrition & metabolism, 9, 8. https://doi.org/10.1186/1743-7075-9-8

269 Uebelhack, R., Busch, R., Alt, F., Beah, Z. M., & Chong, P. W. (2014). Effects of cactus fiber on the excretion of dietary fat in healthy subjects: a double blind, randomized, placebo-controlled, crossover clinical investigation. Current therapeutic research, clinical and experimental, 76, 39–44. https://doi.org/10.1016/j.curtheres.2014.02.001

270 Hall, K. D., Bemis, T., Brychta, R., Chen, K. Y., Courville, A., Crayner, E. J., Goodwin, S., Guo, J., Howard, L., Knuth, N. D., Miller, B. V., 3rd, Prado, C. M., Siervo, M., Skarulis, M. C., Walter, M., Walter, P. J., & Yannai, L. (2015). Calorie for Calorie, Dietary Fat Restriction Results in More Body Fat Loss than Carbohydrate Restriction in People with Obesity. Cell metabolism, 22(3), 427–436. https://doi.org/10.1016/j.cmet.2015.07.021

271 Hall, K. D., Guyenet, S. J., & Leibel, R. L. (2018). The Carbohydrate-Insulin Model of Obesity Is Difficult to Reconcile With Current Evidence. JAMA internal medicine, 178(8), 1103–1105. https://doi.org/10.1001/jamainternmed.2018.2920

272 Gardner, C. D., Trepanowski, J. F., Del Gobbo, L. C., Hauser, M. E., Rigdon, J., Ioannidis, J. P. A., … King, A. C. (2018). Effect of Low-Fat vs Low-Carbohydrate Diet on 12-Month Weight Loss in Overweight Adults and the Association With Genotype Pattern or Insulin Secretion. JAMA, 319(7), 667. doi:10.1001/jama.2018.0245

273 Schoeller, D. A., & Buchholz, A. C. (2005). Energetics of obesity and weight control: does diet composition matter?. Journal of the American Dietetic Association, 105(5 Suppl 1), S24–S28. https://doi.org/10.1016/j.jada.2005.02.025

274 Howell, S., & Kones, R. (2017). "Calories in, calories out" and macronutrient intake: the hope, hype, and science of calories. American journal of physiology. Endocrinology and metabolism, 313(5), E608–E612. https://doi.org/10.1152/ajpendo.00156.2017

275 Bradley, U., Spence, M., Courtney, C. H., McKinley, M. C., Ennis, C. N., McCance, D. R., McEneny, J., Bell, P. M., Young, I. S., & Hunter, S. J. (2009). Low-fat versus low-carbohydrate weight reduction diets: effects on weight loss, insulin resistance, and cardiovascular risk: a randomized control trial. Diabetes, 58(12), 2741–2748. https://doi.org/10.2337/db09-0098

276 Hu, T., Mills, K. T., Yao, L., Demanelis, K., Eloustaz, M., Yancy, W. S., Jr, Kelly, T. N., He, J., & Bazzano, L. A. (2012). Effects of low-carbohydrate diets versus low-fat diets on metabolic risk factors: a meta-analysis of randomized controlled clinical trials. American journal of epidemiology, 176 Suppl 7(Suppl 7), S44–S54. https://doi.org/10.1093/aje/kws264

277 Hall, K. D., Guo, J., Courville, A. B., Boring, J., Brychta, R., Chen, K. Y., Darcey, V., Forde, C. G., Gharib, A. M., Gallagher, I., Howard, R., Joseph, P. V., Milley, L., Ouwerkerk, R., Raisinger, K., Rozga, I., Schick, A., Stagliano, M., Torres, S., Walter, M., … Chung, S. T. (2021). Effect of a plant-based, low-fat diet versus an animal-based, ketogenic diet on ad libitum energy intake. Nature medicine, 27(2), 344–353. https://doi.org/10.1038/s41591-020-01209-1

[278] Putnam et al (2002) 'U.S. Per Capita Food Supply Trends: More Calories, Refined Carbohydrates, and Fats', Food Review/ National Food Review, Vol 25, Issue 3, P 2-15.

279 Page, K. A., Chan, O., Arora, J., Belfort-Deaguiar, R., Dzuira, J., Roehmholdt, B., Cline, G. W., Naik, S., Sinha, R., Constable, R. T., & Sherwin, R. S. (2013). Effects of fructose vs glucose on regional cerebral blood flow in brain regions involved with appetite and reward pathways. JAMA, 309(1), 63–70. https://doi.org/10.1001/jama.2012.116975

280 Teff, K. L., Elliott, S. S., Tschöp, M., Kieffer, T. J., Rader, D., Heiman, M., Townsend, R. R., Keim, N. L., D'Alessio, D., & Havel, P. J. (2004). Dietary fructose reduces circulating insulin and leptin, attenuates postprandial suppression of ghrelin, and increases triglycerides in women. The Journal of clinical endocrinology and metabolism, 89(6), 2963–2972. https://doi.org/10.1210/jc.2003-031855

281 Ma, X., Lin, L., Yue, J., Pradhan, G., Qin, G., Minze, L. J., Wu, H., Sheikh-Hamad, D., Smith, C. W., & Sun, Y. (2013). Ghrelin receptor regulates HFCS-induced adipose inflammation and insulin resistance. Nutrition & diabetes, 3(12), e99. https://doi.org/10.1038/nutd.2013.41

[282] Marantz, P. R., Bird, E. D., & Alderman, M. H. (2008). A call for higher standards of evidence for dietary guidelines. American journal of preventive medicine, 34(3), 234–240. https://doi.org/10.1016/j.amepre.2007.11.017

283 Wardlaw GM, Kessel M. Energy Production and Energy Balance. In: Perspective in Nutrition 2nd Ed. New York, NY: McGraw-Hill Higher Education; 2002. p. 535-537.

284 Hall, K. D., Heymsfield, S. B., Kemnitz, J. W., Klein, S., Schoeller, D. A., & Speakman, J. R. (2012). Energy balance and its components: implications for body weight regulation. The American journal of clinical nutrition, 95(4), 989–994. https://doi.org/10.3945/ajcn.112.036350

285 Jaffe, R.L.; Taylor, W. (2018). The Physics of Energy. Cambridge UK: Cambridge University Press. p. 150,n259, 772, 743.

286 Kiecolt-Glaser, J. K., Habash, D. L., Fagundes, C. P., Andridge, R., Peng, J., Malarkey, W. B., & Belury, M. A. (2015). Daily Stressors, Past Depression, and Metabolic Responses to High-Fat Meals: A Novel Path to Obesity. Biological Psychiatry, 77(7), 653–660. doi:10.1016/j.biopsych.2014.05.018

287 Astrup, A., Buemann, B., Toubro, S., Ranneries, C., & Raben, A. (1996). Low resting metabolic rate in subjects predisposed to obesity: a role for thyroid status. The American journal of clinical nutrition, 63(6), 879–883. https://doi.org/10.1093/ajcn/63.6.879

288 Doucet, E., St-Pierre, S., Alméras, N., Després, J. P., Bouchard, C., & Tremblay, A. (2001). Evidence for the existence of adaptive thermogenesis during weight loss. The British journal of nutrition, 85(6), 715–723. https://doi.org/10.1079/bjn2001348

289 Dulloo, A. G., & Jacquet, J. (1998). Adaptive reduction in basal metabolic rate in response to food deprivation in humans: a role for feedback signals from fat stores. The American Journal of Clinical Nutrition, 68(3), 599–606. doi:10.1093/ajcn/68.3.599

290 Bevilacqua, L., Ramsey, J. J., Hagopian, K., Weindruch, R., & Harper, M.-E. (2004). Effects of short- and medium-term calorie restriction on muscle mitochondrial proton leak and reactive oxygen species production. American Journal of Physiology-Endocrinology and Metabolism, 286(5), E852–E861. doi:10.1152/ajpendo.00367.2003

291 Esterbauer, H., Oberkofler, H., Dallinger, G., Breban, D., Hell, E., Krempler, F., & Patsch, W. (1999). Uncoupling protein-3 gene expression: reduced skeletal muscle mRNA in obese humans during pronounced weight loss. Diabetologia, 42(3), 302–309. doi:10.1007/s001250051155

[292] Axelsson, A. S., Tubbs, E., Mecham, B., Chacko, S., Nenonen, H. A., Tang, Y., Fahey, J. W., Derry, J., Wollheim, C. B., Wierup, N., Haymond, M. W., Friend, S. H., Mulder, H., & Rosengren, A. H. (2017). Sulforaphane reduces hepatic glucose production and improves glucose control in patients with type 2 diabetes. Science translational medicine, 9(394), eaah4477. https://doi.org/10.1126/scitranslmed.aah4477

[293] Mashhadi, N. S., Zakerkish, M., Mohammadiasl, J., Zarei, M., Mohammadshahi, M., & Haghighizadeh, M. H. (2018). Astaxanthin improves glucose metabolism and reduces blood pressure in patients with type 2 diabetes mellitus. Asia Pacific journal of clinical nutrition, 27(2), 341–346. https://doi.org/10.6133/apjcn.052017.11

[294] McCarty, M. F., DiNicolantonio, J. J., & O'Keefe, J. H. (2015). Capsaicin may have important potential for promoting vascular and metabolic health: Table 1. Open Heart, 2(1), e000262. https://doi.org/10.1136/openhrt-2015-000262

[295] Hu, Y., Ehli, E. A., Kittelsrud, J., Ronan, P. J., Munger, K., Downey, T., Bohlen, K., Callahan, L., Munson, V., Jahnke, M., Marshall, L. L., Nelson, K., Huizenga, P., Hansen, R., Soundy, T. J., & Davies, G. E. (2012). Lipid-lowering effect of berberine in human subjects and rats. Phytomedicine : international journal of phytotherapy and phytopharmacology, 19(10), 861–867. https://doi.org/10.1016/j.phymed.2012.05.009

[296] Bhuvaneswari, S., & Anuradha, C. V. (2012). Astaxanthin prevents loss of insulin signaling and improves glucose metabolism in liver of insulin resistant mice. Canadian journal of physiology and pharmacology, 90(11), 1544–1552. https://doi.org/10.1139/y2012-119

[297] Nishida et al (2020) 'Astaxanthin stimulates mitochondrial biogenesis in insulin resistant muscle via activation of AMPK pathway', Journal of Cachexia, Sarcopenia and Muscle, DOI:10.1002/jcsm.12530

[298] Zhao, L., Cang, Z., Sun, H., Nie, X., Wang, N., & Lu, Y. (2017). Berberine improves glucogenesis and lipid metabolism in nonalcoholic fatty liver disease. BMC Endocrine Disorders, 17(1). https://doi.org/10.1186/s12902-017-0165-7

[299] Lee, Y. S., Kim, W. S., Kim, K. H., Yoon, M. J., Cho, H. J., Shen, Y., Ye, J. M., Lee, C. H., Oh, W. K., Kim, C. T., Hohnen-Behrens, C., Gosby, A., Kraegen, E. W., James, D. E., & Kim, J. B. (2006). Berberine, a natural plant product, activates AMP-activated protein kinase with beneficial metabolic effects in diabetic and insulin-resistant states. Diabetes, 55(8), 2256–2264. https://doi.org/10.2337/db06-0006

[300] Yang, J., Yin, J., Gao, H., Xu, L., Wang, Y., Xu, L., & Li, M. (2012). Berberine improves insulin sensitivity by inhibiting fat store and adjusting adipokines profile in human preadipocytes and metabolic syndrome patients. Evidence-based complementary and alternative medicine : eCAM, 2012, 363845. https://doi.org/10.1155/2012/363845

[301] Mashhadi, N. S., Zakerkish, M., Mohammadiasl, J., Zarei, M., Mohammadshahi, M., & Haghighizadeh, M. H. (2018). Astaxanthin improves glucose metabolism and reduces blood pressure in patients with type 2 diabetes mellitus. Asia Pacific journal of clinical nutrition, 27(2), 341–346. https://doi.org/10.6133/apjcn.052017.11

302 2015-2020 Dietary Guidelines 'Appendix 2. Estimated Calorie Needs per Day, by Age, Sex, and Physical Activity Level', Accessed Online: https://health.gov/dietaryguidelines/2015/guidelines/appendix-2/

303 Griggs, R. C., Kingston, W., Jozefowicz, R. F., Herr, B. E., Forbes, G., & Halliday, D. (1989). Effect of testosterone on muscle mass and muscle protein synthesis. Journal of applied physiology (Bethesda, Md. : 1985), 66(1), 498–503. https://doi.org/10.1152/jappl.1989.66.1.498

304 Bhasin, S., Woodhouse, L., Casaburi, R., Singh, A. B., Bhasin, D., Berman, N., … Storer, T. W. (2001). Testosterone dose-response relationships in healthy young men. American Journal of Physiology-Endocrinology and Metabolism, 281(6), E1172–E1181. doi:10.1152/ajpendo.2001.281.6.e1172

305 Bhasin, S., Taylor, W. E., Singh, R., Artaza, J., Sinha-Hikim, I., Jasuja, R., Choi, H., & Gonzalez-Cadavid, N. F. (2003). The mechanisms of androgen effects on body composition: mesenchymal pluripotent cell as the target of androgen action. The journals of gerontology. Series A, Biological sciences and medical sciences, 58(12), M1103–M1110. https://doi.org/10.1093/gerona/58.12.m1103

306 Herbst, K.L. & Bhasin, S. (2004) Testosterone action on skeletal muscle. Curr. Opin. Clin. Nutr. Metab. Care 7, 271–277

307 Grantham, J. P., & Henneberg, M. (2014). The estrogen hypothesis of obesity. PloS one, 9(6), e99776. https://doi.org/10.1371/journal.pone.0099776

[308] Rubinow, K. B. (2017). Estrogens and Body Weight Regulation in Men. Advances in Experimental Medicine and Biology, 285–313. https://doi.org/10.1007/978-3-319-70178-3_14

309 Salter (2018) 'Is "Calories In, Calories Out": A Weight-Loss Myth Or The Truth?', Accessed Online Aug 15 2021: https://www.bodybuilding.com/content/is-calories-in-calories-out-a-weight-loss-myth-or-the-truth.html

310 McClave et al (2001) 'Dissecting the energy needs of the body', Current Opinion in Clinical Nutrition and Metabolic Care: March 2001 - Volume 4 - Issue 2 - p 143-147.

311 Levine J. A. (2005). Measurement of energy expenditure. Public health nutrition, 8(7A), 1123–1132. https://doi.org/10.1079/phn2005800

312 Levine J. A. (2002). Non-exercise activity thermogenesis (NEAT). Best practice & research. Clinical endocrinology & metabolism, 16(4), 679–702. https://doi.org/10.1053/beem.2002.0227

313 Calcagno, M., Kahleova, H., Alwarith, J., Burgess, N. N., Flores, R. A., Busta, M. L., & Barnard, N. D. (2019). The Thermic Effect of Food: A Review. Journal of the American College of Nutrition, 38(6), 547–551. https://doi.org/10.1080/07315724.2018.1552544

314 Westerterp K. R. (2004). Diet induced thermogenesis. Nutrition & metabolism, 1(1), 5. https://doi.org/10.1186/1743-7075-1-5

315 Wycherley, T. P., Moran, L. J., Clifton, P. M., Noakes, M., & Brinkworth, G. D. (2012). Effects of energy-restricted high-protein, low-fat compared with standard-protein, low-fat diets: a meta-analysis of randomized controlled trials. The American journal of clinical nutrition, 96(6), 1281–1298. https://doi.org/10.3945/ajcn.112.044321

316 Halton, T. L., & Hu, F. B. (2004). The effects of high protein diets on thermogenesis, satiety and weight loss: a critical review. Journal of the American College of Nutrition, 23(5), 373–385. https://doi.org/10.1080/07315724.2004.10719381

317 Bray, G. A., Redman, L. M., de Jonge, L., Covington, J., Rood, J., Brock, C., Mancuso, S., Martin, C. K., & Smith, S. R. (2015). Effect of protein overfeeding on energy expenditure measured in a metabolic chamber. The American journal of clinical nutrition, 101(3), 496–505. https://doi.org/10.3945/ajcn.114.091769

318 Crovetti, R., Porrini, M., Santangelo, A., & Testolin, G. (1998). The influence of thermic effect of food on satiety. European journal of clinical nutrition, 52(7), 482–488. https://doi.org/10.1038/sj.ejcn.1600578

319 Weigle, D. S., Breen, P. A., Matthys, C. C., Callahan, H. S., Meeuws, K. E., Burden, V. R., & Purnell, J. Q. (2005). A high-protein diet induces sustained reductions in appetite, ad libitum caloric intake, and body weight despite compensatory changes in diurnal plasma leptin and ghrelin concentrations. The American journal of clinical nutrition, 82(1), 41–48. https://doi.org/10.1093/ajcn.82.1.41

[320] Vander Wal, J. S., Marth, J. M., Khosla, P., Jen, K. L., & Dhurandhar, N. V. (2005). Short-term effect of eggs on satiety in overweight and obese subjects. Journal of the American College of Nutrition, 24(6), 510–515. https://doi.org/10.1080/07315724.2005.10719497

[321] B Keogh, J., & M Clifton, P. (2020). Energy Intake and Satiety Responses of Eggs for Breakfast in Overweight and Obese Adults-A Crossover Study. International journal of environmental research and public health, 17(15), 5583. https://doi.org/10.3390/ijerph17155583

[322] Pombo-Rodrigues, S., Calame, W., & Re, R. (2011). The effects of consuming eggs for lunch on satiety and subsequent food intake. International Journal of Food Sciences and Nutrition, 62(6), 593–599. https://doi.org/10.3109/09637486.2011.566212

323 Taaffe, D. R., Thompson, J., Butterfield, G., & Marcus, R. (1995). Accuracy of equations to predict basal metabolic rate in older women. Journal of the American Dietetic Association, 95(12), 1387–1392. https://doi.org/10.1016/S0002-8223(95)00366-5

324 Frankenfield, D. C., Rowe, W. A., Smith, J. S., & Cooney, R. N. (2003). Validation of several established equations for resting metabolic rate in obese and nonobese people. Journal of the American Dietetic Association, 103(9), 1152–1159. https://doi.org/10.1016/s0002-8223(03)00982-9

325 Frankenfield, D., Roth-Yousey, L., & Compher, C. (2005). Comparison of predictive equations for resting metabolic rate in healthy nonobese and obese adults: a systematic review. Journal of the American Dietetic Association, 105(5), 775–789. https://doi.org/10.1016/j.jada.2005.02.005

326 Daly, J. M., Heymsfield, S. B., Head, C. A., Harvey, L. P., Nixon, D. W., Katzeff, H., & Grossman, G. D. (1985). Human energy requirements: overestimation by widely used prediction equation. The American journal of clinical nutrition, 42(6), 1170–1174. https://doi.org/10.1093/ajcn/42.6.1170

327 Miller, S., Milliron, B. J., & Woolf, K. (2013). Common Prediction Equations Overestimate Measured Resting Metabolic Rate in Young Hispanic Women. Topics in clinical nutrition, 28(2), 120–135. https://doi.org/10.1097/TIN.0b013e31828d7a1b

328 Cunningham J. J. (1980). A reanalysis of the factors influencing basal metabolic rate in normal adults. The American journal of clinical nutrition, 33(11), 2372–2374. https://doi.org/10.1093/ajcn/33.11.2372

329 ten Haaf, T., & Weijs, P. J. (2014). Resting energy expenditure prediction in recreational athletes of 18-35 years: confirmation of Cunningham equation and an improved weight-based alternative. PloS one, 9(9), e108460. https://doi.org/10.1371/journal.pone.0108460

330 Hall K. D. (2008). What is the required energy deficit per unit weight loss?. International journal of obesity (2005), 32(3), 573–576. https://doi.org/10.1038/sj.ijo.0803720

331 McArdle WD. Exercise physiology: energy, nutrition, and human performance. 4th edition edn. Williams & Wilkins; Baltimore: 1996.

332 WISHNOFSKY M. (1958). Caloric equivalents of gained or lost weight. The American journal of clinical nutrition, 6(5), 542–546. https://doi.org/10.1093/ajcn/6.5.542

333 Forbes G. B. (2000). Body fat content influences the body composition response to nutrition and exercise. Annals of the New York Academy of Sciences, 904, 359–365. https://doi.org/10.1111/j.1749-6632.2000.tb06482.x

334 Forbes G. B. (1987). Lean body mass-body fat interrelationships in humans. Nutrition reviews, 45(8), 225–231. https://doi.org/10.1111/j.1753-4887.1987.tb02684.x

335 Forbes G. B. (2000). Body fat content influences the body composition response to nutrition and exercise. Annals of the New York Academy of Sciences, 904, 359–365. https://doi.org/10.1111/j.1749-6632.2000.tb06482.x

336 Forbes G. B. (1987). Lean body mass-body fat interrelationships in humans. Nutrition reviews, 45(8), 225–231. https://doi.org/10.1111/j.1753-4887.1987.tb02684.x

337 Dulloo, A. G., Jacquet, J., & Montani, J. P. (2012). How dieting makes some fatter: from a perspective of human body composition autoregulation. The Proceedings of the Nutrition Society, 71(3), 379–389. https://doi.org/10.1017/S0029665112000225

338 Forbes G. B. (1999). Longitudinal changes in adult fat-free mass: influence of body weight. The American journal of clinical nutrition, 70(6), 1025–1031. https://doi.org/10.1093/ajcn/70.6.1025

339 Vogels, N., & Westerterp-Plantenga, M. S. (2007). Successful Long-term Weight Maintenance: A 2-year Follow-up*. Obesity, 15(5), 1258–1266. doi:10.1038/oby.2007.147

340 Muller, M. J., Bosy-Westphal, A., Kutzner, D., & Heller, M. (2002). Metabolically active components of fat-free mass and resting energy expenditure in humans: recent lessons from imaging technologies. Obesity Reviews, 3(2), 113–122. doi:10.1046/j.1467-789x.2002.00057.x

341 Ravussin, E., Lillioja, S., Knowler, W. C., Christin, L., Freymond, D., Abbott, W. G., Boyce, V., Howard, B. V., & Bogardus, C. (1988). Reduced rate of energy expenditure as a risk factor for body-weight gain. The New England journal of medicine, 318(8), 467–472. https://doi.org/10.1056/NEJM198802253180802

342 Vicente-Rodriguez, G. (2005). Muscular development and physical activity as major determinants of femoral bone mass acquisition during growth. British Journal of Sports Medicine, 39(9), 611–616. doi:10.1136/bjsm.2004.014431

343 Aloia, J. F., Vaswani, A., Ma, R., & Flaster, E. (1995). To what extent is bone mass determined by fat-free or fat mass? The American Journal of Clinical Nutrition, 61(5), 1110–1114. doi:10.1093/ajcn/61.5.1110

344 Marks, B. L., & Rippe, J. M. (1996). The Importance of Fat Free Mass Maintenance in Weight Loss Programmes. Sports Medicine, 22(5), 273–281. doi:10.2165/00007256-199622050-00001

345 Pontzer et al (2021) 'Daily energy expenditure through the human life course', Science, Vol. 373, Issue 6556, pp. 808-812, DOI: 10.1126/science.abe5017

346 Pennington Biomedical Research Center. (2021, August 12). Metabolism changes with age, just not when you might think. ScienceDaily. Retrieved August 13, 2021 from www.sciencedaily.com/releases/2021/08/210812145028.htm

347 Joosen, A. M., & Westerterp, K. R. (2006). Energy expenditure during overfeeding. Nutrition & Metabolism, 3(1). https://doi.org/10.1186/1743-7075-3-25

348 Lowell, B. B., & Spiegelman, B. M. (2000). Towards a molecular understanding of adaptive thermogenesis. Nature, 404(6778), 652–660. https://doi.org/10.1038/35007527

349 Dulloo, A. G., Jacquet, J., Montani, J. P., & Schutz, Y. (2012). Adaptive thermogenesis in human body weight regulation: more of a concept than a measurable entity?. Obesity reviews : an official journal of the International Association for the Study of Obesity, 13 Suppl 2, 105–121. https://doi.org/10.1111/j.1467-789X.2012.01041.x

350 Diaz, E. O., Prentice, A. M., Goldberg, G. R., Murgatroyd, P. R., & Coward, W. A. (1992). Metabolic response to experimental overfeeding in lean and overweight healthy volunteers. The American Journal of Clinical Nutrition, 56(4), 641–655. https://doi.org/10.1093/ajcn/56.4.641

351 Joosen, A. M., Bakker, A. H., & Westerterp, K. R. (2005). Metabolic efficiency and energy expenditure during short-term overfeeding. Physiology & behavior, 85(5), 593–597. https://doi.org/10.1016/j.physbeh.2005.06.006

352 Tremblay, A., Després, J. P., Thériault, G., Fournier, G., & Bouchard, C. (1992). Overfeeding and energy expenditure in humans. The American journal of clinical nutrition, 56(5), 857–862. https://doi.org/10.1093/ajcn/56.5.857

353 Forbes, G. B., Brown, M. R., Welle, S. L., & Lipinski, B. A. (1986). Deliberate overfeeding in women and men: energy cost and composition of the weight gain. The British journal of nutrition, 56(1), 1–9. https://doi.org/10.1079/bjn19860080

354 Jebb et al (1996) 'Changes in macronutrient balance during over- and underfeeding assessed by 12-d continuous whole-body calorimetry', The American Journal of Clinical Nutrition, Volume 64, Issue 3, September 1996, Pages 259–266, https://doi.org/10.1093/ajcn/64.3.259.

355 Levine, J. A., Eberhardt, N. L., & Jensen, M. D. (1999). Role of nonexercise activity thermogenesis in resistance to fat gain in humans. Science (New York, N.Y.), 283(5399), 212–214. https://doi.org/10.1126/science.283.5399.212

356 Pasquet, P., Brigant, L., Froment, A., Koppert, G. A., Bard, D., de Garine, I., & Apfelbaum, M. (1992). Massive overfeeding and energy balance in men: the Guru Walla model. The American journal of clinical nutrition, 56(3), 483–490. https://doi.org/10.1093/ajcn/56.3.483

357 Ravussin, E., Schutz, Y., Acheson, K. J., Dusmet, M., Bourquin, L., & Jéquier, E. (1985). Short-term, mixed-diet overfeeding in man: no evidence for "luxuskonsumption". The American journal of physiology, 249(5 Pt 1), E470–E477. https://doi.org/10.1152/ajpendo.1985.249.5.E470

358 Roberts, S. B., Young, V. R., Fuss, P., Fiatarone, M. A., Richard, B., Rasmussen, H., Wagner, D., Joseph, L., Holehouse, E., & Evans, W. J. (1990). Energy expenditure and subsequent nutrient intakes in overfed young men. American Journal of Physiology-Regulatory, Integrative and Comparative Physiology, 259(3), R461–R469. https://doi.org/10.1152/ajpregu.1990.259.3.r461

359 Zed, C., & James, W. P. (1986). Dietary thermogenesis in obesity: fat feeding at different energy intakes. International journal of obesity, 10(5), 375–390.

360 Tremblay, A., Després, J. P., Thériault, G., Fournier, G., & Bouchard, C. (1992). Overfeeding and energy expenditure in humans. The American journal of clinical nutrition, 56(5), 857–862. https://doi.org/10.1093/ajcn/56.5.857

361 Ravussin, E., Schutz, Y., Acheson, K. J., Dusmet, M., Bourquin, L., & Jéquier, E. (1985). Short-term, mixed-diet overfeeding in man: no evidence for "luxuskonsumption". The American journal of physiology, 249(5 Pt 1), E470–E477. https://doi.org/10.1152/ajpendo.1985.249.5.E470

362 Roberts, S. B., Young, V. R., Fuss, P., Fiatarone, M. A., Richard, B., Rasmussen, H., Wagner, D., Joseph, L., Holehouse, E., & Evans, W. J. (1990). Energy expenditure and subsequent nutrient intakes in overfed young men. American Journal of Physiology-Regulatory, Integrative and Comparative Physiology, 259(3), R461–R469. https://doi.org/10.1152/ajpregu.1990.259.3.r461

363 Norgan, N. G., & Durnin, J. V. (1980). The effect of 6 weeks of overfeeding on the body weight, body composition, and energy metabolism of young men. The American journal of clinical nutrition, 33(5), 978–988. https://doi.org/10.1093/ajcn/33.5.978

364 Joosen, A. M., Bakker, A. H., & Westerterp, K. R. (2005). Metabolic efficiency and energy expenditure during short-term overfeeding. Physiology & behavior, 85(5), 593–597. https://doi.org/10.1016/j.physbeh.2005.06.006

365 Bouchard, C., Tremblay, A., Després, J. P., Nadeau, A., Lupien, P. J., Thériault, G., Dussault, J., Moorjani, S., Pinault, S., & Fournier, G. (1990). The response to long-term overfeeding in identical twins. The New England journal of medicine, 322(21), 1477–1482. https://doi.org/10.1056/NEJM199005243222101

366 Bouchard, C., Tremblay, A., Després, J. P., Nadeau, A., Lupien, P. J., Thériault, G., Dussault, J., Moorjani, S., Pinault, S., & Fournier, G. (1990). The response to long-term overfeeding in identical twins. The New England journal of medicine, 322(21), 1477–1482. https://doi.org/10.1056/NEJM199005243222101

367 Levine, J. A., Eberhardt, N. L., & Jensen, M. D. (1999). Role of nonexercise activity thermogenesis in resistance to fat gain in humans. Science (New York, N.Y.), 283(5399), 212–214. https://doi.org/10.1126/science.283.5399.212

368 Levine, J. A., Eberhardt, N. L., & Jensen, M. D. (1999). Role of nonexercise activity thermogenesis in resistance to fat gain in humans. Science (New York, N.Y.), 283(5399), 212–214. https://doi.org/10.1126/science.283.5399.212

369 Joosen, A. M., & Westerterp, K. R. (2006). Energy expenditure during overfeeding. Nutrition & Metabolism, 3(1). https://doi.org/10.1186/1743-7075-3-25

370 Horton, T. J., Drougas, H., Brachey, A., Reed, G. W., Peters, J. C., & Hill, J. O. (1995). Fat and carbohydrate overfeeding in humans: different effects on energy storage. The American journal of clinical nutrition, 62(1), 19–29. https://doi.org/10.1093/ajcn/62.1.19

371 DeLany, J. P., Windhauser, M. M., Champagne, C. M., & Bray, G. A. (2000). Differential oxidation of individual dietary fatty acids in humans. The American Journal of Clinical Nutrition, 72(4), 905–911. https://doi.org/10.1093/ajcn/72.4.905

372 Lasekan, J. B., Rivera, J., Hirvonen, M. D., Keesey, R. E., & Ney, D. M. (1992). Energy expenditure in rats maintained with intravenous or intragastric infusion of total parenteral nutrition solutions containing medium- or long-chain triglyceride emulsions. The Journal of nutrition, 122(7), 1483–1492. https://doi.org/10.1093/jn/122.7.1483

373 Horton, T. J., Drougas, H., Brachey, A., Reed, G. W., Peters, J. C., & Hill, J. O. (1995). Fat and carbohydrate overfeeding in humans: different effects on energy storage. The American journal of clinical nutrition, 62(1), 19–29. https://doi.org/10.1093/ajcn/62.1.19

374 Piers, L. S., Walker, K. Z., Stoney, R. M., Soares, M. J., & O'Dea, K. (2003). Substitution of saturated with monounsaturated fat in a 4-week diet affects body weight and composition of overweight and obese men. The British journal of nutrition, 90(3), 717–727. https://doi.org/10.1079/bjn2003948

253

[375] Holt, S. H., Miller, J. C., Petocz, P., & Farmakalidis, E. (1995). A satiety index of common foods. European journal of clinical nutrition, 49(9), 675–690.

376 Lindqvist, A., de la Cour, C. D., Stegmark, A., Håkanson, R., & Erlanson-Albertsson, C. (2005). Overeating of palatable food is associated with blunted leptin and ghrelin responses. Regulatory Peptides, 130(3), 123–132. doi:10.1016/j.regpep.2005.05.002

377 Friedman, J. M., & Halaas, J. L.·(1998). Leptin and the regulation of body weight in mammals. Nature, 395(6704), 763–770. doi:10.1038/27376

378 Margetic, S., Gazzola, C., Pegg, G. G., & Hill, R. A. (2002). Leptin: a review of its peripheral actions and interactions. International journal of obesity and related metabolic disorders : journal of the International Association for the Study of Obesity, 26(11), 1407–1433. https://doi.org/10.1038/sj.ijo.0802142

379 Montague, C. T., Farooqi, I. S., Whitehead, J. P., Soos, M. A., Rau, H., Wareham, N. J., Sewter, C. P., Digby, J. E., Mohammed, S. N., Hurst, J. A., Cheetham, C. H., Earley, A. R., Barnett, A. H., Prins, J. B., & O'Rahilly, S. (1997). Congenital leptin deficiency is associated with severe early-onset obesity in humans. Nature, 387(6636), 903–908. https://doi.org/10.1038/43185

380 Farooqi, I. S., Matarese, G., Lord, G. M., Keogh, J. M., Lawrence, E., Agwu, C., Sanna, V., Jebb, S. A., Perna, F., Fontana, S., Lechler, R. I., DePaoli, A. M., & O'Rahilly, S. (2002). Beneficial effects of leptin on obesity, T cell hyporesponsiveness, and neuroendocrine/metabolic dysfunction of human congenital leptin deficiency. The Journal of clinical investigation, 110(8), 1093–1103. https://doi.org/10.1172/JCI15693

381 Gibson, W. T., Farooqi, I. S., Moreau, M., DePaoli, A. M., Lawrence, E., O'Rahilly, S., & Trussell, R. A. (2004). Congenital leptin deficiency due to homozygosity for the Delta133G mutation: report of another case and evaluation of response to four years of leptin therapy. The Journal of clinical endocrinology and metabolism, 89(10), 4821–4826. https://doi.org/10.1210/jc.2004-0376

382 Farooqi, I. S., Jebb, S. A., Langmack, G., Lawrence, E., Cheetham, C. H., Prentice, A. M., Hughes, I. A., McCamish, M. A., & O'Rahilly, S. (1999). Effects of recombinant leptin therapy in a child with congenital leptin deficiency. The New England journal of medicine, 341(12), 879–884. https://doi.org/10.1056/NEJM199909163411204

383 Knight, Z. A., Hannan, K. S., Greenberg, M. L., & Friedman, J. M. (2010). Hyperleptinemia Is Required for the Development of Leptin Resistance. PLoS ONE, 5(6), e11376. doi:10.1371/journal.pone.0011376

384 Haas, V. K., Gaskin, K. J., Kohn, M. R., Clarke, S. D., & Müller, M. J. (2010). Different thermic effects of leptin in adolescent females with varying body fat content. Clinical nutrition (Edinburgh, Scotland), 29(5), 639–645. https://doi.org/10.1016/j.clnu.2010.03.013

385 Maffei, M., Halaas, J., Ravussin, E., Pratley, R. E., Lee, G. H., Zhang, Y., ... Friedman, J. M. (1995). Leptin levels in human and rodent: Measurement of plasma leptin and ob RNA in obese and weight-reduced subjects. Nature Medicine, 1(11), 1155–1161. doi:10.1038/nm1195-1155

386 Jung, C. H., & Kim, M. S. (2013). Molecular mechanisms of central leptin resistance in obesity. Archives of pharmacal research, 36(2), 201–207. https://doi.org/10.1007/s12272-013-0020-y

387 Knudsen, N., Laurberg, P., Perrild, H., Bülow, I., Ovesen, L., & Jørgensen, T. (2002). Risk factors for goiter and thyroid nodules. Thyroid : official journal of the American Thyroid Association, 12(10), 879–888. https://doi.org/10.1089/105072502761016502

388 Schomburg L. (2011). Selenium, selenoproteins and the thyroid gland: interactions in health and disease. Nature reviews. Endocrinology, 8(3), 160–171. https://doi.org/10.1038/nrendo.2011.174

389 Schomburg, L. (2011). Selenium, selenoproteins and the thyroid gland: interactions in health and disease. Nature Reviews Endocrinology, 8(3), 160–171. doi:10.1038/nrendo.2011.174

390 Milanesi and Brent (2017) 'Chapter 12 - Iodine and Thyroid Hormone Synthesis, Metabolism, and Action', Molecular, Genetic, and Nutritional Aspects of Major and Trace Minerals, Pages 143-150, DOI: https://doi.org/10.1016/B978-0-12-802168-2.00012-9

391 Hennemann, G., Docter, R., Friesema, E. C. H., de Jong, M., Krenning, E. P., & Visser, T. J. (2001). Plasma Membrane Transport of Thyroid Hormones and Its Role inThyroid Hormone Metabolism and Bioavailability. Endocrine Reviews, 22(4), 451–476. doi:10.1210/edrv.22.4.0435

392 Krenning, E., Docter, R., Bernard, B., Visser, T., & Hennemann, G. (1981). Characteristics of active transport of thyroid hormone into rat hepatocytes. Biochimica et biophysica acta, 676(3), 314–320. https://doi.org/10.1016/0304-4165(81)90165-3

393 Centanni, M., & Robbins, J. (1987). Role of sodium in thyroid hormone uptake by rat skeletal muscle. The Journal of clinical investigation, 80(4), 1068–1072. https://doi.org/10.1172/JCI113162

394 de Jong, M., Visser, T. J., Bernard, B. F., Docter, R., Vos, R. A., Hennemann, G., & Krenning, E. P. (1993). Transport and metabolism of iodothyronines in cultured human hepatocytes. The Journal of clinical endocrinology and metabolism, 77(1), 139–143. https://doi.org/10.1210/jcem.77.1.8392080

395 Krenning, E., Docter, R., Bernard, B., Visser, T., & Hennemann, G. (1980). Regulation of the active transport of 3,3',5-triiodothyronine (T3) into primary cultured rat hepatocytes by ATP. FEBS letters, 119(2), 279–282. https://doi.org/10.1016/0014-5793(80)80271-7

396 Osty, J., Valensi, P., Samson, M., Francon, J., & Blondeau, J. P. (1990). Transport of thyroid hormones by human erythrocytes: kinetic characterization in adults and newborns. The Journal of clinical endocrinology and metabolism, 71(6), 1589–1595. https://doi.org/10.1210/jcem-71-6-1589

397 Winther, K. H., Rayman, M. P., Bonnema, S. J., & Hegedüs, L. (2020). Selenium in thyroid disorders - essential knowledge for clinicians. Nature reviews. Endocrinology, 16(3), 165–176. https://doi.org/10.1038/s41574-019-0311-6

398 Mehran, L., Amouzegar, A., Rahimabad, P. K., Tohidi, M., Tahmasebinejad, Z., & Azizi, F. (2017). Thyroid Function and Metabolic Syndrome: A Population-Based Thyroid Study. Hormone and metabolic research = Hormon- und Stoffwechselforschung = Hormones et metabolisme, 49(3), 192–200. https://doi.org/10.1055/s-0042-117279

399 Cappola, A. R., Desai, A. S., Medici, M., Cooper, L. S., Egan, D., Sopko, G., ... Wassner, A. J. (2019). Thyroid and Cardiovascular Disease. Circulation, 139(25), 2892–2909. doi:10.1161/circulationaha.118.036859

400 Laurberg, P., Knudsen, N., Andersen, S., Carlé, A., Pedersen, I. B., & Karmisholt, J. (2012). Thyroid Function and Obesity. European Thyroid Journal, 1(3), 159–167. doi:10.1159/000342994

401 Samuels, M. H. (2014). Psychiatric and cognitive manifestations of hypothyroidism. Current Opinion in Endocrinology & Diabetes and Obesity, 21(5), 377–383. doi:10.1097/med.0000000000000089

402 Bennett, W. E., & Heuckeroth, R. O. (2012). Hypothyroidism Is a Rare Cause of Isolated Constipation. Journal of Pediatric Gastroenterology and Nutrition, 54(2), 285–287. doi:10.1097/mpg.0b013e318239714f

403 (2013). International Journal of Geriatric Psychiatry, 28(2). doi:10.1002/gps.v28.2

404 Wolf, F. (2003). Cell physiology of magnesium. Molecular Aspects of Medicine, 24(1-3), 11–26. doi:10.1016/s0098-2997(02)00088-2

405 Takaya, J., Higashino, H., & Kobayashi, Y. (2004). Intracellular magnesium and insulin resistance. Magnesium research, 17(2), 126–136.

[406] Pittler, M. H., Stevinson, C., & Ernst, E. (2003). Chromium picolinate for reducing body weight: meta-analysis of randomized trials. International journal of obesity and related metabolic disorders : journal of the International Association for the Study of Obesity, 27(4), 522–529. https://doi.org/10.1038/sj.ijo.0802262

[407] Onakpoya, I., Posadzki, P., & Ernst, E. (2013). Chromium supplementation in overweight and obesity: a systematic review and meta-analysis of randomized clinical trials. Obesity reviews : an official journal of the International Association for the Study of Obesity, 14(6), 496–507. https://doi.org/10.1111/obr.12026

[408] Willoughby, D., Hewlings, S., & Kalman, D. (2018). Body Composition Changes in Weight Loss: Strategies and Supplementation for Maintaining Lean Body Mass, a Brief Review. Nutrients, 10(12), 1876. https://doi.org/10.3390/nu10121876

[409] Tian, H., Guo, X., Wang, X., He, Z., Sun, R., Ge, S., & Zhang, Z. (2013). Chromium picolinate supplementation for overweight or obese adults. The Cochrane database of systematic reviews, 2013(11), CD010063. https://doi.org/10.1002/14651858.CD010063.pub2

[410] Tsang, C., Taghizadeh, M., Aghabagheri, E., Asemi, Z., & Jafarnejad, S. (2019). A meta-analysis of the effect of chromium supplementation on anthropometric indices of subjects with overweight or obesity. Clinical obesity, 9(4), e12313. https://doi.org/10.1111/cob.12313

[411] Anton, S. D., Morrison, C. D., Cefalu, W. T., Martin, C. K., Coulon, S., Geiselman, P., Han, H., White, C. L., & Williamson, D. A. (2008). Effects of chromium picolinate on food intake and satiety. Diabetes technology & therapeutics, 10(5), 405–412. https://doi.org/10.1089/dia.2007.0292

[412] Manore M. M. (2012). Dietary supplements for improving body composition and reducing body weight: where is the evidence?. International journal of sport nutrition and exercise metabolism, 22(2), 139–154. https://doi.org/10.1123/ijsnem.22.2.139

413 Fothergill, E., Guo, J., Howard, L., Kerns, J.C., Knuth, N.D., Brychta, R., Chen, K.Y., Skarulis, M.C., Walter, M., Walter, P.J. and Hall, K.D. (2016), Persistent metabolic adaptation 6 years after "The Biggest Loser" competition. Obesity, 24: 1612-1619. https://doi.org/10.1002/oby.21538

[414] Piers, L. S., Walker, K. Z., Stoney, R. M., Soares, M. J., & O'Dea, K. (2003). Substitution of saturated with monounsaturated fat in a 4-week diet affects body weight and composition of overweight and obese men. The British journal of nutrition, 90(3), 717–727. https://doi.org/10.1079/bjn2003948

[415] Moeller, L. C., & Broecker-Preuss, M. (2011). Transcriptional regulation by nonclassical action of thyroid hormone. Thyroid research, 4 Suppl 1(Suppl 1), S6. https://doi.org/10.1186/1756-6614-4-S1-S6

[416] Yen P. M. (2001). Physiological and molecular basis of thyroid hormone action. Physiological reviews, 81(3), 1097–1142. https://doi.org/10.1152/physrev.2001.81.3.1097

[417] Knudsen, N., Laurberg, P., Rasmussen, L. B., Bülow, I., Perrild, H., Ovesen, L., & Jørgensen, T. (2005). Small Differences in Thyroid Function May Be Important for Body Mass Index and the Occurrence of Obesity in the Population. The Journal of Clinical Endocrinology & Metabolism, 90(7), 4019–4024. doi:10.1210/jc.2004-2225

[418] Fox, C. S., Pencina, M. J., D'Agostino, R. B., Murabito, J. M., Seely, E. W., Pearce, E. N., & Vasan, R. S. (2008). Relations of thyroid function to body weight: cross-sectional and longitudinal observations in a community-based sample. Archives of internal medicine, 168(6), 587–592. https://doi.org/10.1001/archinte.168.6.587

[419] Laurberg, P., Knudsen, N., Andersen, S., Carlé, A., Pedersen, I. B., & Karmisholt, J. (2012). Thyroid Function and Obesity. European Thyroid Journal, 1(3), 159–167. doi:10.1159/000342994

[420] Samuels, M. H. (2014). Psychiatric and cognitive manifestations of hypothyroidism. Current Opinion in Endocrinology & Diabetes and Obesity, 21(5), 377–383. doi:10.1097/med.0000000000000089

[421] Bennett, W. E., & Heuckeroth, R. O. (2012). Hypothyroidism Is a Rare Cause of Isolated Constipation. Journal of Pediatric Gastroenterology and Nutrition, 54(2), 285–287. doi:10.1097/mpg.0b013e318239714f

[422] Joffe, R.T., Pearce, E.N., Hennessey, J.V., Ryan, J.J. and Stern, R.A. (2013), Subclinical hypothyroidism, mood, and cognition in older adults: a review. Int J Geriatr Psychiatry, 28: 111-118. doi:10.1002/gps.3796

[423] Dons, Robert F.; Jr, Frank H. Wians (2009). *Endocrine and metabolic disorders clinical lab testing manual* (4th ed.). Boca Raton: CRC Press. p. 10. ISBN 9781420079364.

[424] Nordio, M., & Basciani, S. (2017). Myo-inositol plus selenium supplementation restores euthyroid state in Hashimoto's patients with subclinical hypothyroidism. European review for medical and pharmacological sciences, 21(2 Suppl), 51–59.

[425] Ongphiphadhanakul, B., Fang, S. L., Tang, K.-T., Patwardhan, N. A., & Braverman, L. E. (1994). Tumor necrosis factor-α decreases thyrotropin-induced 5'-deiodinase activity in FRTL-5 thyroid cells. European Journal of Endocrinology, 130(5), 502–507. doi:10.1530/eje.0.1300502

[426] Abdullatif, H. D., & Ashraf, A. P. (2006). REVERSIBLE SUBCLINICAL HYPOTHYROIDISM IN THE PRESENCE OF ADRENAL INSUFFICIENCY. Endocrine Practice, 12(5), 572–575. doi:10.4158/ep.12.5.572

[427] Wajner, S. M., Goemann, I. M., Bueno, A. L., Larsen, P. R., & Maia, A. L. (2011). IL-6 promotes nonthyroidal illness syndrome by blocking thyroxine activation while promoting thyroid hormone inactivation in human cells. Journal of Clinical Investigation, 121(5), 1834–1845. doi:10.1172/jci44678

[428] Bartalena, L., Brogioni, S., Grasso, L., Velluzzi, F., & Martino, E. (1994). Relationship of the increased serum interleukin-6 concentration to changes of thyroid function in nonthyroidal illness. Journal of Endocrinological Investigation, 17(4), 269–274. doi:10.1007/bf03348974

[429] Corssmit, E. P., Heyligenberg, R., Endert, E., Sauerwein, H. P., & Romijn, J. A. (1995). Acute effects of interferon-alpha administration on thyroid hormone metabolism in healthy men. The Journal of Clinical Endocrinology & Metabolism, 80(11), 3140–3144. doi:10.1210/jcem.80.11.7593416

[430] Bohr et al (1904) 'Concerning a Biologically Important Relationship - The Influence of the Carbon Dioxide Content of Blood on its Oxygen Binding', Skand. Arch. Physiol. 16, 401-412 (1904) by Ulf Marquardt for CHEM-342, January 1997, Accessed Online: https://www1.udel.edu/chem/white/C342/Bohr(1904).html

[431] Stegen, K., De Bruyne, K., Rasschaert, W., Van de Woestijne, K. P., & Van den Bergh, O. (1999). Fear-relevant images as conditioned stimuli for somatic complaints, respiratory behavior, and reduced end-tidal pCO_2. Journal of Abnormal Psychology, 108(1), 143–152. doi:10.1037/0021-843x.108.1.143

[432] Lee and Levine (1999) 'Acute respiratory alkalosis associated with low minute ventilation in a patient with severe hypothyroidism', Can J Anaesth. 1999 Feb;46(2):185-9.

[433] Ellis, Amy C; Hyatt, Tanya C; Gower, Barbara A; Hunter, Gary R (2017-05-02). "Respiratory Quotient Predicts Fat Mass Gain in Premenopausal Women". *Obesity (Silver Spring, Md.)*. 18 (12): 2255–2259.

[434] al-Saady et al (1989) 'High fat, low carbohydrate, enteral feeding lowers PaCO2 and reduces the period of ventilation in artificially ventilated patients', Intensive Care Med. 1989;15(5):290-5.

[435] Fade, J. V., Franklyn, J. A., Cross, K. W., Jones, S. C., & Sheppard, M. C. (1991). Prevalence and follow-up of abnormal thyrotrophin (TSH) concentrations in the elderly in the United Kingdom. Clinical Endocrinology, 34(1), 77–84. doi:10.1111/j.1365-2265.1991.tb01739.x

[436] Åsvold, B. O., Vatten, L. J., & Bjøro, T. (2013). Changes in the prevalence of hypothyroidism: the HUNT Study in Norway. European Journal of Endocrinology, 169(5), 613–620. doi:10.1530/eje-13-0459

[437] Canaris, G. J., Manowitz, N. R., Mayor, G., & Ridgway, E. C. (2000). The Colorado Thyroid Disease Prevalence Study. Archives of Internal Medicine, 160(4), 526. doi:10.1001/archinte.160.4.526

[438] McGrogan, A., Seaman, H. E., Wright, J. W., & de Vries, C. S. (2008). The incidence of autoimmune thyroid disease: a systematic review of the literature. Clinical endocrinology, 69(5), 687–696. https://doi.org/10.1111/j.1365-2265.2008.03338.x

[439] Garmendia Madariaga, A., Santos Palacios, S., Guillén-Grima, F., & Galofré, J. C. (2014). The Incidence and Prevalence of Thyroid Dysfunction in Europe: A Meta-Analysis. The Journal of Clinical Endocrinology & Metabolism, 99(3), 923–931. doi:10.1210/jc.2013-2409

[440] Protsiv, M., Ley, C., Lankester, J., Hastie, T., & Parsonnet, J. (2020). Decreasing human body temperature in the United States since the Industrial Revolution. eLife, 9. doi:10.7554/elife.49555

[441] Landsberg, L., Young, J. B., Leonard, W. R., Linsenmeier, R. A., & Turek, F. W. (2009). Is obesity associated with lower body temperatures? Core temperature: a forgotten variable in energy balance. Metabolism, 58(6), 871–876. doi:10.1016/j.metabol.2009.02.017

[442] Asvold, B. O., Bjøro, T., & Vatten, L. J. (2009). Association of serum TSH with high body mass differs between smokers and never-smokers. The Journal of clinical endocrinology and metabolism, 94(12), 5023–5027. https://doi.org/10.1210/jc.2009-1180

[443] De Pergola, G., Ciampolillo, A., Paolotti, S., Trerotoli, P., & Giorgino, R. (2007). Free triiodothyronine and thyroid stimulating hormone are directly associated with waist circumference, independently of insulin resistance, metabolic parameters and blood pressure in overweight and obese women. Clinical endocrinology, 67(2), 265–269. https://doi.org/10.1111/j.1365-2265.2007.02874.x

[444] Iacobellis, G., Ribaudo, M. C., Zappaterreno, A., Iannucci, C. V., & Leonetti, F. (2005). Relationship of thyroid function with body mass index, leptin, insulin sensitivity and adiponectin in euthyroid obese women. Clinical endocrinology, 62(4), 487–491. https://doi.org/10.1111/j.1365-2265.2005.02247.x

[445] Radetti, G., Kleon, W., Buzi, F., Crivellaro, C., Pappalardo, L., di Iorgi, N., & Maghnie, M. (2008). Thyroid function and structure are affected in childhood obesity. The Journal of clinical endocrinology and metabolism, 93(12), 4749–4754. https://doi.org/10.1210/jc.2008-0823

[446] Moulin de Moraes, C. M., Mancini, M. C., de Melo, M. E., Figueiredo, D. A., Villares, S. M., Rascovski, A., Zilberstein, B., & Halpern, A. (2005). Prevalence of subclinical hypothyroidism in a morbidly obese population and improvement after weight loss induced by Roux-en-Y gastric bypass. Obesity surgery, 15(9), 1287–1291. https://doi.org/10.1381/096089205774512537

[447] Bastemir, M., Akin, F., Alkis, E., & Kaptanoglu, B. (2007). Obesity is associated with increased serum TSH level, independent of thyroid function. Swiss medical weekly, 137(29-30), 431–434.

[448] Nyrnes, A., Jorde, R., & Sundsfjord, J. (2005). Serum TSH is positively associated with BMI. International Journal of Obesity, 30(1), 100–105. https://doi.org/10.1038/sj.ijo.0803112

[449] Fox, C. S., Pencina, M. J., D'Agostino, R. B., Murabito, J. M., Seely, E. W., Pearce, E. N., & Vasan, R. S. (2008). Relations of thyroid function to body weight: cross-sectional and longitudinal observations in a community-based sample. Archives of internal medicine, 168(6), 587–592. https://doi.org/10.1001/archinte.168.6.587

[450] Alevizaki, M., Saltiki, K., Voidonikola, P., Mantzou, E., Papamichael, C., & Stamatelopoulos, K. (2009). Free thyroxine is an independent predictor of subcutaneous fat in euthyroid individuals. European journal of endocrinology, 161(3), 459–465. https://doi.org/10.1530/EJE-09-0441

[451] Knudsen, N., Laurberg, P., Rasmussen, L. B., Bülow, I., Perrild, H., Ovesen, L., & Jørgensen, T. (2005). Small differences in thyroid function may be important for body mass index and the occurrence of obesity in the population. The Journal of clinical endocrinology and metabolism, 90(7), 4019–4024. https://doi.org/10.1210/jc.2004-2225

[452] Knudsen, N., Laurberg, P., Rasmussen, L. B., Bülow, I., Perrild, H., Ovesen, L., & Jørgensen, T. (2005). Small differences in thyroid function may be important for body mass index and the occurrence of obesity in the population. The Journal of clinical endocrinology and metabolism, 90(7), 4019–4024. https://doi.org/10.1210/jc.2004-2225

[453] Reinehr, T., de Sousa, G., & Andler, W. (2006). Hyperthyrotropinemia in obese children is reversible after weight loss and is not related to lipids. The Journal of clinical endocrinology and metabolism, 91(8), 3088–3091. https://doi.org/10.1210/jc.2006-0095

[454] Kok, P., Roelfsema, F., Langendonk, J. G., Frölich, M., Burggraaf, J., Meinders, A. E., & Pijl, H. (2005). High circulating thyrotropin levels in obese women are reduced after body weight loss induced by caloric restriction. The Journal of clinical endocrinology and metabolism, 90(8), 4659–4663. https://doi.org/10.1210/jc.2005-0920

[455] Santini, F., Galli, G., Maffei, M., Fierabracci, P., Pelosini, C., Marsili, A., Giannetti, M., Castagna, M. G., Checchi, S., Molinaro, E., Piaggi, P., Pacini, F., Elisei, R., Vitti, P., & Pinchera, A. (2010). Acute exogenous TSH administration stimulates leptin secretion in vivo. European journal of endocrinology, 163(1), 63–67. https://doi.org/10.1530/EJE-10-0138

[456] Oge, A., Bayraktar, F., Saygili, F., Guney, E., & Demir, S. (2005). TSH influences serum leptin levels independent of thyroid hormones in hypothyroid and hyperthyroid patients. Endocrine journal, 52(2), 213–217. https://doi.org/10.1507/endocrj.52.213

[457] Menendez, C., Baldelli, R., Camiña, J. P., Escudero, B., Peino, R., Dieguez, C., & Casanueva, F. F. (2003). TSH stimulates leptin secretion by a direct effect on adipocytes. The Journal of endocrinology, 176(1), 7–12. https://doi.org/10.1677/joe.0.1760007

[458] Iacobellis, G., Ribaudo, M. C., Zappaterreno, A., Iannucci, C. V., & Leonetti, F. (2005). Relationship of thyroid function with body mass index, leptin, insulin sensitivity and adiponectin in euthyroid obese women. Clinical endocrinology, 62(4), 487–491. https://doi.org/10.1111/j.1365-2265.2005.02247.x

[459] Zimmermann-Belsing, T., Brabant, G., Holst, J. J., & Feldt-Rasmussen, U. (2003). Circulating leptin and thyroid dysfunction. European journal of endocrinology, 149(4), 257–271. https://doi.org/10.1530/eje.0.1490257

[460] Reinehr T. (2010). Obesity and thyroid function. Molecular and cellular endocrinology, 316(2), 165–171. https://doi.org/10.1016/j.mce.2009.06.005

[461] Reinehr, T., de Sousa, G., & Andler, W. (2006). Hyperthyrotropinemia in obese children is reversible after weight loss and is not related to lipids. The Journal of clinical endocrinology and metabolism, 91(8), 3088–3091. https://doi.org/10.1210/jc.2006-0095

[462] Nannipieri, M., Cecchetti, F., Anselmino, M., Camastra, S., Niccolini, P., Lamacchia, M., Rossi, M., Iervasi, G., & Ferrannini, E. (2009). Expression of thyrotropin and thyroid hormone receptors in adipose tissue of patients with morbid obesity and/or type 2 diabetes: effects of weight loss. International journal of obesity (2005), 33(9), 1001–1006. https://doi.org/10.1038/ijo.2009.140

[463] De Pergola, G., Ciampolillo, A., Paolotti, S., Trerotoli, P., & Giorgino, R. (2007). Free triiodothyronine and thyroid stimulating hormone are directly associated with waist circumference, independently of insulin resistance, metabolic parameters and blood pressure in overweight and obese women. Clinical endocrinology, 67(2), 265–269. https://doi.org/10.1111/j.1365-2265.2007.02874.x

[464] Cusin, I., Rouru, J., Visser, T., Burger, A. G., & Rohner-Jeanrenaud, F. (2000). Involvement of thyroid hormones in the effect of intracerebroventricular leptin infusion on uncoupling protein-3 expression in rat muscle. Diabetes, 49(7), 1101–1105. https://doi.org/10.2337/diabetes.49.7.1101

[465] Gong, D. W., He, Y., Karas, M., & Reitman, M. (1997). Uncoupling protein-3 is a mediator of thermogenesis regulated by thyroid hormone, beta3-adrenergic agonists, and leptin. The Journal of biological chemistry, 272(39), 24129–24132. https://doi.org/10.1074/jbc.272.39.24129

[466] Nannipieri, M., Cecchetti, F., Anselmino, M., Camastra, S., Niccolini, P., Lamacchia, M., Rossi, M., Iervasi, G., & Ferrannini, E. (2009). Expression of thyrotropin and thyroid hormone receptors in adipose tissue of patients with morbid obesity and/or type 2 diabetes: effects of weight loss. International journal of obesity (2005), 33(9), 1001–1006. https://doi.org/10.1038/ijo.2009.140

[467] Kok, P., Roelfsema, F., Langendonk, J. G., Frölich, M., Burggraaf, J., Meinders, A. E., & Pijl, H. (2005). High circulating thyrotropin levels in obese women are reduced after body weight loss induced by caloric restriction. The Journal of clinical endocrinology and metabolism, 90(8), 4659–4663. https://doi.org/10.1210/jc.2005-0920

[468] Bray, G. A., Fisher, D. A., & Chopra, I. J. (1976). Relation of thyroid hormones to body-weight. Lancet (London, England), 1(7971), 1206–1208. https://doi.org/10.1016/s0140-6736(76)92158-9

[469] Vadiveloo, T., Donnan, P. T., Murphy, M. J., & Leese, G. P. (2013). Age- and Gender-Specific TSH Reference Intervals in People With No Obvious Thyroid Disease in Tayside, Scotland: The Thyroid Epidemiology, Audit, and Research Study (TEARS). The Journal of Clinical Endocrinology & Metabolism, 98(3), 1147–1153. doi:10.1210/jc.2012-3191

[470] Leung, A. M., & Braverman, L. E. (2014). Consequences of excess iodine. Nature reviews. Endocrinology, 10(3), 136–142. https://doi.org/10.1038/nrendo.2013.251

[471] Laurberg, P., Cerqueira, C., Ovesen, L., Rasmussen, L. B., Perrild, H., Andersen, S., Pedersen, I. B., & Carlé, A. (2010). Iodine intake as a determinant of thyroid disorders in populations. Best practice & research. Clinical endocrinology & metabolism, 24(1), 13–27. https://doi.org/10.1016/j.beem.2009.08.013

[472] Teng, W., Shan, Z., Teng, X., Guan, H., Li, Y., Teng, D., … Li, C. (2006). Effect of Iodine Intake on Thyroid Diseases in China. New England Journal of Medicine, 354(26), 2783–2793. doi:10.1056/nejmoa054022

[473] Farebrother, J., Zimmermann, M. B., & Andersson, M. (2019). Excess iodine intake: sources, assessment, and effects on thyroid function. Annals of the New York Academy of Sciences, 1446(1), 44–65. https://doi.org/10.1111/nyas.14041

[474] Flores-Rebollar, A., Moreno-Castañeda, L., Vega-Servín, N. S., López-Carrasco, G., & Ruiz-Juvera, A. (2015). PREVALENCE OF AUTOIMMUNE THYROIDITIS AND THYROID DYSFUNCTION IN HEALTHY ADULT MEXICANS WITH A SLIGHTLY EXCESSIVE IODINE INTAKE. Nutricion hospitalaria, 32(2), 918–924. https://doi.org/10.3305/nh.2015.32.2.9246

[475] Luo, Y., Kawashima, A., Ishido, Y., Yoshihara, A., Oda, K., Hiroi, N., Ito, T., Ishii, N., & Suzuki, K. (2014). Iodine excess as an environmental risk factor for autoimmune thyroid disease. International journal of molecular sciences, 15(7), 12895–12912. https://doi.org/10.3390/ijms150712895

[476] NIH (2020) 'Iodine: Fact Sheet for Health Professionals', Dietary Supplement Fact Sheets, Accessed Online Dec 20 2020: https://ods.od.nih.gov/factsheets/Iodine-HealthProfessional/

[477] World Health Organization & Food and Agriculture Organization of the United Nations. (2004). 'Vitamin and mineral requirements in human nutrition'. Geneva, Switzerland: WHO. Accessed Online Dec 20 2020: https://www.who.int/nutrition/publications/micronutrients/9241546123/en/

[478] Institute of Medicine (US) Panel on Micronutrients (2001) 'Dietary Reference Intakes for Vitamin A, Vitamin K, Arsenic, Boron, Chromium, Copper, Iodine, Iron, Manganese, Molybdenum, Nickel, Silicon, Vanadium, and Zinc', Washington (DC): National Academies Press (US); 2001.

[479] Gardner, D. F., Centor, R. M., & Utiger, R. D. (1988). Effects of low dose oral iodide supplementation on thyroid function in normal men. Clinical endocrinology, 28(3), 283–288. https://doi.org/10.1111/j.1365-2265.1988.tb01214.x

[480] World Health Organization. 1989. Toxological evaluation of certain food additives and contaminants. WHO Food Additives Series 24. Prepared by: The 33rd Meeting of the Joint FAO/WHO Expert Committee on Food Additives (JECFA). Geneva, Switzerland: World Health Organization.

[481] World Health Organization (2013) 'Urinary iodine concentrations for determining iodine status in populations', WHO/NMH/NHD/EPG/13.1, Accessed Online March 30th 2022: https://www.who.int/vmnis/indicators/urinaryiodine/en/

[482] Zava, T. T., & Zava, D. T. (2011). Assessment of Japanese iodine intake based on seaweed consumption in Japan: A literature-based analysis. Thyroid research, 4, 14. https://doi.org/10.1186/1756-6614-4-14

[483] Pennington JAT, Schoen SA, Salmon GD, Young B, Johnson RD, Marts RW. Composition of Core Foods of the U.S. Food Supply, 1982-1991. III. Copper, Manganese, Selenium, and Iodine. J Food Comp Anal. 1995;8(2):171-217.

[484] Meikle, A. W. (2004). The Interrelationships Between Thyroid Dysfunction and Hypogonadism in Men and Boys. Thyroid, 14(supplement 1), 17–25. doi:10.1089/105072504323024552

[485] Endocrine Society. (2012, June 25). Overweight men can boost low testosterone levels by losing weight. ScienceDaily. Retrieved March 17, 2022 from www.sciencedaily.com/releases/2012/06/120625124914.htm

[486] Allan, C. A., & McLachlan, R. I. (2010). Androgens and obesity. Current opinion in endocrinology, diabetes, and obesity, 17(3), 224–232. https://doi.org/10.1097/MED.0b013e3283398ee2

[487] Fui, M. N., Dupuis, P., & Grossmann, M. (2014). Lowered testosterone in male obesity: mechanisms, morbidity and management. Asian journal of andrology, 16(2), 223–231. https://doi.org/10.4103/1008-682X.122365

[488] Traish, A. M. (2014). Testosterone and weight loss. Current Opinion in Endocrinology, Diabetes & Obesity, 21(5), 313–322. https://doi.org/10.1097/med.0000000000000086

[489] Laughlin, G. A., Barrett-Connor, E., & Bergstrom, J. (2008). Low Serum Testosterone and Mortality in Older Men. The Journal of Clinical Endocrinology & Metabolism, 93(1), 68–75. doi:10.1210/jc.2007-1792

[490] De Pergola G. (2000). The adipose tissue metabolism: role of testosterone and dehydroepiandrosterone. International journal of obesity and related metabolic disorders : journal of the International Association for the Study of Obesity, 24 Suppl 2, S59–S63. https://doi.org/10.1038/sj.ijo.0801280

[491] Singh, R., Artaza, J. N., Taylor, W. E., Braga, M., Yuan, X., Gonzalez-Cadavid, N. F., & Bhasin, S. (2006). Testosterone inhibits adipogenic differentiation in 3T3-L1 cells: nuclear translocation of androgen receptor complex with beta-catenin and T-cell factor 4 may

bypass canonical Wnt signaling to down-regulate adipogenic transcription factors. Endocrinology, 147(1), 141–154. https://doi.org/10.1210/en.2004-1649

[492] Singh, R., Artaza, J. N., Taylor, W. E., Gonzalez-Cadavid, N. F., & Bhasin, S. (2003). Androgens stimulate myogenic differentiation and inhibit adipogenesis in C3H 10T1/2 pluripotent cells through an androgen receptor-mediated pathway. Endocrinology, 144(11), 5081–5088. https://doi.org/10.1210/en.2003-0741

[493] Sattler et al (2010) 'Testosterone Threshold Levels and Lean Tissue Mass Targets Needed to Enhance Skeletal Muscle Strength and Function: The HORMA Trial', The Journals of Gerontology: Series A, Volume 66A, Issue 1, January 2011, Pages 122–129, https://doi.org/10.1093/gerona/glq183

[494] Santosa, S., Khosla, S., McCready, L. K., & Jensen, M. D. (2010). Effects of estrogen and testosterone on resting energy expenditure in older men. Obesity (Silver Spring, Md.), 18(12), 2392–2394. https://doi.org/10.1038/oby.2010.98

[495] Zurlo, F., Larson, K., Bogardus, C., & Ravussin, E. (1990). Skeletal muscle metabolism is a major determinant of resting energy expenditure. The Journal of clinical investigation, 86(5), 1423–1427. https://doi.org/10.1172/JCI114857

[496] Yuki, A., Otsuka, R., Kozakai, R. et al. Relationship between Low Free Testosterone Levels and Loss of Muscle Mass. Sci Rep 3, 1818 (2013). https://doi.org/10.1038/srep01818

[497] Meikle A. W. (2004). The interrelationships between thyroid dysfunction and hypogonadism in men and boys. Thyroid : official journal of the American Thyroid Association, 14 Suppl 1, S17–S25. https://doi.org/10.1089/105072504323024552

[498] Chen, D., Yan, Y., Huang, H., Dong, Q., & Tian, H. (2018). The association between subclinical hypothyroidism and erectile dysfunction. Pakistan journal of medical sciences, 34(3), 621–625. https://doi.org/10.12669/pjms.343.14330

[499] Thomas L. Lemke; David A. Williams (2008). Foye's Principles of Medicinal Chemistry. Lippincott Williams & Wilkins. pp. 883–. ISBN 978-0-7817-6879-5.

[500] Sinha, R. A., Singh, B. K., & Yen, P. M. (2018). Direct effects of thyroid hormones on hepatic lipid metabolism. Nature reviews. Endocrinology, 14(5), 259–269. https://doi.org/10.1038/nrendo.2018.10

[501] Marx et al (2011). Pregnenolone as a novel therapeutic candidate in schizophrenia: emerging preclinical and clinical evidence. Neuroscience, 191, 78–90. https://doi.org/10.1016/j.neuroscience.2011.06.076

[502] HENDERSON, E., WEINBERG, M., & WRIGHT, W. A. (1950). Pregnenolone. The Journal of clinical endocrinology and metabolism, 10(4), 455–474. https://doi.org/10.1210/jcem-10-4-455

[503] Tagawa, N., Tamanaka, J., Fujinami, A., Kobayashi, Y., Takano, T., Fukata, S., Kuma, K., Tada, H., & Amino, N. (2000). Serum dehydroepiandrosterone, dehydroepiandrosterone sulfate, and pregnenolone sulfate concentrations in patients with hyperthyroidism and hypothyroidism. Clinical chemistry, 46(4), 523–528.

[504] Japundzic, M., Bastomsky, C. h., & Japundzic, I. (1975). Effet de la pregnenolone-16 alpha-carbonitrile sur l'activité de la glande thyroïde et l'antéhypophyse du rat [Effect of pregnenolone-16 alpha-carbonitrile on the activity of the rat thyroid gland and anterior pituitary]. Bulletin de l'Association des anatomistes, 59(165), 419–426.

[505] Kleine B, Rossmanith WG (11 February 2016). Hormones and the Endocrine System: Textbook of Endocrinology. Springer. pp. 264–265. ISBN 978-3-319-15060-4.

[506] Rainey, W. E., & Nakamura, Y. (2008). Regulation of the adrenal androgen biosynthesis. The Journal of steroid biochemistry and molecular biology, 108(3-5), 281–286. https://doi.org/10.1016/j.jsbmb.2007.09.015

[507] Pearce (2012) 'Update in Lipid Alterations in Subclinical Hypothyroidism', The Journal of Clinical Endocrinology & Metabolism, Volume 97, Issue 2, 1 February 2012, Pages 326–333, https://doi.org/10.1210/jc.2011-2532

[508] Abrams and Grundy (1981) 'Cholesterol metabolism in hypothyroidism and hyperthyroidism in man', J Lipid Res 1981 Feb;22(2):323-38.

[509] O'Donnell, A. B., Araujo, A. B., & McKinlay, J. B. (2004). The health of normally aging men: The Massachusetts Male Aging Study (1987–2004). Experimental Gerontology, 39(7), 975–984. doi:10.1016/j.exger.2004.03.023

[510] Travison et al (2007) 'A Population-Level Decline in Serum Testosterone Levels in American Men', Journal of Clinical Endocrinology & Metabolism 92(1):196-202, DOI: 10.1210/jc.2006-1375.

[511] https://www.ncbi.nlm.nih.gov/pmc/articles/PMC3880087/

[512] Pilz et al (2010) 'Effect of Vitamin D Supplementation on Testosterone Levels in Men', Hormone and Metabolic Research 43(3):223-5, DOI: 10.1055/s-0030-1269854

[513] Schooling, C. M., Au Yeung, S. L., Freeman, G., & Cowling, B. J. (2013). The effect of statins on testosterone in men and women, a systematic review and meta-analysis of randomized controlled trials. BMC Medicine, 11(1). doi:10.1186/1741-7015-11-57

[514] Frias, J. (2002). EFFECTS OF ACUTE ALCOHOL INTOXICATION ON PITUITARY-GONADAL AXIS HORMONES, PITUITARY-ADRENAL AXIS HORMONES, beta-ENDORPHIN AND PROLACTIN IN HUMAN ADULTS OF BOTH SEXES. Alcohol and Alcoholism, 37(2), 169–173. doi:10.1093/alcalc/37.2.169

[515] Meeker, J. D., & Ferguson, K. K. (2014). Urinary Phthalate Metabolites Are Associated With Decreased Serum Testosterone in Men, Women, and Children From NHANES 2011–2012. The Journal of Clinical Endocrinology & Metabolism, 99(11), 4346–4352. doi:10.1210/jc.2014-2555

[516] Purohit, V. (2000). Can alcohol promote aromatization of androgens to estrogens? A review. Alcohol, 22(3), 123–127. doi:10.1016/s0741-8329(00)00124-5

[517] Wang, C., Jackson, G., Jones, T. H., Matsumoto, A. M., Nehra, A., Perelman, M. A., … Cunningham, G. (2011). Low Testosterone Associated With Obesity and the Metabolic Syndrome Contributes to Sexual Dysfunction and Cardiovascular Disease Risk in Men With Type 2 Diabetes. Diabetes Care, 34(7), 1669–1675. doi:10.2337/dc10-2339

[518] Vermeulen, A., Kaufman, J. M., Goemaere, S., & van Pottelberg, I. (2002). Estradiol in elderly men. The aging male : the official journal of the International Society for the Study of the Aging Male, 5(2), 98–102.

[519] Hayes, F. J., DeCruz, S., Seminara, S. B., Boepple, P. A., & Crowley, W. F., Jr (2001). Differential regulation of gonadotropin secretion by testosterone in the human male: absence of a negative feedback effect of testosterone on follicle-stimulating hormone secretion. The Journal of clinical endocrinology and metabolism, 86(1), 53–58. https://doi.org/10.1210/jcem.86.1.7101

[520] George, J. T., Millar, R. P., & Anderson, R. A. (2010). Hypothesis: kisspeptin mediates male hypogonadism in obesity and type 2 diabetes. Neuroendocrinology, 91(4), 302–307. https://doi.org/10.1159/000299767

[521] Pellitero, S., Olaizola, I., Alastrue, A., Martínez, E., Granada, M. L., Balibrea, J. M., Moreno, P., Serra, A., Navarro-Díaz, M., Romero, R., & Puig-Domingo, M. (2012). Hypogonadotropic hypogonadism in morbidly obese males is reversed after bariatric surgery. Obesity surgery, 22(12), 1835–1842. https://doi.org/10.1007/s11695-012-0734-9

[522] Tajar, A., Forti, G., O'Neill, T. W., Lee, D. M., Silman, A. J., Finn, J. D., Bartfai, G., Boonen, S., Casanueva, F. F., Giwercman, A., Han, T. S., Kula, K., Labrie, F., Lean, M. E., Pendleton, N., Punab, M., Vanderschueren, D., Huhtaniemi, I. T., Wu, F. C., & EMAS Group

(2010). Characteristics of secondary, primary, and compensated hypogonadism in aging men: evidence from the European Male Ageing Study. The Journal of clinical endocrinology and metabolism, 95(4), 1810–1818. https://doi.org/10.1210/jc.2009-1796

[523] Grossmann, M., Tang Fui, M., & Dupuis, P. (2014). Lowered testosterone in male obesity: Mechanisms, morbidity and management. Asian Journal of Andrology, 16(2), 223. doi:10.4103/1008-682x.122365

[524] Grossmann, M., Cheung, A. S., & Zajac, J. D. (2013). Androgens and prostate cancer; pathogenesis and deprivation therapy. Best Practice & Research Clinical Endocrinology & Metabolism, 27(4), 603–616. doi:10.1016/j.beem.2013.05.001

[525] Frayn, K. N. (2000). Visceral fat and insulin resistance — causative or correlative? British Journal of Nutrition, 83(S1), S71–S77. doi:10.1017/s0007114500000982

[526] Ali Deb, A., Okechukwu, C. E., Emara, S., Gillott, L., & Abbas, S. A. (2019). Central obesity and erectile dysfunction in men. International Journal of Family & Community Medicine, 3(6). https://doi.org/10.15406/ijfcm.2019.03.00171

[527] Bergman, R. N., Kim, S. P., Catalano, K. J., Hsu, I. R., Chiu, J. D., Kabir, M. , Hucking, K. and Ader, M. (2006), Why Visceral Fat is Bad: Mechanisms of the Metabolic Syndrome. Obesity, 14: 16S-19S.

[528] Anderson, K. E., Rosner, W., Khan, M. S., New, M. I., Pang, S., Wissel, P. S., & Kappas, A. (1987). Diet-hormone interactions: Protein/carbohydrate ratio alters reciprocally the plasma levels of testosterone and cortisol and their respective binding globulins in man. Life Sciences, 40(18), 1761–1768. doi:10.1016/0024-3205(87)90086-5

[529] Whittaker, J., & Harris, M. (2022). Low-carbohydrate diets and men's cortisol and testosterone: Systematic review and meta-analysis. Nutrition and health, 2601060221083079. Advance online publication. https://doi.org/10.1177/02601060221083079

[530] Cignarelli, A., Conte, E., Genchi, V. A., Giordano, F., Leo, S. D., Perrini, S., Natalicchio, A., Laviola, L., & Giorgino, F. (2021). Effects of a very low-calorie ketogenic diet on androgen levels in overweight/obese men: a single-arm uncontrolled study. Endocrine Abstracts. https://doi.org/10.1530/endoabs.73.pep4.3

[531] Spaulding, S. W., Chopra, I. J., Sherwin, R. S., & Lyall, S. S. (1976). EFFECT OF CALORIC RESTRICTION AND DIETARY COMPOSITION ON SERUM T3 AND REVERSE T3 IN MAN. The Journal of Clinical Endocrinology & Metabolism, 42(1), 197–200. doi:10.1210/jcem-42-1-197

[532] Elmquist, J. K., Maratos-Flier, E., Saper, C. B., & Flier, J. S. (1998). Unraveling the central nervous system pathways underlying responses to leptin. Nature neuroscience, 1(6), 445–450. https://doi.org/10.1038/2164

[533] Paz-Filho, G., Wong, M.-L., Licinio, J., & Mastronardi, C. (2012). Leptin therapy, insulin sensitivity, and glucose homeostasis. Indian Journal of Endocrinology and Metabolism, 16(9), 549. doi:10.4103/2230-8210.105571

[534] Berglund, E. D., Vianna, C. R., Donato, J., Kim, M. H., Chuang, J.-C., Lee, C. E., … Elmquist, J. K. (2012). Direct leptin action on POMC neurons regulates glucose homeostasis and hepatic insulin sensitivity in mice. Journal of Clinical Investigation, 122(3), 1000–1009. doi:10.1172/jci59816

535 Brownlee, K. K., Moore, A. W., & Hackney, A. C. (2005). Relationship between circulating cortisol and testosterone: influence of physical exercise. Journal of sports science & medicine, 4(1), 76–83.

536 Bambino, T. H., & Hsueh, A. J. (1981). Direct inhibitory effect of glucocorticoids upon testicular luteinizing hormone receptor and steroidogenesis in vivo and in vitro. Endocrinology, 108(6), 2142–2148. https://doi.org/10.1210/endo-108-6-2142

[537] Meeker, J. D., & Ferguson, K. K. (2014). Urinary phthalate metabolites are associated with decreased serum testosterone in men, women, and children from NHANES 2011-2012. The Journal of clinical endocrinology and metabolism, 99(11), 4346 4352. https://doi.org/10.1210/jc.2014-2555

[538] Chang, W. H., Li, S. S., Wu, M. H., Pan, H. A., & Lee, C. C. (2015). Phthalates might interfere with testicular function by reducing testosterone and insulin-like factor 3 levels. Human reproduction (Oxford, England), 30(11), 2658–2670. https://doi.org/10.1093/humrep/dev225

[539] Axelsson, J., Ingre, M., Åkerstedt, T., & Holmbäck, U. (2005). Effects of Acutely Displaced Sleep on Testosterone. The Journal of Clinical Endocrinology & Metabolism, 90(8), 4530–4535. doi:10.1210/jc.2005-0520

[540] Leproult and Van Cauter (2015) 'Effect of 1 Week of Sleep Restriction on Testosterone Levels in Young Healthy MenFREE', JAMA. 2011 Jun 1; 305(21): 2173–2174.

[541] Andersen, M. L., & Tufik, S. (2008). The effects of testosterone on sleep and sleep-disordered breathing in men: Its bidirectional interaction with erectile function. Sleep Medicine Reviews, 12(5), 365–379. doi:10.1016/j.smrv.2007.12.003

[542] Wittert, G. (2014). The relationship between sleep disorders and testosterone in men. Asian Journal of Andrology, 16(2), 262. doi:10.4103/1008-682x.122586

[543] Leproult, R. (2011). Effect of 1 Week of Sleep Restriction on Testosterone Levels in Young Healthy Men. JAMA, 305(21), 2173. doi:10.1001/jama.2011.710

[544] Penev, P. D. (2007). Association Between Sleep and Morning Testosterone Levels In Older Men. Sleep, 30(4), 427–432. doi:10.1093/sleep/30.4.427

[545] Broussard JL, Ehrmann DA, Van Cauter E, Tasali E, Brady MJ. Impaired Insulin Signaling in Human Adipocytes After Experimental Sleep Restriction: A Randomized, Crossover Study. Ann Intern Med. 2012;157:549–557. doi: 10.7326/0003-4819-157-8-201210160-00005

[546] Cheung IN et al (2016) 'Morning and Evening Blue-Enriched Light Exposure Alters Metabolic Function in Normal Weight Adults', PLoS One. 2016 May 18;11(5):e0155601.

[547] Obayashi, K., Saeki, K., Iwamoto, J., Ikada, Y., & Kurumatani, N. (2014). Independent associations of exposure to evening light and nocturnal urinary melatonin excretion with diabetes in the elderly. Chronobiology international, 31(3), 394–400. https://doi.org/10.3109/07420528.2013.864299

[548] Obayashi, K., Saeki, K., Iwamoto, J., Okamoto, N., Tomioka, K., Nezu, S., Ikada, Y., & Kurumatani, N. (2013). Exposure to light at night, nocturnal urinary melatonin excretion, and obesity/dyslipidemia in the elderly: a cross-sectional analysis of the HEIJO-KYO study. The Journal of clinical endocrinology and metabolism, 98(1), 337–344. https://doi.org/10.1210/jc.2012-2874

[549] Nedeltcheva et al (2010) 'Insufficient sleep undermines dietary efforts to reduce adiposity', Ann Intern Med. 2010 Oct 5; 153(7): 435–441.

[550] https://www.ncbi.nlm.nih.gov/pubmed/20357041

[551] Jones (2013) 'In U.S., 40% Get Less Than Recommended Amount of Sleep', Gallup, WELL-BEING, DECEMBER 19, 2013, Accessed Online: https://news.gallup.com/poll/166553/less-recommended-amount-sleep.aspx

552 Vaamonde, D., Da Silva-Grigoletto, M. E., García-Manso, J. M., Barrera, N., & Vaamonde-Lemos, R. (2012). Physically active men show better semen parameters and hormone values than sedentary men. European journal of applied physiology, 112(9), 3267–3273. https://doi.org/10.1007/s00421-011-2304-6

259

553 Craig, B. W., Brown, R., & Everhart, J. (1989). Effects of progressive resistance training on growth hormone and testosterone levels in young and elderly subjects. Mechanisms of ageing and development, 49(2), 159–169. https://doi.org/10.1016/0047-6374(89)90099-7

554 Timón Andrada, R., Maynar Mariño, M., Muñoz Marín, D., Olcina Camacho, G. J., Caballero, M. J., & Maynar Mariño, J. I. (2007). Variations in urine excretion of steroid hormones after an acute session and after a 4-week programme of strength training. European journal of applied physiology, 99(1), 65–71. https://doi.org/10.1007/s00421-006-0319-1

555 Shaner, A. A., Vingren, J. L., Hatfield, D. L., Budnar, R. G., Jr, Duplanty, A. A., & Hill, D. W. (2014). The acute hormonal response to free weight and machine weight resistance exercise. Journal of strength and conditioning research, 28(4), 1032–1040. https://doi.org/10.1519/JSC.0000000000000317

556 Wilk, M., Petr, M., Krzysztofik, M., Zajac, A., & Stastny, P. (2018). Endocrine response to high intensity barbell squats performed with constant movement tempo and variable training volume. Neuro endocrinology letters, 39(4), 342–348.

557 Barnes, M. J., Miller, A., Reeve, D., & Stewart, R. (2019). Acute Neuromuscular and Endocrine Responses to Two Different Compound Exercises: Squat vs. Deadlift. Journal of strength and conditioning research, 33(9), 2381–2387. https://doi.org/10.1519/JSC.0000000000002140

558 Mangine, G. T., Hoffman, J. R., Gonzalez, A. M., Townsend, J. R., Wells, A. J., Jajtner, A. R., ... Stout, J. R. (2015). The effect of training volume and intensity on improvements in muscular strength and size in resistance-trained men. Physiological Reports, 3(8), e12472. doi:10.14814/phy2.12472

559 Kraemer, W. J., Marchitelli, L., Gordon, S. E., Harman, E., Dziados, J. E., Mello, R., Frykman, P., McCurry, D., & Fleck, S. J. (1990). Hormonal and growth factor responses to heavy resistance exercise protocols. Journal of applied physiology (Bethesda, Md. : 1985), 69(4), 1442–1450. https://doi.org/10.1152/jappl.1990.69.4.1442

560 Hackney, A. C., Hosick, K. P., Myer, A., Rubin, D. A., & Battaglini, C. L. (2012). Testosterone responses to intensive interval versus steady-state endurance exercise. Journal of endocrinological investigation, 35(11), 947–950. https://doi.org/10.1007/BF03346740

561 Hämäläinen EK, et al (1983) 'Decrease of serum total and free testosterone during a low-fat high-fibre diet', J Steroid Biochem. 1983 Mar;18(3):369-70.

562 Chang, C. S., Choi, J. B., Kim, H. J., & Park, S. B. (2011). Correlation Between Serum Testosterone Level and Concentrations of Copper and Zinc in Hair Tissue. Biological Trace Element Research, 144(1-3), 264–271. doi:10.1007/s12011-011-9085-y

563 Anderson, K. E., Rosner, W., Khan, M. S., New, M. I., Pang, S., Wissel, P. S., & Kappas, A. (1987). Diet-hormone interactions: Protein/carbohydrate ratio alters reciprocally the plasma levels of testosterone and cortisol and their respective binding globulins in man. Life Sciences, 40(18), 1761–1768. doi:10.1016/0024-3205(87)90086-5

[564] Nielsen, F. H., Hunt, C. D., Mullen, L. M., & Hunt, J. R. (1987). Effect of dietary boron on mineral, estrogen, and testosterone metabolism in postmenopausal women. FASEB journal : official publication of the Federation of American Societies for Experimental Biology, 1(5), 394–397.

565 Murrell (2018) 'Typical testosterone levels in males and females', Medical News Today, Accessed Online July 23 2021: https://www.medicalnewstoday.com/articles/323085#typical-testosterone-levels

566 Selby C. (1990). Sex hormone binding globulin: origin, function and clinical significance. Annals of clinical biochemistry, 27 (Pt 6), 532–541. https://doi.org/10.1177/000456329002700603

[567] Hammond, G.L. (2017). Sex Hormone-Binding Globulin and the Metabolic Syndrome. In: Winters, S., Huhtaniemi, I. (eds) Male Hypogonadism. Contemporary Endocrinology. Humana Press, Cham. https://doi.org/10.1007/978-3-319-53298-1_15

[568] Jandikova, H., Duskova, M., Simunkova, K., Racz, B., Hill, M., Kralikova, E., Vondra, K., & Starka, L. (2015). The steroid spectrum during and after quitting smoking. Physiological research, 64(Suppl 2), S211–S218. https://doi.org/10.33549/physiolres.933068

[569] Hirko, K. A., Spiegelman, D., Willett, W. C., Hankinson, S. E., & Eliassen, A. H. (2014). Alcohol consumption in relation to plasma sex hormones, prolactin, and sex hormone-binding globulin in premenopausal women. Cancer epidemiology, biomarkers & prevention : a publication of the American Association for Cancer Research, cosponsored by the American Society of Preventive Oncology, 23(12), 2943–2953. https://doi.org/10.1158/1055-9965.EPI-14-0982

[570] De Besi, L., Zucchetta, P., Zotti, S., & Mastrogiacomo, I. (1989). Sex hormones and sex hormone binding globulin in males with compensated and decompensated cirrhosis of the liver. Acta endocrinologica, 120(3), 271–276. https://doi.org/10.1530/acta.0.1200271

[571] Tanskanen, M. M., Kyröläinen, H., Uusitalo, A. L., Huovinen, J., Nissilä, J., Kinnunen, H., Atalay, M., & Häkkinen, K. (2011). Serum sex hormone-binding globulin and cortisol concentrations are associated with overreaching during strenuous military training. Journal of strength and conditioning research, 25(3), 787–797. https://doi.org/10.1519/JSC.0b013e3181c1fa5d

[572] Stomati, M., Hartmann, B., Spinetti, A. et al. Effects of hormonal replacement therapy on plasma sex hormone-binding globulin, androgen and insulin-like growth factor-1 levels in postmenopausal women. J Endocrinol Invest 19, 535–541 (1996). https://doi.org/10.1007/BF03349013

[573] Ford, H.C., Cooke, R.R., Kelghtley, E.A. and Feek, C.M. (1992), Serum levels of free and bound testosterone in hyperthyroidism. Clinical Endocrinology, 36: 187-192. https://doi.org/10.1111/j.1365-2265.1992.tb00956.x

[574] Panzer, C., Wise, S., Fantini, G.V., Kang, D., Munarriz, R.M., Guay, A.T., & Goldstein, I. (2006). Impact of oral contraceptives on sex hormone-binding globulin and androgen levels: a retrospective study in women with sexual dysfunction. The journal of sexual medicine, 3 1, 104-13 .

[575] Zimmerman, Y., Eijkemans, M. J., Coelingh Bennink, H. J., Blankenstein, M. A., & Fauser, B. C. (2014). The effect of combined oral contraception on testosterone levels in healthy women: a systematic review and meta-analysis. Human reproduction update, 20(1), 76–105. https://doi.org/10.1093/humupd/dmt038

[576] Cangemi, R., Friedmann, J.A., Holloszy, J. O., & Fontana, L. (2010). Long-term effects of calorie restriction on serum sex-hormone concentrations in men. Aging cell, 9(2), 236–242. https://doi.org/10.1111/j.1474-9726.2010.00553.x

[577] Estour, B., Pugeat, M., Lang, F., Dechaud, H., Pellet, J., & Rousset, H. (1986). Sex hormone binding globulin in women with anorexia nervosa. Clinical endocrinology, 24(5), 571–576. https://doi.org/10.1111/j.1365-2265.1986.tb03287.x

[578] Longcope, C., Feldman, H. A., McKinlay, J. B., & Araujo, A. B. (2000). Diet and sex hormone-binding globulin. The Journal of clinical endocrinology and metabolism, 85(1), 293–296. https://doi.org/10.1210/jcem.85.1.6291

[579] Vermeulen, A., Kaufman, J. M., Goemaere, S., & van Pottelberg, I. (2002). Estradiol in elderly men. The aging male : the official journal of the International Society for the Study of the Aging Male, 5(2), 98–102.

[580] Janssen, I., Powell, L. H., Kazlauskaite, R., & Dugan, S. A. (2010). Testosterone and visceral fat in midlife women: the Study of Women's Health Across the Nation (SWAN) fat patterning study. Obesity (Silver Spring, Md.), 18(3), 604–610. https://doi.org/10.1038/oby.2009.251

[581] Brown, L. M., Gent, L., Davis, K., & Clegg, D. J. (2010). Metabolic impact of sex hormones on obesity. Brain research, 1350, 77–85. https://doi.org/10.1016/j.brainres.2010.04.056

[582] Frank, A. P., de Souza Santos, R., Palmer, B. F., & Clegg, D. J. (2019). Determinants of body fat distribution in humans may provide insight about obesity-related health risks. Journal of lipid research, 60(10), 1710–1719. https://doi.org/10.1194/jlr.R086975

[583] Lombardi, G., Zarrilli, S., Colao, A., Paesano, L., Di Somma, C., Rossi, F., & De Rosa, M. (2001). Estrogens and health in males. Molecular and cellular endocrinology, 178(1-2), 51–55. https://doi.org/10.1016/s0303-7207(01)00420-8

[584] Burger H. G. (2002). Androgen production in women. Fertility and sterility, 77 Suppl 4, S3–S5. https://doi.org/10.1016/s0015-0282(02)02985-0

[585] Baker, L., Meldrum, K. K., Wang, M., Sankula, R., Vanam, R., Raiesdana, A., Tsai, B., Hile, K., Brown, J. W., & Meldrum, D. R. (2003). The role of estrogen in cardiovascular disease. The Journal of surgical research, 115(2), 325–344. https://doi.org/10.1016/s0022-4804(03)00215-4

[586] Almeida et al (2016) 'Estrogens and Androgens in Skeletal Physiology and Pathophysiology', Physiol Rev. 2017;97(1):135–187. doi:10.1152/physrev.00033.2015

[587] Pérez-López, F. R., Larrad-Mur, L., Kallen, A., Chedraui, P., & Taylor, H. S. (2010). Review: Gender Differences in Cardiovascular Disease: Hormonal and Biochemical Influences. Reproductive Sciences, 17(6), 511–531. https://doi.org/10.1177/1933719110367829

[588] Schulster et al (2016) 'The role of estradiol in male reproductive function', Asian J Androl. 2016 May-Jun;18(3):435-40. doi:10.4103/1008-682X.173932

[589] Luglio H. F. (2014). Estrogen and body weight regulation in women: the role of estrogen receptor alpha (ER-α) on adipocyte lipolysis. Acta medica Indonesiana, 46(4), 333–338.

[590] Lizcano, F., & Guzmán, G. (2014). Estrogen Deficiency and the Origin of Obesity during Menopause. BioMed research international, 2014, 757461. https://doi.org/10.1155/2014/757461

[591] Santosa, S., & Jensen, M. D. (2013). Adipocyte fatty acid storage factors enhance subcutaneous fat storage in postmenopausal women. Diabetes, 62(3), 775–782. https://doi.org/10.2337/db12-0912

[592] Davis, S. R., Castelo-Branco, C., Chedraui, P., Lumsden, M. A., Nappi, R. E., Shah, D., & Villaseca, P. (2012). Understanding weight gain at menopause. Climacteric, 15(5), 419–429. https://doi.org/10.3109/13697137.2012.707385

[593] Schorr, M., & Miller, K. K. (2017). The endocrine manifestations of anorexia nervosa: mechanisms and management. Nature reviews. Endocrinology, 13(3), 174–186. https://doi.org/10.1038/nrendo.2016.175

[594] Resulaj, M., Polineni, S., Meenaghan, E., Eddy, K., Lee, H., & Fazeli, P. K. (2019). Transdermal Estrogen in Women With Anorexia Nervosa: An Exploratory Pilot Study. JBMR plus, 4(1), e10251. https://doi.org/10.1002/jbm4.10251

[595] Gourgari, E., Lodish, M., Keil, M., Sinaii, N., Turkbey, E., Lyssikatos, C., Nesterova, M., de la Luz Sierra, M., Xekouki, P., Khurana, D., Ten, S., Dobs, A., & Stratakis, C. A. (2016). Bilateral Adrenal Hyperplasia as a Possible Mechanism for Hyperandrogenism in Women With Polycystic Ovary Syndrome. The Journal of Clinical Endocrinology & Metabolism, 101(9), 3353–3360. https://doi.org/10.1210/jc.2015-4019

[596] Witchel, S. F., Oberfield, S. E., & Peña, A. S. (2019). Polycystic Ovary Syndrome: Pathophysiology, Presentation, and Treatment With Emphasis on Adolescent Girls. Journal of the Endocrine Society, 3(8), 1545–1573. https://doi.org/10.1210/js.2019-00078

[597] Cassar, S., Misso, M. L., Hopkins, W. G., Shaw, C. S., Teede, H. J., & Stepto, N. K. (2016). Insulin resistance in polycystic ovary syndrome: a systematic review and meta-analysis of euglycaemic-hyperinsulinaemic clamp studies. Human reproduction (Oxford, England), 31(11), 2619–2631. https://doi.org/10.1093/humrep/dew243

[598] Diamanti-Kandarakis, E., & Dunaif, A. (2012). Insulin resistance and the polycystic ovary syndrome revisited: an update on mechanisms and implications. Endocrine reviews, 33(6), 981–1030. https://doi.org/10.1210/er.2011-1034

[599] Randolph, J. F., Jr, Kipersztok, S., Ayers, J. W., Ansbacher, R., Peegel, H., & Menon, K. M. (1987). The effect of insulin on aromatase activity in isolated human endometrial glands and stroma. American journal of obstetrics and gynecology, 157(6), 1534–1539. https://doi.org/10.1016/s0002-9378(87)80258-2

[600] Chen, J., Shen, S., Tan, Y., Xia, D., Xia, Y., Cao, Y., Wang, W., Wu, X., Wang, H., Yi, L., Gao, Q., & Wang, Y. (2015). The correlation of aromatase activity and obesity in women with or without polycystic ovary syndrome. Journal of ovarian research, 8, 11. https://doi.org/10.1186/s13048-015-0139-1

[601] la Marca, A., Morgante, G., Palumbo, M., Cianci, A., Petraglia, F., & De Leo, V. (2002). Insulin-lowering treatment reduces aromatase activity in response to follicle-stimulating hormone in women with polycystic ovary syndrome. Fertility and sterility, 78(6), 1234–1239. https://doi.org/10.1016/s0015-0282(02)04346-7

[602] DiNicolantonio, J. J., & H O'Keefe, J. (2022). Myo-inositol for insulin resistance, metabolic syndrome, polycystic ovary syndrome and gestational diabetes. Open heart, 9(1), e001989. https://doi.org/10.1136/openhrt-2022-001989

[603] Cao, X., Xu, P., Oyola, M. G., Xia, Y., Yan, X., Saito, K., Zou, F., Wang, C., Yang, Y., Hinton, A., Jr, Yan, C., Ding, H., Zhu, L., Yu, L., Yang, B., Feng, Y., Clegg, D. J., Khan, S., DiMarchi, R., Mani, S. K., … Xu, Y. (2014). Estrogens stimulate serotonin neurons to inhibit binge-like eating in mice. The Journal of clinical investigation, 124(10), 4351–4362. https://doi.org/10.1172/JCI74726

[604] Edler, C., Lipson, S. F., & Keel, P. K. (2007). Ovarian hormones and binge eating in bulimia nervosa. Psychological medicine, 37(1), 131–141. https://doi.org/10.1017/S0033291706008956

[605] Klump, K. L., Racine, S. E., Hildebrandt, B., Burt, S. A., Neale, M., Sisk, C. L., Boker, S., & Keel, P. K. (2014). Ovarian Hormone Influences on Dysregulated Eating: A Comparison of Associations in Women with versus without Binge Episodes. Clinical psychological science : a journal of the Association for Psychological Science, 2(4), 545–559. https://doi.org/10.1177/2167702614521794

[606] Gordon et al (2017) 'Functional Hypothalamic Amenorrhea: An Endocrine Society Clinical Practice Guideline', The Journal of Clinical Endocrinology & Metabolism, Volume 102, Issue 5, 1 May 2017, Pages 1413–1439, https://doi.org/10.1210/jc.2017-00131

[607] Christiansen (2021) 'What Women Should Know About Having Low Estrogen', Verywell Health, Accessed Online April 19th 2022: https://www.verywellhealth.com/low-estrogen-levels-4588661

[608] Dikshit, A., Hales, K., & Hales, D. B. (2017). Whole flaxseed diet alters estrogen metabolism to promote 2-methoxtestradiol-induced apoptosis in hen ovarian cancer. The Journal of nutritional biochemistry, 42, 117–125. https://doi.org/10.1016/j.jnutbio.2017.01.002

[609] El Wakf, A. M., Hassan, H. A., & Gharib, N. S. (2014). Osteoprotective effect of soybean and sesame oils in ovariectomized rats via estrogen-like mechanism. Cytotechnology, 66(2), 335–343. https://doi.org/10.1007/s10616-013-9580-4

[610] Gangula, P. R., Dong, Y. L., Al-Hendy, A., Richard-Davis, G., Montgomery-Rice, V., Haddad, G., Millis, R., Nicholas, S. B., & Moseberry, D. (2013). Protective cardiovascular and renal actions of vitamin D and estrogen. Frontiers in bioscience (Scholar edition), 5(1), 134–148. https://doi.org/10.2741/s362

[611] Agnoli, C., Grioni, S., Krogh, V., Pala, V., Allione, A., Matullo, G., Di Gaetano, C., Tagliabue, G., Pedraglio, S., Garrone, G., Cancarini, I., Cavalleri, A., & Sieri, S. (2016). Plasma Riboflavin and Vitamin B-6, but Not Homocysteine, Folate, or Vitamin B-12, Are Inversely Associated with Breast Cancer Risk in the European Prospective Investigation into Cancer and Nutrition-Varese Cohort. The Journal of nutrition, 146(6), 1227–1234. https://doi.org/10.3945/jn.115.225433

[612] Gentry-Maharaj, A., Karpinskyj, C., Glazer, C., Burnell, M., Ryan, A., Fraser, L., Lanceley, A., Jacobs, I., Hunter, M. S., & Menon, U. (2015). Use and perceived efficacy of complementary and alternative medicines after discontinuation of hormone therapy: a nested United Kingdom Collaborative Trial of Ovarian Cancer Screening cohort study. Menopause (New York, N.Y.), 22(4), 384–390. https://doi.org/10.1097/GME.0000000000000330

[613] Powers, C. N., & Setzer, W. N. (2015). A molecular docking study of phytochemical estrogen mimics from dietary herbal supplements. In silico pharmacology, 3, 4. https://doi.org/10.1186/s40203-015-0008-z

[614] Ghazanfarpour, M., Sadeghi, R., Latifnejad Roudsari, R., Mirzaii Najmabadi, K., Mousavi Bazaz, M., Abdolahian, S., & Khadivzadeh, T. (2015). Effects of red clover on hot flash and circulating hormone concentrations in menopausal women: a systematic review and meta-analysis. Avicenna journal of phytomedicine, 5(6), 498–511.

[615] Rani, A., & Sharma, A. (2013). The genus Vitex: A review. Pharmacognosy reviews, 7(14), 188–198. https://doi.org/10.4103/0973-7847.120522

[616] Leach, M. J., & Moore, V. (2012). Black cohosh (Cimicifuga spp.) for menopausal symptoms. The Cochrane database of systematic reviews, 2012(9), CD007244. https://doi.org/10.1002/14651858.CD007244.pub2

[617] Nielsen, F. H., Hunt, C. D., Mullen, L. M., & Hunt, J. R. (1987). Effect of dietary boron on mineral, estrogen, and testosterone metabolism in postmenopausal women. FASEB journal : official publication of the Federation of American Societies for Experimental Biology, 1(5), 394–397.

[618] Kolan (2014) 'Estrogen Dominance', US Department of Veteran Affairs, Accessed Online April 16th 2022: https://www.va.gov/WHOLEHEALTHLIBRARY/tools/estrogen-dominance.asp

[619] Lee, J.R.; Hopkins, V. (2004). What Your Doctor May Not Tell You About(TM): Menopause: The Breakthrough Book on Natural Progesterone. Grand Central Publishing. ISBN 978-0-7595-1004-3.

[620] Johnson, R. E., & Murad, M. H. (2009). Gynecomastia: pathophysiology, evaluation, and management. Mayo Clinic proceedings, 84(11), 1010–1015. https://doi.org/10.1016/S0025-6196(11)60671-X

[621] Niewoehner, C. B., & Schorer, A. E. (2008). Gynaecomastia and breast cancer in men. BMJ (Clinical research ed.), 336(7646), 709–713. https://doi.org/10.1136/bmj.39511.493391.BE

[622] Cuhaci, N., Polat, S. B., Evranos, B., Ersoy, R., & Cakir, B. (2014). Gynecomastia: Clinical evaluation and management. Indian journal of endocrinology and metabolism, 18(2), 150–158. https://doi.org/10.4103/2230-8210.129104

[623] Narula, H. S., & Carlson, H. E. (2014). Gynaecomastia--pathophysiology, diagnosis and treatment. Nature reviews. Endocrinology, 10(11), 684–698. https://doi.org/10.1038/nrendo.2014.139

[624] Restrepo, R., Cervantes, L. F., Swirsky, A. M., & Diaz, A. (2021). Breast development in pediatric patients from birth to puberty: physiology, pathology and imaging correlation. Pediatric radiology, 51(11), 1959–1969. https://doi.org/10.1007/s00247-021-05099-4

[625] Poon, S., Siu, K. K., & Tsang, A. (2020). Isoniazid-induced gynaecomastia: report of a paediatric case and review of literature. BMC endocrine disorders, 20(1), 160. https://doi.org/10.1186/s12902-020-00639-9

[626] Cuhaci, N., Polat, S. B., Evranos, B., Ersoy, R., & Cakir, B. (2014). Gynecomastia: Clinical evaluation and management. Indian journal of endocrinology and metabolism, 18(2), 150–158. https://doi.org/10.4103/2230-8210.129104

[627] Devalia, H. L., & Layer, G. T. (2009). Current concepts in gynaecomastia. The surgeon : journal of the Royal Colleges of Surgeons of Edinburgh and Ireland, 7(2), 114–119. https://doi.org/10.1016/s1479-666x(09)80026-7

[628] Deepinder, F., & Braunstein, G. D. (2012). Drug-induced gynecomastia: an evidence-based review. Expert opinion on drug safety, 11(5), 779–795. https://doi.org/10.1517/14740338.2012.712109

[629] Millenium Wellness Center (2014), Accessed Online April 20th 2022: https://hormonebalance.org/userfiles/file/Medications%20that%20increase%20aromatase.pdf

[630] Aiman, U., Haseeen, M. A., & Rahman, S. Z. (2009). Gynecomastia: An ADR due to drug interaction. Indian journal of pharmacology, 41(6), 286–287. https://doi.org/10.4103/0253-7613.59929

[631] Iglesias, P., Carrero, J. J., & Díez, J. J. (2012). Gonadal dysfunction in men with chronic kidney disease: clinical features, prognostic implications and therapeutic options. Journal of nephrology, 25(1), 31–42. https://doi.org/10.5301/JN.2011.8481

[632] Delgado, B. J., & Lopez-Ojeda, W. (2021). Estrogen. In StatPearls. StatPearls Publishing.

[633] Renton (2022) 'Health Risks of High Estrogen in Men and Women', Verywell Health, Accessed Online April 19th 2022: https://www.verywellhealth.com/high-estrogen-5217149

[634] Campbell, K. L., Foster-Schubert, K. E., Alfano, C. M., Wang, C. C., Wang, C. Y., Duggan, C. R., Mason, C., Imayama, I., Kong, A., Xiao, L., Bain, C. E., Blackburn, G. L., Stanczyk, F. Z., & McTiernan, A. (2012). Reduced-calorie dietary weight loss, exercise, and sex hormones in postmenopausal women: randomized controlled trial. Journal of clinical oncology : official journal of the American Society of Clinical Oncology, 30(19), 2314–2326. https://doi.org/10.1200/JCO.2011.37.9792

[635] Hildebrand, J. S., Gapstur, S. M., Campbell, P. T., Gaudet, M. M., & Patel, A. V. (2013). Recreational physical activity and leisure-time sitting in relation to postmenopausal breast cancer risk. Cancer epidemiology, biomarkers & prevention : a publication of the American Association for Cancer Research, cosponsored by the American Society of Preventive Oncology, 22(10), 1906–1912. https://doi.org/10.1158/1055-9965.EPI-13-0407

[636] Gorbach, S. L., & Goldin, B. R. (1987). Diet and the excretion and enterohepatic cycling of estrogens. Preventive medicine, 16(4), 525–531. https://doi.org/10.1016/0091-7435(87)90067-3

[637] Michnovicz, J. J., Adlercreutz, H., & Bradlow, H. L. (1997). Changes in levels of urinary estrogen metabolites after oral indole-3-carbinol treatment in humans. Journal of the National Cancer Institute, 89(10), 718–723. https://doi.org/10.1093/jnci/89.10.718

[638] Higdon, J. V., Delage, B., Williams, D. E., & Dashwood, R. H. (2007). Cruciferous vegetables and human cancer risk: epidemiologic evidence and mechanistic basis. Pharmacological research, 55(3), 224–236. https://doi.org/10.1016/j.phrs.2007.01.009

[639] Purohit V. (1998). Moderate alcohol consumption and estrogen levels in postmenopausal women: a review. Alcoholism, clinical and experimental research, 22(5), 994–997. https://doi.org/10.1111/j.1530-0277.1998.tb03694.x

[640] NIH (2018) 'Insulin Resistance & Prediabetes', NIDDK, Accessed Online March 29th 2022: https://www.niddk.nih.gov/health-information/diabetes/overview/what-is-diabetes/prediabetes-insulin-resistance

[641] Roden, M., Price, T. B., Perseghin, G., Petersen, K. F., Rothman, D. L., Cline, G. W., & Shulman, G. I. (1996). Mechanism of free fatty acid-induced insulin resistance in humans. The Journal of clinical investigation, 97(12), 2859–2865. https://doi.org/10.1172/JCI118742

[642] Koyama, K., Chen, G., Lee, Y., & Unger, R. H. (1997). Tissue triglycerides, insulin resistance, and insulin production: implications for hyperinsulinemia of obesity. The American journal of physiology, 273(4), E708–E713. https://doi.org/10.1152/ajpendo.1997.273.4.E708

[643] Schinner, S., Scherbaum, W. A., Bornstein, S. R., & Barthel, A. (2005). Molecular mechanisms of insulin resistance. Diabetic medicine : a journal of the British Diabetic Association, 22(6), 674–682. https://doi.org/10.1111/j.1464-5491.2005.01566.x

[644] Isganaitis, E., & Lustig, R. H. (2005). Fast food, central nervous system insulin resistance, and obesity. Arteriosclerosis, thrombosis, and vascular biology, 25(12), 2451–2462. https://doi.org/10.1161/01.ATV.0000186208.06964.91

[645] Michael H et al (2008) 'Insulin Resistance and Hyperinsulinemia', Diabetes Care Feb 2008, 31 (Supplement 2) S262-S268.

[646] Wang G. (2014). Raison d'être of insulin resistance: the adjustable threshold hypothesis. Journal of the Royal Society, Interface, 11(101), 20140892. https://doi.org/10.1098/rsif.2014.0892

[647] Taylor, R. (2012). Insulin Resistance and Type 2 Diabetes. Diabetes, 61(4), 778–779. https://doi.org/10.2337/db12-0073

[648] Modan, M., Halkin, H., Almog, S., Lusky, A., Eshkol, A., Shefi, M., Shitrit, A., ... Fuchs, Z. (1985). Hyperinsulinemia. A link between hypertension obesity and glucose intolerance. The Journal of clinical investigation, 75(3), 809-17.

[649] Rizza, R.A., Mandarino, L.J., Genest, J. et al. Diabetologia (1985) 28: 70.

[650] Del Prato S et al (1994) 'Effect of sustained physiologic hyperinsulinaemia and hyperglycaemia on insulin secretion and insulin sensitivity in man', Diabetologia. 1994 Oct;37(10):1025-35.

[651] Chiu, K. C., Chu, A., Go, V. L., & Saad, M. F. (2004). Hypovitaminosis D is associated with insulin resistance and beta cell dysfunction. The American journal of clinical nutrition, 79(5), 820–825. https://doi.org/10.1093/ajcn/79.5.820

[652] Ivy J. L. (1997). Role of exercise training in the prevention and treatment of insulin resistance and non-insulin-dependent diabetes mellitus. Sports medicine (Auckland, N.Z.), 24(5), 321–336. https://doi.org/10.2165/00007256-199724050-00004

[653] Reutrakul, S., & Van Cauter, E. (2018). Sleep influences on obesity, insulin resistance, and risk of type 2 diabetes. Metabolism: clinical and experimental, 84, 56–66. https://doi.org/10.1016/j.metabol.2018.02.010

[654] Mesarwi, O., Polak, J., Jun, J., & Polotsky, V. Y. (2013). Sleep disorders and the development of insulin resistance and obesity. Endocrinology and metabolism clinics of North America, 42(3), 617–634. https://doi.org/10.1016/j.ecl.2013.05.001

[655] Stenvers, D. J., Scheer, F., Schrauwen, P., la Fleur, S. E., & Kalsbeek, A. (2019). Circadian clocks and insulin resistance. Nature reviews. Endocrinology, 15(2), 75–89. https://doi.org/10.1038/s41574-018-0122-1

[656] Isganaitis, E., & Lustig, R. H. (2005). Fast food, central nervous system insulin resistance, and obesity. Arteriosclerosis, thrombosis, and vascular biology, 25(12), 2451–2462. https://doi.org/10.1161/01.ATV.0000186208.06964.91

[657] Fantry L. E. (2003). Protease inhibitor-associated diabetes mellitus: a potential cause of morbidity and mortality. Journal of acquired immune deficiency syndromes (1999), 32(3), 243–244. https://doi.org/10.1097/00126334-200303010-00001

[658] Burghardt, K. J., Seyoum, B., Mallisho, A., Burghardt, P. R., Kowluru, R. A., & Yi, Z. (2018). Atypical antipsychotics, insulin resistance and weight; a meta-analysis of healthy volunteer studies. Progress in neuro-psychopharmacology & biological psychiatry, 83, 55–63. https://doi.org/10.1016/j.pnpbp.2018.01.004

[659] Joseph, J. J., & Golden, S. H. (2017). Cortisol dysregulation: the bidirectional link between stress, depression, and type 2 diabetes mellitus. Annals of the New York Academy of Sciences, 1391(1), 20–34. https://doi.org/10.1111/nyas.13217

[660] King (2005). Lange Q&A USMLE Step 1 (6th ed.). New York: McGraw-Hill Medical. p. 82. ISBN 978-0-07-144578-8.

[661] Piroli, G. G., Grillo, C. A., Reznikov, L. R., Adams, S., McEwen, B. S., Charron, M. J., & Reagan, L. P. (2007). Corticosterone impairs insulin-stimulated translocation of GLUT4 in the rat hippocampus. Neuroendocrinology, 85(2), 71–80. https://doi.org/10.1159/000101694

[662] Peraldi, P., & Spiegelman, B. (1998). TNF-alpha and insulin resistance: summary and future prospects. Molecular and cellular biochemistry, 182(1-2), 169–175.

[663] Brown, A. E., & Walker, M. (2016). Genetics of Insulin Resistance and the Metabolic Syndrome. Current cardiology reports, 18(8), 75. https://doi.org/10.1007/s11886-016-0755-4

[664] Kapadia, K. B., Bhatt, P. A., & Shah, J. S. (2012). Association between altered thyroid state and insulin resistance. Journal of pharmacology & pharmacotherapeutics, 3(2), 156–160. https://doi.org/10.4103/0976-500X.95517

[665] B, U. U., Mn, S., Km, S., Prashant, A., Doddamani, P., & Sv, S. (2015). Effect of insulin resistance in assessing the clinical outcome of clinical and subclinical hypothyroid patients. Journal of clinical and diagnostic research : JCDR, 9(2), OC01–OC4. https://doi.org/10.7860/JCDR/2015/9754.5513

[666] Vyakaranam, S., Vanaparthy, S., Nori, S., Palarapu, S., & Bhongir, A. V. (2014). Study of Insulin Resistance in Subclinical Hypothyroidism. International journal of health sciences and research, 4(9), 147–153.

[667] Luna-Vazquez, F., Cruz-Lumbreras, R., Rodríguez-Castelán, J., Cervantes-Rodríguez, M., Rodríguez-Antolín, J., Arroyo-Helguera, O., Castelán, F., Martínez-Gómez, M., & Cuevas, E. (2014). Association between the serum concentration of triiodothyronine with components of metabolic syndrome, cardiovascular risk, and diet in euthyroid post-menopausal women without and with metabolic syndrome. SpringerPlus, 3(1). https://doi.org/10.1186/2193-1801-3-266

[668] Kapadia, K. B., Bhatt, P. A., & Shah, J. S. (2012). Association between altered thyroid state and insulin resistance. Journal of pharmacology & pharmacotherapeutics, 3(2), 156–160. https://doi.org/10.4103/0976-500X.95517

[669] Bilgin, H., & Pirgon, Ö. (2014). Thyroid Function in Obese Children with Non-Alcoholic Fatty Liver Disease. Journal of Clinical Research in Pediatric Endocrinology, 152–157. https://doi.org/10.4274/jcrpe.1488

[670] Dimitriadis, G., Baker, B., Marsh, H., Mandarino, L., Rizza, R., Bergman, R., Haymond, M., & Gerich, J. (1985). Effect of thyroid hormone excess on action, secretion, and metabolism of insulin in humans. The American journal of physiology, 248(5 Pt 1), E593–E601. https://doi.org/10.1152/ajpendo.1985.248.5.E593

[671] Férnandez-Real et al (2006) 'Thyroid Function Is Intrinsically Linked to Insulin Sensitivity and Endothelium-Dependent Vasodilation in Healthy Euthyroid Subjects', The Journal of Clinical Endocrinology & Metabolism, Volume 91, Issue 9, 1 September 2006, Pages 3337–3343, https://doi.org/10.1210/jc.2006-0841

[672] Ortega, E., Koska, J., Pannacciulli, N., Bunt, J. C., & Krakoff, J. (2008). Free triiodothyronine plasma concentrations are positively associated with insulin secretion in euthyroid individuals. European Journal of Endocrinology, 158(2), 217–221. https://doi.org/10.1530/eje-07-0592

[673] Ren, R., Jiang, X., Zhang, X., Guan, Q., Yu, C., Li, Y., Gao, L., Zhang, H. and Zhao, J. (2014), Association between thyroid hormones and body fat in euthyroid subjects. Clin Endocrinol, 80: 585-590. https://doi.org/10.1111/cen.12311

[674] Roos et al (2007) 'Thyroid Function Is Associated with Components of the Metabolic Syndrome in Euthyroid Subjects ', The Journal of Clinical Endocrinology & Metabolism, Volume 92, Issue 2, 1 February 2007, Pages 491–496, https://doi.org/10.1210/jc.2006-1718

[675] Prats-Puig, A., Sitjar, C., Ribot, R., Calvo, M., Clausell-Pomés, N., Soler-Roca, M., Soriano-Rodríguez, P., Osiniri, I., Ros-Miquel, M., Bassols, J., de Zegher, F., Ibáñez, L. and López-Bermejo, A. (2012), Relative Hypoadiponectinemia, Insulin Resistance, and Increased Visceral Fat in Euthyroid Prepubertal Girls With Low-Normal Serum Free Thyroxine. Obesity, 20: 1455-1461. https://doi.org/10.1038/oby.2011.206

[676] Kouidhi, S., Berhouma, R., Ammar, M., Rouissi, K., Jarboui, S., Clerget-Froidevaux, M.-S., Seugnet, I., Abid, H., Bchir, F., Demeneix, B., Guissouma, H., & Elgaaied, A. B. (2012). Relationship of Thyroid Function with Obesity and Type 2 Diabetes in Euthyroid Tunisian Subjects. Endocrine Research, 38(1), 15–23. https://doi.org/10.3109/07435800.2012.699987

[677] Lin, Y. and Sun, Z. (2011), Thyroid hormone potentiates insulin signaling and attenuates hyperglycemia and insulin resistance in a mouse model of type 2 diabetes. British Journal of Pharmacology, 162: 597-610. https://doi.org/10.1111/j.1476-5381.2010.01056.x

[678] Bollinger, S. S., Weltman, N. Y., Gerdes, A. M., & Schlenker, E. H. (2015). T3 supplementation affects ventilatory timing & glucose levels in type 2 diabetes mellitus model. Respiratory Physiology & Neurobiology, 205, 92–98. https://doi.org/10.1016/j.resp.2014.10.020

[679] Krysiak, R., Gilowska, M., Szkróbka, W., & Okopień, B. (2016). The effect of metformin on the hypothalamic-pituitary-thyroid axis in patients with type 2 diabetes and amiodarone-induced hypothyroidism. Pharmacological Reports, 68(2), 490–494. https://doi.org/10.1016/j.pharep.2015.11.010

[680] Dimitriadis, G., Baker, B., Marsh, H., Mandarino, L., Rizza, R., Bergman, R., Haymond, M., & Gerich, J. (1985). Effect of thyroid hormone excess on action, secretion, and metabolism of insulin in humans. American Journal of Physiology-Endocrinology and Metabolism, 248(5), E593–E601. https://doi.org/10.1152/ajpendo.1985.248.5.e593

[681] CAVALLO-PERIN, P., BRUNO, A., BOINE, L., CASSADER, M., LENTI, G. and PAGANO, G. (1988), Insulin resistance in Graves' disease: a quantitative in-vivo evaluation. European Journal of Clinical Investigation, 18: 607-613. https://doi.org/10.1111/j.1365-2362.1988.tb01275.x

[682] Brenta G. (2011). Why can insulin resistance be a natural consequence of thyroid dysfunction?. Journal of thyroid research, 2011, 152850. https://doi.org/10.4061/2011/152850

[683] Beylot M. (1996). Regulation of in vivo ketogenesis: role of free fatty acids and control by epinephrine, thyroid hormones, insulin and glucagon. Diabetes & metabolism, 22(5), 299–304.

[684] Dai, G., Levy, O., & Carrasco, N. (1996). Cloning and characterization of the thyroid iodide transporter. Nature, 379(6564), 458–460. https://doi.org/10.1038/379458a0

[685] Hennemann, G., Docter, R., Friesema, E. C. H., de Jong, M., Krenning, E. P., & Visser, T. J. (2001). Plasma Membrane Transport of Thyroid Hormones and Its Role inThyroid Hormone Metabolism and Bioavailability. Endocrine Reviews, 22(4), 451–476. doi:10.1210/edrv.22.4.0435

[686] Krenning, E., Docter, R., Bernard, B., Visser, T., & Hennemann, G. (1981). Characteristics of active transport of thyroid hormone into rat hepatocytes. Biochimica et biophysica acta, 676(3), 314–320. https://doi.org/10.1016/0304-4165(81)90165-3

[687] Centanni, M., & Robbins, J. (1987). Role of sodium in thyroid hormone uptake by rat skeletal muscle. The Journal of clinical investigation, 80(4), 1068–1072. https://doi.org/10.1172/JCI113162

[688] de Jong, M., Visser, T. J., Bernard, B. F., Docter, R., Vos, R. A., Hennemann, G., & Krenning, E. P. (1993). Transport and metabolism of iodothyronines in cultured human hepatocytes. The Journal of clinical endocrinology and metabolism, 77(1), 139–143. https://doi.org/10.1210/jcem.77.1.8392080

[689] Krenning, E., Docter, R., Bernard, B., Visser, T., & Hennemann, G. (1980). Regulation of the active transport of 3,3',5-triiodothyronine (T3) into primary cultured rat hepatocytes by ATP. FEBS letters, 119(2), 279–282. https://doi.org/10.1016/0014-5793(80)80271-7

[690] Osty, J., Valensi, P., Samson, M., Francon, J., & Blondeau, J. P. (1990). Transport of thyroid hormones by human erythrocytes: kinetic characterization in adults and newborns. The Journal of clinical endocrinology and metabolism, 71(6), 1589–1595. https://doi.org/10.1210/jcem-71-6-1589

[691] Dohán, O., De la Vieja, A., Paroder, V., Riedel, C., Artani, M., Reed, M., Ginter, C. S., & Carrasco, N. (2003). The sodium/iodide Symporter (NIS): characterization, regulation, and medical significance. Endocrine reviews, 24(1), 48–77. https://doi.org/10.1210/er.2001-0029

[692] https://www.ncbi.nlm.nih.gov/pubmed/21036373

[693] Iwaoka, T., Umeda, T., Inoue, J., Naomi, S., Sasaki, M., Fujimoto, Y., Gui, C., Ideguchi, Y., & Sato, T. (1994). Dietary NaCl restriction deteriorates oral glucose tolerance in hypertensive patients with impairment of glucose tolerance. American journal of hypertension, 7(5), 460–463. https://doi.org/10.1093/ajh/7.5.460

[694] Iwaoka, T., Umeda, T., Ohno, M., Inoue, J., Naomi, S., Sato, T., & Kawakami, I. (1988). The effect of low and high NaCl diets on oral glucose tolerance. Klinische Wochenschrift, 66(16), 724–728. https://doi.org/10.1007/BF01726415

[695] Garg, R., Williams, G. H., Hurwitz, S., Brown, N. J., Hopkins, P. N., & Adler, G. K. (2011). Low-salt diet increases insulin resistance in healthy subjects. Metabolism: clinical and experimental, 60(7), 965–968. https://doi.org/10.1016/j.metabol.2010.09.005

[696] Garg, R., Sun, B., & Williams, J. (2014). Effect of low salt diet on insulin resistance in salt-sensitive versus salt-resistant hypertension. Hypertension (Dallas, Tex. : 1979), 64(6), 1384–1387. https://doi.org/10.1161/HYPERTENSIONAHA.114.03880

[697] Gomi, T., Shibuya, Y., Sakurai, J., Hirawa, N., Hasegawa, K., & Ikeda, T. (1998). Strict dietary sodium reduction worsens insulin sensitivity by increasing sympathetic nervous activity in patients with primary hypertension. American journal of hypertension, 11(9), 1048–1055. https://doi.org/10.1016/s0895-7061(98)00126-5

[698] Townsend, R. R., Kapoor, S., & McFadden, C. B. (2007). Salt intake and insulin sensitivity in healthy human volunteers. Clinical science (London, England : 1979), 113(3), 141–148. https://doi.org/10.1042/CS20060361

[699] Perry, C. G., Palmer, T., Cleland, S. J., Morton, I. J., Salt, I. P., Petrie, J. R., Gould, G. W., & Connell, J. M. (2003). Decreased insulin sensitivity during dietary sodium restriction is not mediated by effects of angiotensin II on insulin action. Clinical science (London, England : 1979), 105(2), 187–194. https://doi.org/10.1042/CS20020320

[700] Egan, B. M., Weder, A. B., Petrin, J., & Hoffman, R. G. (1991). Neurohumoral and metabolic effects of short-term dietary NaCl restriction in men. Relationship to salt-sensitivity status. American journal of hypertension, 4(5 Pt 1), 416–421. https://doi.org/10.1093/ajh/4.5.416

[701] Ruppert, M., Diehl, J., Kolloch, R., Overlack, A., Kraft, K., Göbel, B., Hittel, N., & Stumpe, K. O. (1991). Short-term dietary sodium restriction increases serum lipids and insulin in salt-sensitive and salt-resistant normotensive adults. Klinische Wochenschrift, 69 Suppl 25, 51–57.

[702] Weder, A. B., & Egan, B. M. (1991). Potential deleterious impact of dietary salt restriction on cardiovascular risk factors. Klinische Wochenschrift, 69 Suppl 25, 45–50.

[703] Egan, B. M., Stepniakowski, K., & Goodfriend, T. L. (1994). Renin and aldosterone are higher and the hyperinsulinemic effect of salt restriction greater in subjects with risk factors clustering. American journal of hypertension, 7(10 Pt 1), 886–893. https://doi.org/10.1016/0895-7061(94)P1710-H

[704] Del Río, A., & Rodríguez-Villamil, J. L. (1993). Metabolic effects of strict salt restriction in essential hypertensive patients. Journal of internal medicine, 233(5), 409–414. https://doi.org/10.1111/j.1365-2796.1993.tb00692.x

[705] Meland, E., Laerum, E., Aakvaag, A., & Ulvik, R. J. (1994). Salt restriction and increased insulin production in hypertensive patients. Scandinavian journal of clinical and laboratory investigation, 54(5), 405–409. https://doi.org/10.3109/00365519409088441

[706] Feldman, R. D., & Schmidt, N. D. (1999). Moderate dietary salt restriction increases vascular and systemic insulin resistance. American journal of hypertension, 12(6), 643–647. https://doi.org/10.1016/s0895-7061(99)00016-3

[707] https://www.ncbi.nlm.nih.gov/pubmed/20226958

[708] Brands, M. W., & Manhiani, M. M. (2012). Sodium-retaining effect of insulin in diabetes. American journal of physiology. Regulatory, integrative and comparative physiology, 303(11), R1101–R1109. https://doi.org/10.1152/ajpregu.00390.2012

[709] Yatabe, M. S., Yatabe, J., Yoneda, M., Watanabe, T., Otsuki, M., Felder, R. A., Jose, P. A., & Sanada, H. (2010). Salt sensitivity is associated with insulin resistance, sympathetic overactivity, and decreased suppression of circulating renin activity in lean patients with essential hypertension. The American journal of clinical nutrition, 92(1), 77–82. https://doi.org/10.3945/ajcn.2009.29028

[710] Sullivan, J. M. (1991). Salt sensitivity. Definition, conception, methodology, and long-term issues. Hypertension, 17(1_Suppl), I61–I61. doi:10.1161/01.hyp.17.1_suppl.i61

[711] Young, D. B., Lin, H., & McCabe, R. D. (1995). Potassium's cardiovascular protective mechanisms. The American journal of physiology, 268(4 Pt 2), R825–R837. https://doi.org/10.1152/ajpregu.1995.268.4.R825

[712] Haddy, F. J., Vanhoutte, P. M., & Feletou, M. (2006). Role of potassium in regulating blood flow and blood pressure. American journal of physiology. Regulatory, integrative and comparative physiology, 290(3), R546–R552. https://doi.org/10.1152/ajpregu.00491.2005

[713] Houston M. C. (2011). The importance of potassium in managing hypertension. Current hypertension reports, 13(4), 309–317. https://doi.org/10.1007/s11906-011-0197-8

[714] SAGILD, U., ANDERSEN, V., & ANDREASEN, P. B. (1961). Glucose tolerance and insulin responsiveness in experimental potassium depletion. Acta medica Scandinavica, 169, 243–251. https://doi.org/10.1111/j.0954-6820.1961.tb07829.x

[715] Rowe, J. W., Tobin, J. D., Rosa, R. M., & Andres, R. (1980). Effect of experimental potassium deficiency on glucose and insulin metabolism. Metabolism, 29(6), 498–502. doi:10.1016/0026-0495(80)90074-8

[716] Ekmekcioglu, C., Elmadfa, I., Meyer, A. L., & Moeslinger, T. (2016). The role of dietary potassium in hypertension and diabetes. Journal of physiology and biochemistry, 72(1), 93–106. https://doi.org/10.1007/s13105-015-0449-1

[717] Oria-Hernández, J., Cabrera, N., Pérez-Montfort, R., & Ramírez-Silva, L. (2005). Pyruvate kinase revisited: the activating effect of K+. The Journal of biological chemistry, 280(45), 37924–37929. https://doi.org/10.1074/jbc.M508490200

[718] Lee, H., Lee, J., Hwang, S. S., Kim, S., Chin, H. J., Han, J. S., & Heo, N. J. (2013). Potassium intake and the prevalence of metabolic syndrome: the Korean National Health and Nutrition Examination Survey 2008-2010. PloS one, 8(1), e55106. https://doi.org/10.1371/journal.pone.0055106

[719] Colditz, G. A., Manson, J. E., Stampfer, M. J., Rosner, B., Willett, W. C., & Speizer, F. E. (1992). Diet and risk of clinical diabetes in women. The American journal of clinical nutrition, 55(5), 1018–1023. https://doi.org/10.1093/ajcn/55.5.1018

[720] Chatterjee, R., Colangelo, L. A., Yeh, H. C., Anderson, C. A., Daviglus, M. L., Liu, K., & Brancati, F. L. (2012). Potassium intake and risk of incident type 2 diabetes mellitus: the Coronary Artery Risk Development in Young Adults (CARDIA) Study. Diabetologia, 55(5), 1295–1303. https://doi.org/10.1007/s00125-012-2487-3

[721] Chatterjee, R., Yeh, H. C., Shafi, T., Selvin, E., Anderson, C., Pankow, J. S., Miller, E., & Brancati, F. (2010). Serum and dietary potassium and risk of incident type 2 diabetes mellitus: The Atherosclerosis Risk in Communities (ARIC) study. Archives of internal medicine, 170(19), 1745–1751. https://doi.org/10.1001/archinternmed.2010.362

[722] NIH (2021) 'Potassium', Fact Sheet for Health Professionals, Accessed Online March 30th 2022: https://ods.od.nih.gov/factsheets/Potassium-HealthProfessional/

[723] World Health Organization (WHO). Guideline: Potassium Intake for Adults and Children; WHO: Geneva, Switzerland, 2012.

[724] Chobanian, A. V., Bakris, G. L., Black, H. R., Cushman, W. C., Green, L. A., Izzo, J. L., Jr, Jones, D. W., Materson, B. J., Oparil, S., Wright, J. T., Jr, Roccella, E. J., Joint National Committee on Prevention, Detection, Evaluation, and Treatment of High Blood Pressure. National Heart, Lung, and Blood Institute, & National High Blood Pressure Education Program Coordinating Committee (2003). Seventh report of the Joint National Committee on Prevention, Detection, Evaluation, and Treatment of High Blood Pressure. Hypertension (Dallas, Tex. : 1979), 42(6), 1206–1252. https://doi.org/10.1161/01.HYP.0000107251.49515.c2

[725] Fulgoni, V. L., 3rd, Keast, D. R., Bailey, R. L., & Dwyer, J. (2011). Foods, fortificants, and supplements: Where do Americans get their nutrients?. The Journal of nutrition, 141(10), 1847–1854. https://doi.org/10.3945/jn.111.142257

[726] DeSalvo, K. B., Olson, R., & Casavale, K. O. (2016). Dietary Guidelines for Americans. JAMA, 315(5), 457–458. https://doi.org/10.1001/jama.2015.18396

[727] Kyu, H. H., Bachman, V. F., Alexander, L. T., Mumford, J. E., Afshin, A., Estep, K., Veerman, J. L., Delwiche, K., Iannarone, M. L., Moyer, M. L., Cercy, K., Vos, T., Murray, C. J., & Forouzanfar, M. H. (2016). Physical activity and risk of breast cancer, colon cancer, diabetes, ischemic heart disease, and ischemic stroke events: systematic review and dose-response meta-analysis for the Global Burden of Disease Study 2013. BMJ (Clinical research ed.), 354, i3857. https://doi.org/10.1136/bmj.i3857

[728] Balkau, B., Mhamdi, L., Oppert, J. M., Nolan, J., Golay, A., Porcellati, F., Laakso, M., Ferrannini, E., EGIR-RISC Study Group (2008). Physical activity and insulin sensitivity: the RISC study. Diabetes, 57(10), 2613-8.

[729] Lund, S., Holman, G. D., Schmitz, O., & Pedersen, O. (1995). Contraction stimulates translocation of glucose transporter GLUT4 in skeletal muscle through a mechanism distinct from that of insulin. Proceedings of the National Academy of Sciences of the United States of America, 92(13), 5817-21.

[730] Ishiguro, H., Kodama, S., Horikawa, C., Fujihara, K., Hirose, A. S., Hirasawa, R., Yachi, Y., Ohara, N., Shimano, H., Hanyu, O., & Sone, H. (2016). In Search of the Ideal Resistance Training Program to Improve Glycemic Control and its Indication for Patients with Type 2 Diabetes Mellitus: A Systematic Review and Meta-Analysis. Sports medicine (Auckland, N.Z.), 46(1), 67–77. https://doi.org/10.1007/s40279-015-0379-7

[731] Stöckli, J., Fazakerley, D. J., & James, D. E. (2011). GLUT4 exocytosis. Journal of Cell Science, 124(24), 4147–4159. https://doi.org/10.1242/jcs.097063

[732] Leto, D., Saltiel, A. Regulation of glucose transport by insulin: traffic control of GLUT4. Nat Rev Mol Cell Biol 13, 383–396 (2012). https://doi.org/10.1038/nrm3351

[733] Shiloah E et al (2003) 'Effect of Acute Psychotic Stress in Nondiabetic Subjects on β-Cell Function and Insulin Sensitivity', Diabetes Care 2003 May; 26(5): 1462-1467.

[734] Piroli GG et al (2007) 'Corticosterone Impairs Insulin-Stimulated Translocation of GLUT4 in the Rat Hippocampus', Neuroendocrinology 2007;85:71–80.

[735] Paul-Labrador M. et al (2006) 'Effects of a randomized controlled trial of transcendental meditation on components of the metabolic syndrome in subjects with coronary heart disease', Arch Intern Med. 2006 Jun 12;166(11):1218-24.

[736] Taylor, P. N., Albrecht, D., Scholz, A., Gutierrez-Buey, G., Lazarus, J. H., Dayan, C. M., & Okosieme, O. E. (2018). Global epidemiology of hyperthyroidism and hypothyroidism. Nature reviews. Endocrinology, 14(5), 301–316. https://doi.org/10.1038/nrendo.2018.18

[737] Garmendia Madariaga, A., Santos Palacios, S., Guillén-Grima, F., & Galofré, J. C. (2014). The Incidence and Prevalence of Thyroid Dysfunction in Europe: A Meta-Analysis. The Journal of Clinical Endocrinology & Metabolism, 99(3), 923–931. doi:10.1210/jc.2013-2409

[738] Bülow Pedersen, I., Laurberg, P., Knudsen, N., Jørgensen, T., Perrild, H., Ovesen, L., & Rasmussen, L. B. (2007). An Increased Incidence of Overt Hypothyroidism after Iodine Fortification of Salt in Denmark: A Prospective Population Study. The Journal of Clinical Endocrinology & Metabolism, 92(8), 3122–3127. doi:10.1210/jc.2007-0732

[739] Boelaert, K., Newby, P. R., Simmonds, M. J., Holder, R. L., Carr-Smith, J. D., Heward, J. M., Manji, N., Allahabadia, A., Armitage, M., Chatterjee, K. V., Lazarus, J. H., Pearce, S. H., Vaidya, B., Gough, S. C., & Franklyn, J. A. (2010). Prevalence and relative risk of other autoimmune diseases in subjects with autoimmune thyroid disease. The American journal of medicine, 123(2), 183.e1–183.e1839. https://doi.org/10.1016/j.amjmed.2009.06.030

[740] Schultheiss, U. T., Teumer, A., Medici, M., Li, Y., Daya, N., Chaker, L., Homuth, G., Uitterlinden, A. G., Nauck, M., Hofman, A., Selvin, E., Völzke, H., Peeters, R. P., & Köttgen, A. (2015). A genetic risk score for thyroid peroxidase antibodies associates with clinical thyroid disease in community-based populations. The Journal of clinical endocrinology and metabolism, 100(5), E799–E807. https://doi.org/10.1210/jc.2014-4352

[741] Marinò, M., Latrofa, F., Menconi, F., Chiovato, L., & Vitti, P. (2015). Role of genetic and non-genetic factors in the etiology of Graves' disease. Journal of endocrinological investigation, 38(3), 283–294. https://doi.org/10.1007/s40618-014-0214-2

[742] Bülow Pedersen, I., Knudsen, N., Carlé, A., Schomburg, L., Köhrle, J., Jørgensen, T., … Laurberg, P. (2013). Serum selenium is low in newly diagnosed Graves' disease: a population-based study. Clinical Endocrinology, 79(4), 584–590. doi:10.1111/cen.12185

[743] Tomer, Y. & Davies, T. F. (1993) Infection, thyroid disease, and autoimmunity. Endocr. Rev. 14, 107–120.

[744] Kaptein EM 1986 Thyroid hormone metabolism in illness. In: Hennemann G, ed. Thyroid hormone metabolism. New York: Marcel Dekker; 297–333

[745] Kaptein, E. M., Feinstein, E. I., Nicoloff, J. T., & Massry, S. G. (1983). Serum reverse triiodothyronine and thyroxine kinetics in patients with chronic renal failure. The Journal of clinical endocrinology and metabolism, 57(1), 181–189. https://doi.org/10.1210/jcem-57-1-181

[746] Hue, L., & Taegtmeyer, H. (2009). The Randle cycle revisited: a new head for an old hat. American journal of physiology. Endocrinology and metabolism, 297 3, E578-91 .

[747] Bevilacqua et al (1990) 'Operation of Randle's cycle in patients with NIDDM', Diabetes. 1990 Mar;39(3):383-9.

[748] Randle et al (1963) 'THE GLUCOSE FATTY-ACID CYCLE ITS ROLE IN INSULIN SENSITIVITY AND THE METABOLIC DISTURBANCES OF DIABETES MELLITUS', The Lancet, ORIGINAL ARTICLES| VOLUME 281, ISSUE 7285, P785-789, APRIL 13, 1963.

[749] Delarue and Magnan (2007) 'Free fatty acids and insulin resistance', Curr Opin Clin Nutr Metab Care. 2007 Mar;10(2):142-8.

[750] Shuldiner and McLenithan (2004) 'Genes and pathophysiology of type 2 diabetes: more than just the Randle cycle all over again', J Clin Invest. 2004 Nov;114(10):1414-7.

[751] Frayn et al (2006) 'Fatty acid metabolism in adipose tissue, muscle and liver in health and disease', Essays Biochem. 2006;42:89-103.

[752] Randle et al (1963) 'The glucose fatty-acid cycle. Its role in insulin sensitivity and the metabolic disturbances of diabetes mellitus', Lancet. 1963 Apr 13;1(7285):785-9.

[753] Lucidi, P., Rossetti, P., Porcellati, F., Pampanelli, S., Candeloro, P., Andreoli, A. M., Perriello, G., Bolli, G. B., & Fanelli, C. G. (2010). Mechanisms of insulin resistance after insulin-induced hypoglycemia in humans: the role of lipolysis. Diabetes, 59(6), 1349–1357. https://doi.org/10.2337/db09-0745

[754] Storlien LH et al (1991) 'Influence of Dietary Fat Composition on Development of Insulin Resistance in Rats: Relationship to Muscle Triglyceride and ω-3 Fatty Acids in Muscle Phospholipid', Diabetes 1991 Feb; 40(2): 280-289.

[755] Isganaitis E and Lustig R.H. (2005) 'Fast Food, Central Nervous System Insulin Resistance, and Obesity', Arteriosclerosis, Thrombosis, and Vascular Biology. 2005;25:2451–2462.

[756] Clément L et al (2002) 'Dietary trans-10,cis-12 conjugated linoleic acid induces hyperinsulinemia and fatty liver in the mouse', J Lipid Res. 2002 Sep;43(9):1400-9.

[757] DiNicolantonio, J. J., O'Keefe, J. H., & Lucan, S. C. (2015). Added fructose: a principal driver of type 2 diabetes mellitus and its consequences. Mayo Clinic proceedings, 90(3), 372–381. https://doi.org/10.1016/j.mayocp.2014.12.019

[758] DiNicolantonio, J. J., Subramonian, A. M., & O'Keefe, J. H. (2017). Added fructose as a principal driver of non-alcoholic fatty liver disease: a public health crisis. Open heart, 4(2), e000631. https://doi.org/10.1136/openhrt-2017-000631

[759] DiNicolantonio, J. J., Mehta, V., Onkaramurthy, N., & O'Keefe, J. H. (2018). Fructose-induced inflammation and increased cortisol: A new mechanism for how sugar induces visceral adiposity. Progress in Cardiovascular Diseases, 61(1), 3–9. https://doi.org/10.1016/j.pcad.2017.12.001

[760] Goodwin et al (1998) 'Regulation of energy metabolism of the heart during acute increase in heart work', J Biol Chem. 1998 Nov 6;273(45):29530-9.

[761] Stanley, K., Fraser, R. and Bruce, C. (1998), Physiological changes in insulin resistance in human pregnancy: longitudinal study with the hyperinsulinaemic euglycaemic clamp technique. BJOG: An International Journal of Obstetrics & Gynaecology, 105: 756-759. https://doi.org/10.1111/j.1471-0528.1998.tb10207.x

[762] Sonagra, A. D., Biradar, S. M., K, D., & Murthy D S, J. (2014). Normal pregnancy- a state of insulin resistance. Journal of clinical and diagnostic research : JCDR, 8(11), CC01–CC3. https://doi.org/10.7860/JCDR/2014/10068.5081

[763] Newbern, D., & Freemark, M. (2011). Placental hormones and the control of maternal metabolism and fetal growth. Current opinion in endocrinology, diabetes, and obesity, 18(6), 409–416. https://doi.org/10.1097/MED.0b013e32834c800d

[764] Wang, G (2014) 'Raison d'être of insulin resistance: the adjustable threshold hypothesis', Journal of the Royal Society, Vol 11(101).

[765] Unger RH et al (2012) 'Gluttony, sloth and the metabolic syndrome: a roadmap to lipotoxicity', Trends in Endocrinology and Metabolism 21 (2010) 345–352.

[766] Kraegen, EW et al (1991) 'Development of Muscle Insulin Resistance After Liver Insulin Resistance in High-Fat–Fed Rats', Diabetes Nov 1991, 40 (11) 1397-1403.

[767] Sierra, S., Lara-Villoslada, F., Comalada, M., Olivares, M., & Xaus, J. (2006). Dietary fish oil n−3 fatty acids increase regulatory cytokine production and exert anti-inflammatory effects in two murine models of inflammation. Lipids, 41(12), 1115–1125. doi:10.1007/s11745-006-5061-2

[768] Huang YJ et al (1997) 'Amelioration of insulin resistance and hypertension in a fructose-fed rat model with fish oil supplementation', Metabolism Clinical and Experimental, November 1997Volume 46, Issue 11, Pages 1252–1258.

[769] Hill JO, Peters JC, Lin D, et al. Lipid accumulation and body fat distribution is influenced by type of dietary fat fed to rats. Int J Obes Relat Metab Disord. 1993 Apr;17(4):223-36.

[770] Flachs, P., Rossmeisl, M., Kuda, O., & Kopecky, J. (2013). Stimulation of mitochondrial oxidative capacity in white fat independent of UCP1: A key to lean phenotype. Biochimica et Biophysica Acta (BBA) - Molecular and Cell Biology of Lipids, 1831(5), 986–1003. doi:10.1016/j.bbalip.2013.02.003

[771] Flachs, P., Mohamed-Ali, V., Horakova, O., Rossmeisl, M., Hosseinzadeh-Attar, M. J., Hensler, M., … Kopecky, J. (2006). Polyunsaturated fatty acids of marine origin induce adiponectin in mice fed a high-fat diet. Diabetologia, 49(2), 394–397. doi:10.1007/s00125-005-0053-y

[772] Hensler, M., Bardova, K., Jilkova, Z. M., Wahli, W., Meztger, D., Chambon, P., Kopecky, J., & Flachs, P. (2011). The inhibition of fat cell proliferation by n-3 fatty acids in dietary obese mice. Lipids in health and disease, 10, 128. https://doi.org/10.1186/1476-511X-10-128

[773] Ruzickova, J., Rossmeisl, M., Prazak, T., Flachs, P., Sponarova, J., Veck, M., Tvrzicka, E., Bryhn, M., & Kopecky, J. (2004). Omega-3 PUFA of marine origin limit diet-induced obesity in mice by reducing cellularity of adipose tissue. Lipids, 39(12), 1177–1185. https://doi.org/10.1007/s11745-004-1345-9

[774] Gago-Dominguez, M., Jiang, X., & Castelao, J. E. (2007). Lipid peroxidation, oxidative stress genes and dietary factors in breast cancer protection: a hypothesis. Breast cancer research : BCR, 9(1), 201. https://doi.org/10.1186/bcr1628

[775] Kew, S., Banerjee, T., Minihane, A. M., Finnegan, Y. E., Williams, C. M., & Calder, P. C. (2003). Relation between the fatty acid composition of peripheral blood mononuclear cells and measures of immune cell function in healthy, free-living subjects aged 25–72 y. The American Journal of Clinical Nutrition, 77(5), 1278–1286. doi:10.1093/ajcn/77.5.1278

[776] Kanner J. (2007). Dietary advanced lipid oxidation endproducts are risk factors to human health. Molecular nutrition & food research, 51(9), 1094–1101. https://doi.org/10.1002/mnfr.200600303

[777] Tan, E., & Scott, E. M. (2014). Circadian rhythms, insulin action, and glucose homeostasis. Current opinion in clinical nutrition and metabolic care, 17(4), 343–348. https://doi.org/10.1097/MCO.0000000000000061

[778] Willi, C., Bodenmann, P., Ghali, W. A., Faris, P. D., & Cornuz, J. (2007). Active smoking and the risk of type 2 diabetes: a systematic review and meta-analysis. JAMA, 298(22), 2654–2664. https://doi.org/10.1001/jama.298.22.2654

[779] Attvall S et al (1993) 'Smoking induces insulin resistance--a potential link with the insulin resistance syndrome', J Intern Med. 1993 Apr;233(4):327-32.

[780] Koppes, L. L. J., Dekker, J. M., Hendriks, H. F. J., Bouter, L. M., & Heine, R. J. (2005). Moderate Alcohol Consumption Lowers the Risk of Type 2 Diabetes: A meta-analysis of prospective observational studies. Diabetes Care, 28(3), 719–725. doi:10.2337/diacare.28.3.719

[781] Brien, S. E., Ronksley, P. E., Turner, B. J., Mukamal, K. J., & Ghali, W. A. (2011). Effect of alcohol consumption on biological markers associated with risk of coronary heart disease: systematic review and meta-analysis of interventional studies. BMJ, 342(feb22 1), d636–d636. doi:10.1136/bmj.d636

[782] Joosten, M. M., Beulens, J. W. J., Kersten, S., & Hendriks, H. F. J. (2008). Moderate alcohol consumption increases insulin sensitivity and ADIPOQ expression in postmenopausal women: a randomised, crossover trial. Diabetologia, 51(8), 1375–1381. doi:10.1007/s00125-008-1031-y

[783] Ken C Chiu, Audrey Chu, Vay Liang W Go, Mohammed F Saad; Hypovitaminosis D is associated with insulin resistance and β cell dysfunction, The American Journal of Clinical Nutrition, Volume 79, Issue 5, 1 May 2004, Pages 820–825.

[784] Rosique-Esteban, N., Guasch-Ferré, M., Hernández-Alonso, P., & Salas-Salvadó, J. (2018). Dietary Magnesium and Cardiovascular Disease: A Review with Emphasis in Epidemiological Studies. Nutrients, 10(2), 168. doi:10.3390/nu10020168

[785] De Baaij, J. H. F., Hoenderop, J. G. J., & Bindels, R. J. M. (2015). Magnesium in Man: Implications for Health and Disease. Physiological Reviews, 95(1), 1–46. doi:10.1152/physrev.00012.2014

[786] El-Aal, A. A., El-Ghffar, E. A. A., Ghali, A. A., Zughbur, M. R., & Sirdah, M. M. (2018). The effect of vitamin C and/or E supplementations on type 2 diabetic adult males under metformin treatment: A single-blinded randomized controlled clinical trial. Diabetes & Metabolic Syndrome: Clinical Research & Reviews, 12(4), 483–489. doi:10.1016/j.dsx.2018.03.013

[787] Feng, W., Ding, Y., Zhang, W., Chen, Y., Li, Q., Wang, W., … Wu, X. (2018). Chromium malate alleviates high-glucose and insulin resistance in L6 skeletal muscle cells by regulating glucose uptake and insulin sensitivity signaling pathways. BioMetals, 31(5), 891–908. doi:10.1007/s10534-018-0132-4

[788] Mayo Clinic (2022) 'Prediabetes', Accessed Online March 30th 2022: https://www.mayoclinic.org/diseases-conditions/prediabetes/diagnosis-treatment/drc-20355284

[789] WHO (2006) 'Definition and Diagnosis of Diabetes Mellitus and Intermediate Hyperglycemia', Accessed Online March 30 2022: https://www.who.int/diabetes/publications/Definition%20and%20diagnosis%20of%20diabetes_new.pdf

[790] Buppajarntham et al (2021) 'Insulin', Medscape, Accessed Online March 29, 2022: https://emedicine.medscape.com/article/2089224-overview

[791] Mayo Clinic (2022) 'Glucose Tolerance Test', Accessed Online March 30th 2022: https://www.mayoclinic.org/tests-procedures/glucose-tolerance-test/about/pac-20394296

[792] Roy Moxham (7 February 2002). The Great Hedge of India: The Search for the Living Barrier that Divided a People. Basic Books. ISBN 978-0-7867-0976-2.

[793] Rolph, George (1873). Something about sugar: its history, growth, manufacture and distribution. San Francisco: J.J. Newbegin.

[794] Adas, Michael (January 2001). Agricultural and Pastoral Societies in Ancient and Classical History. Temple University Press. ISBN 1-56639-832-0. p. 311.

[795] Sen, Tansen. (2003). Buddhism, Diplomacy, and Trade: The Realignment of Sino-Indian Relations, 600–1400. Manoa: Asian Interactions and Comparisons, a joint publication of the University of Hawaii Press and the Association for Asian Studies. ISBN 0-8248-2593-4. pp. 38–40.

[796] Jean-Pierre (1990) 'Jean Meyer. Histoire du Sucre', Annales de Démographie Historique, Année 1990, pp. 507-509.

[797] Manning, Patrick (2006). "Slavery & Slave Trade in West Africa 1450-1930". Themes in West Africa's history. Akyeampong, Emmanuel Kwaku. Athens: Ohio University. pp. 102–103. ISBN 978-0-8214-4566-2.

[798] Strong, Roy (2002), Feast: A History of Grand Eating, Jonathan Cape, ISBN 0224061380

[799] Antonio Benítez Rojo (1996). The Repeating: The Caribbean and the Postmodern Perspective. James E. Maraniss (translation). Duke University Press. p. 93. ISBN 0-8223-1865-2.

[800] Abreu y Galindo, J. de (1977). A. Cioranescu (ed.). Historia de la conquista de las siete islas de Canarias. Tenerife: Goya ediciones.

[801] Marggraf (1747) "Experiences chimiques faites dans le dessein de tirer un veritable sucre de diverses plantes, qui croissent dans nos contrées" [Chemical experiments made with the intention of extracting real sugar from diverse plants that grow in our lands], Histoire de l'académie royale des sciences et belles-lettres de Berlin, pages 79–90.

[802] Hill, G.; Langer, R. H. M. (1991). Agricultural plants. Cambridge, UK: Cambridge University Press. pp. 197–199. ISBN 978-0-521-40563-8.

[803] Zucker-Museum im Haus Amrumer Straße(2004) 'Festveranstaltung zum 100jährigen Bestehen des Berliner Institut für Zuckerindustrie', Accessed Online April 10th 2022: https://web.archive.org/web/20070824035034/http://www2.tu-berlin.de/~zuckerinstitut/museum.html

[804] Otter, Chris (2020). Diet for a large planet. USA: University of Chicago Press. p. 73. ISBN 978-0-226-69710-9.

[805] The Sugar Association Inc (2015) 'Refining and Processing Sugar', Consumer Fact Sheet, Accessed Online April 10th 2022: https://web.archive.org/web/20150221031555/http://westernsugar.com/pdf/Refining%20and%20Processing%20Sugar.pdf

[806] Ludwig, D. S. (2002). The Glycemic Index. JAMA, 287(18), 2414. https://doi.org/10.1001/jama.287.18.2414

[807] DiNicolantonio JJ, Lucan SC. Sugar season. It's everywhere and addictive. The New York Times. 12 Dec 2014.

[808] Snow HL. Refined sugar: its use and misuse. The Improvement Era Magazine 1948;51.

[809] Moose (1944) 'SUGAR A "DILUTING" AGENT', JAMA. 1944;125(10):738-739. doi:10.1001/jama.1944.02850280054021

[810] Br Med J (1933) 'RELATION OF EXCESSIVE CARBOHYDRATE INGESTION TO CATARRHS AND OTHER DISEASES', 1:738, doi: https://doi.org/10.1136/bmj.1.3773.738

[811] Lonsdale and Marrs (2017) 'Thiamine Deficiency Disease, Dysautonomia, and High Calorie Malnutrition', Academic Press 2017

[812] Feinman, R. D., & Volek, J. S. (2008). Carbohydrate restriction as the default treatment for type 2 diabetes and metabolic syndrome. Scandinavian Cardiovascular Journal, 42(4), 256–263. https://doi.org/10.1080/14017430802014838

[813] Volek, J. S., & Feinman, R. D. (2005). Carbohydrate restriction improves the features of Metabolic Syndrome. Metabolic Syndrome may be defined by the response to carbohydrate restriction. Nutrition & metabolism, 2, 31. https://doi.org/10.1186/1743-7075-2-31

[814] Feinman, R. D., Pogozelski, W. K., Astrup, A., Bernstein, R. K., Fine, E. J., Westman, E. C., Accurso, A., Frassetto, L., Gower, B. A., McFarlane, S. I., Nielsen, J. V., Krarup, T., Saslow, L., Roth, K. S., Vernon, M. C., Volek, J. S., Wilshire, G. B., Dahlqvist, A., Sundberg, R., … Worm, N. (2015). Dietary carbohydrate restriction as the first approach in diabetes management: Critical review and evidence base. Nutrition, 31(1), 1–13. https://doi.org/10.1016/j.nut.2014.06.011

[815] Glushakova, O., Kosugi, T., Roncal, C., Mu, W., Heinig, M., Cirillo, P., Sánchez-Lozada, L. G., Johnson, R. J., & Nakagawa, T. (2008). Fructose Induces the Inflammatory Molecule ICAM-1 in Endothelial Cells. Journal of the American Society of Nephrology, 19(9), 1712–1720. https://doi.org/10.1681/asn.2007121304

[816] Nair, S., P Chacko, V., Arnold, C., & Diehl, A. M. (2003). Hepatic ATP reserve and efficiency of replenishing: comparison between obese and nonobese normal individuals. The American journal of gastroenterology, 98(2), 466–470. https://doi.org/10.1111/j.1572-0241.2003.07221.x

[817] Bode, J.C., Zelder, O., Rumpelt, H.J. and Wittkampy, U. (1973), Depletion of Liver Adenosine Phosphates and Metabolic Effects of Intravenous Infusion of Fructose or Sorbitol in Man and in the Rat,. European Journal of Clinical Investigation, 3: 436-441. https://doi.org/10.1111/j.1365-2362.1973.tb02211.x

[818] Bray, G. A. (2013). Energy and Fructose From Beverages Sweetened With Sugar or High-Fructose Corn Syrup Pose a Health Risk for Some People. Advances in Nutrition, 4(2), 220–225. https://doi.org/10.3945/an.112.002816

[819] Cannon, J. R., Harvison, P. J., & Rush, G. F. (1991). The effects of fructose on adenosine triphosphate depletion following mitochondrial dysfunction and lethal cell injury in isolated rat hepatocytes. Toxicology and applied pharmacology, 108(3), 407–416. https://doi.org/10.1016/0041-008x(91)90087-u

[820] Latta et al (1999) 'Metabolic Depletion of Atp by Fructose Inversely Controls Cd95- and Tumor Necrosis Factor Receptor 1–Mediated Hepatic Apoptosis', J Exp Med (2000) 191 (11): 1975–1986.

[821] Abdelmalek, M. F., Lazo, M., Horska, A., Bonekamp, S., Lipkin, E. W., Balasubramanyam, A., Bantle, J. P., Johnson, R. J., Diehl, A. M., Clark, J. M., & Fatty Liver Subgroup of Look AHEAD Research Group (2012). Higher dietary fructose is associated with impaired hepatic adenosine triphosphate homeostasis in obese individuals with type 2 diabetes. Hepatology (Baltimore, Md.), 56(3), 952–960. https://doi.org/10.1002/hep.25741

[822] Page, K. A., Chan, O., Arora, J., Belfort-DeAguiar, R., Dzuira, J., Roehmholdt, B., Cline, G. W., Naik, S., Sinha, R., Constable, R. T., & Sherwin, R. S. (2013). Effects of Fructose vs Glucose on Regional Cerebral Blood Flow in Brain Regions Involved With Appetite and Reward Pathways. JAMA, 309(1), 63. https://doi.org/10.1001/jama.2012.116975

[823] Bernadette P. Marriott, Lauren Olsho, Louise Hadden & Patty Connor (2010) Intake of Added Sugars and Selected Nutrients in the United States, National Health and Nutrition Examination Survey (NHANES) 2003—2006, Critical Reviews in Food Science and Nutrition, 50:3, 228-258, DOI: 10.1080/10408390903626223

[824] Walker, R. W., Dumke, K. A., & Goran, M. I. (2014). Fructose content in popular beverages made with and without high-fructose corn syrup. Nutrition, 30(7–8), 928–935. https://doi.org/10.1016/j.nut.2014.04.003

[825] Ventura, E. E., Davis, J. N., & Goran, M. I. (2011). Sugar Content of Popular Sweetened Beverages Based on Objective Laboratory Analysis: Focus on Fructose Content. Obesity, 19(4), 868–874. Portico. https://doi.org/10.1038/oby.2010.255

[826] Michael I. Goran, Stanley J. Ulijaszek & Emily E. Ventura (2013) High fructose corn syrup and diabetes prevalence: A global perspective, Global Public Health, 8:1, 55-64, DOI: 10.1080/17441692.2012.736257

[827] Bes-Rastrollo, M., Schulze, M. B., Ruiz-Canela, M., & Martinez-Gonzalez, M. A. (2013). Financial conflicts of interest and reporting bias regarding the association between sugar-sweetened beverages and weight gain: a systematic review of systematic reviews. PLoS medicine, 10(12), e1001578. https://doi.org/10.1371/journal.pmed.1001578

[828] Raben, A., Vasilaras, T. H., Møller, A. C., & Astrup, A. (2002). Sucrose compared with artificial sweeteners: different effects on ad libitum food intake and body weight after 10 wk of supplementation in overweight subjects. The American journal of clinical nutrition, 76(4), 721–729. https://doi.org/10.1093/ajcn/76.4.721

[829] Tordoff, M. G., & Alleva, A. M. (1990). Effect of drinking soda sweetened with aspartame or high-fructose corn syrup on food intake and body weight. The American journal of clinical nutrition, 51(6), 963–969. https://doi.org/10.1093/ajcn/51.6.963

[830] Ludwig, D. S., Peterson, K. E., & Gortmaker, S. L. (2001). Relation between consumption of sugar-sweetened drinks and childhood obesity: a prospective, observational analysis. The Lancet, 357(9255), 505–508. https://doi.org/10.1016/s0140-6736(00)04041-1

[831] Perez-Pozo, S. E., Schold, J., Nakagawa, T., Sánchez-Lozada, L. G., Johnson, R. J., & Lillo, J. L. (2009). Excessive fructose intake induces the features of metabolic syndrome in healthy adult men: role of uric acid in the hypertensive response. International Journal of Obesity, 34(3), 454–461. https://doi.org/10.1038/ijo.2009.259

[832] Reiser, S., Handler, H. B., Gardner, L. B., Hallfrisch, J. G., Michaelis, O. E., 4th, & Prather, E. S. (1979). Isocaloric exchange of dietary starch and sucrose in humans. II. Effect on fasting blood insulin, glucose, and glucagon and on insulin and glucose response to a sucrose load. The American journal of clinical nutrition, 32(11), 2206–2216. https://doi.org/10.1093/ajcn/32.11.2206

[833] Reiser, S., Michaelis, O. E., 4th, Cataland, S., & O'Dorisio, T. M. (1980). Effect of isocaloric exchange of dietary starch and sucrose in humans on the gastric inhibitory polypeptide response to a sucrose load. The American journal of clinical nutrition, 33(9), 1907–1911. https://doi.org/10.1093/ajcn/33.9.1907

[834] Hallfrisch, J., Ellwood, K. C., Michaelis, O. E., Reiser, S., O'Dorisio, T. M., & Prather, E. S. (1983). Effects of Dietary Fructose on Plasma Glucose and Hormone Responses in Normal and Hyperinsulinemic Men. The Journal of Nutrition, 113(9), 1819–1826. https://doi.org/10.1093/jn/113.9.1819

[835] Te Morenga et al (2014) 'Dietary sugars and cardiometabolic risk: systematic review and meta-analyses of randomized controlled trials of the effects on blood pressure and lipids', The American Journal of Clinical Nutrition, Volume 100, Issue 1, July 2014, Pages 65–79, https://doi.org/10.3945/ajcn.113.081521

[836] McCarty, M. F., & DiNicolantonio, J. J. (2014). The cardiometabolic benefits of glycine: Is glycine an 'antidote' to dietary fructose? Open Heart, 1(1), e000103. https://doi.org/10.1136/openhrt-2014-000103

[837] Basu, S., Yoffe, P., Hills, N., & Lustig, R. H. (2013). The Relationship of Sugar to Population-Level Diabetes Prevalence: An Econometric Analysis of Repeated Cross-Sectional Data. PLoS ONE, 8(2), e57873. https://doi.org/10.1371/journal.pone.0057873

[838] Bray, G. A., Nielsen, S. J., & Popkin, B. M. (2004). Consumption of high-fructose corn syrup in beverages may play a role in the epidemic of obesity. The American journal of clinical nutrition, 79(4), 537–543. https://doi.org/10.1093/ajcn/79.4.537

[839] YUDKIN, J. Sugar and Disease. Nature 239, 197–199 (1972). https://doi.org/10.1038/239197a0

[840] Shapiro, A., Mu, W., Roncal, C., Cheng, K.-Y., Johnson, R. J., & Scarpace, P. J. (2008). Fructose-induced leptin resistance exacerbates weight gain in response to subsequent high-fat feeding. American Journal of Physiology-Regulatory, Integrative and Comparative Physiology, 295(5), R1370–R1375. https://doi.org/10.1152/ajpregu.00195.2008

[841] DiNicolantonio, J. J., O'Keefe, J. H., & Lucan, S. C. (2014). An Unsavory Truth: Sugar, More than Salt, Predisposes to Hypertension and Chronic Disease. The American Journal of Cardiology, 114(7), 1126–1128. https://doi.org/10.1016/j.amjcard.2014.07.002

[842] Bray, G. A., & Popkin, B. M. (2014). Dietary Sugar and Body Weight: Have We Reached a Crisis in the Epidemic of Obesity and Diabetes? Diabetes Care, 37(4), 950–956. https://doi.org/10.2337/dc13-2085

[843] Welsh, J. A., Sharma, A. J., Grellinger, L., & Vos, M. B. (2011). Consumption of added sugars is decreasing in the United States. American Journal of Clinical Nutrition, 94(3), 726–734. https://doi.org/10.3945/ajcn.111.018366

[844] Cordain et al (2003) 'Hyperinsulinemic diseases of civilization: more than just Syndrome X', Comparative Biochemistry and Physiology Part A: Molecular & Integrative Physiology, Volume 136, Issue 1, September 2003, Pages 95-112.

[845] Malnik E. World Health Organisation advises halving sugar intake. The Telegraph. March 2014.

[846] Ahrens R. A. (1974). Sucrose, hypertension, and heart disease an historical perspective. The American journal of clinical nutrition, 27(4), 403–422. https://doi.org/10.1093/ajcn/27.4.403

[847] MacDonald and Thomas (1956) 'Studies on the genesis of experimental diffuse hepatic fibrosis.', Clinical Science, 01 Aug 1956, 15(3):373-387.

[848] Durand, A. M., Fisher, M., & Adams, M. (1968). The influence of type of dietary carbohydrate. Effect on histological findings in two strains of rats. Archives of pathology, 85(3), 318–324.

[849] DALDERUP, L. M., & VISSER, W. (1969). Influence of Extra Sucrose in the Daily Food on the Life-span of Wistar Albino Rats. Nature, 222(5198), 1050–1052. https://doi.org/10.1038/2221050a0

[850] DiNicolantonio, J. J., & Berger, A. (2016). Added sugars drive nutrient and energy deficit in obesity: a new paradigm. Open heart, 3(2), e000469. https://doi.org/10.1136/openhrt-2016-000469

[851] Vartanian, L. R., Schwartz, M. B., & Brownell, K. D. (2007). Effects of Soft Drink Consumption on Nutrition and Health: A Systematic Review and Meta-Analysis. American Journal of Public Health, 97(4), 667–675. https://doi.org/10.2105/ajph.2005.083782

[852] Nguyen, T. Q., Maalouf, N. M., Sakhaee, K., & Moe, O. W. (2011). Comparison of Insulin Action on GlucoseversusPotassium Uptake in Humans. Clinical Journal of the American Society of Nephrology, 6(7), 1533–1539. https://doi.org/10.2215/cjn.00750111

[853] Ludwig, D. S., Aronne, L. J., Astrup, A., de Cabo, R., Cantley, L. C., Friedman, M. I., Heymsfield, S. B., Johnson, J. D., King, J. C., Krauss, R. M., Lieberman, D. E., Taubes, G., Volek, J. S., Westman, E. C., Willett, W. C., Yancy, W. S., & Ebbeling, C. B. (2021). The carbohydrate-insulin model: a physiological perspective on the obesity pandemic. The American Journal of Clinical Nutrition, 114(6), 1873–1885. https://doi.org/10.1093/ajcn/nqab270

[854] Buu, L.-M., & Chen, Y.-C. (2014). Impact of glucose levels on expression of hypha-associated secreted aspartyl proteinases in Candida albicans. Journal of Biomedical Science, 21(1). https://doi.org/10.1186/1423-0127-21-22

[855] Vidotto, V., Sinicco, A., Accattatis, G., & Aoki, S. (1996). Influence of fructose on Candida albicans germ tube production. Mycopathologia, 135(2), 85–88. https://doi.org/10.1007/bf00436456

[856] Satokari, R. (2020). High Intake of Sugar and the Balance between Pro- and Anti-Inflammatory Gut Bacteria. Nutrients, 12(5), 1348. https://doi.org/10.3390/nu12051348

[857] Vargas, S. L., Patrick, C. C., Ayers, G. D., & Hughes, W. T. (1993). Modulating effect of dietary carbohydrate supplementation on Candida albicans colonization and invasion in a neutropenic mouse model. Infection and immunity, 61(2), 619–626. https://doi.org/10.1128/iai.61.2.619-626.1993

[858] Weig, M., Werner, E., Frosch, M., & Kasper, H. (1999). Limited effect of refined carbohydrate dietary supplementation on colonization of the gastrointestinal tract of healthy subjects by Candida albicans. The American journal of clinical nutrition, 69(6), 1170–1173. https://doi.org/10.1093/ajcn/69.6.1170

[859] Brown, V., Sexton, J. A., & Johnston, M. (2006). A Glucose Sensor in Candida albicans. Eukaryotic Cell, 5(10), 1726–1737. https://doi.org/10.1128/ec.00186-06

[860] Bäckhed, F., Ley, R. E., Sonnenburg, J. L., Peterson, D. A., & Gordon, J. I. (2005). Host-Bacterial Mutualism in the Human Intestine. Science, 307(5717), 1915–1920. https://doi.org/10.1126/science.1104816

[861] Rodaki et al (2009) 'Glucose Promotes Stress Resistance in the Fungal Pathogen Candida albicans', Molecular Biology of the Cell, Vol 20, No 22.

[862] Guo, P., Wang, H., Ji, L., Song, P., & Ma, X. (2021). Impacts of Fructose on Intestinal Barrier Function, Inflammation and Microbiota in a Piglet Model. Nutrients, 13(10), 3515. https://doi.org/10.3390/nu13103515

[863] Johnson, R. J., Rivard, C., Lanaspa, M. A., Otabachian-Smith, S., Ishimoto, T., Cicerchi, C., Cheeke, P. R., Macintosh, B., & Hess, T. (2013). Fructokinase, Fructans, Intestinal Permeability, and Metabolic Syndrome: An Equine Connection?. Journal of equine veterinary science, 33(2), 120–126. https://doi.org/10.1016/j.jevs.2012.05.004

[864] Zhang, D. M., Jiao, R. Q., & Kong, L. D. (2017). High Dietary Fructose: Direct or Indirect Dangerous Factors Disturbing Tissue and Organ Functions. Nutrients, 9(4), 335. https://doi.org/10.3390/nu9040335

[865] Cho, Y. E., Kim, D. K., Seo, W., Gao, B., Yoo, S. H., & Song, B. J. (2021). Fructose Promotes Leaky Gut, Endotoxemia, and Liver Fibrosis Through Ethanol-Inducible Cytochrome P450-2E1-Mediated Oxidative and Nitrative Stress. Hepatology (Baltimore, Md.), 73(6), 2180–2195. https://doi.org/10.1002/hep.30652

[866] Yu, R., Wen, S., Wang, Q., Wang, C., Zhang, L., Wu, X., Li, J., & Kong, L. (2021). Mulberroside A repairs high fructose diet-induced damage of intestinal epithelial and blood-brain barriers in mice: A potential for preventing hippocampal neuroinflammatory injury. Journal of neurochemistry, 157(6), 1979–1991. https://doi.org/10.1111/jnc.15242

[867] Cheng, H., Zhou, J., Sun, Y., Zhan, Q., & Zhang, D. (2022). High fructose diet: A risk factor for immune system dysregulation. Human immunology, S0198-8859(22)00067-2. Advance online publication. https://doi.org/10.1016/j.humimm.2022.03.007

[868] DiNicolantonio, J. J., & Berger, A. (2016). Added sugars drive nutrient and energy deficit in obesity: a new paradigm. Open Heart, 3(2), e000469. https://doi.org/10.1136/openhrt-2016-000469

[869] KAUFMAN, R. E. (1940). INFLUENCE OF THIAMINE ON BLOOD SUGAR LEVELS IN DIABETIC PATIENTS. Archives of Internal Medicine, 66(5), 1079. https://doi.org/10.1001/archinte.1940.00190170070004

[870] Page, G. L., Laight, D., & Cummings, M. H. (2011). Thiamine deficiency in diabetes mellitus and the impact of thiamine replacement on glucose metabolism and vascular disease. International journal of clinical practice, 65(6), 684–690. https://doi.org/10.1111/j.1742-1241.2011.02680.x

[871] Williams, R.D., Mason, H.L., & Smith, B.F. (1939). Induced vitamin B1 deficiency in human subjects. Proc Staff Meet. Mayo Clin. 1939:14:787-793.

[872] Williams et al (1940) 'OBSERVATIONS ON INDUCED THIAMINE (VITAMIN B1) DEFICIENCY IN MAN', Arch Intern Med (Chic). 1940;66(4):785-799. doi:10.1001/archinte.1940.00190160002001

[873] Wang, J., Persuitte, G., Olendzki, B. C., Wedick, N. M., Zhang, Z., Merriam, P. A., Fang, H., Carmody, J., Olendzki, G. F., & Ma, Y. (2013). Dietary magnesium improves insulin resistance among non-diabetic individuals with metabolic syndrome participating in a dietary trial. Nutrients, 5(10), 3910–3919. https://doi.org/10.3390/nu5103910

[874] Humphries, S. (1999). Low dietary magnesium is associated with insulin resistance in a sample of young, nondiabetic black Americans. American Journal of Hypertension, 12(8), 747–756. doi:10.1016/s0895-7061(99)00041-2

[875] Huerta, M. G., Roemmich, J. N., Kington, M. L., Bovbjerg, V. E., Weltman, A. L., Holmes, V. F., … Nadler, J. L. (2005). Magnesium Deficiency Is Associated With Insulin Resistance in Obese Children. Diabetes Care, 28(5), 1175–1181. doi:10.2337/diacare.28.5.1175

[876] Rodríguez-Morán, M., Simental Mendía, L. E., Zambrano Galván, G., & Guerrero-Romero, F. (2011). The role of magnesium in type 2 diabetes: a brief based-clinical review. Magnesium research, 24(4), 156–162. https://doi.org/10.1684/mrh.2011.0299

[877] Hata, A., Doi, Y., Ninomiya, T., Mukai, N., Hirakawa, Y., Hata, J., … Kiyohara, Y. (2013). Magnesium intake decreases Type 2 diabetes risk through the improvement of insulin resistance and inflammation: the Hisayama Study. Diabetic Medicine, 30(12), 1487–1494. doi:10.1111/dme.12250

[878] Evangelopoulos, A. A., Vallianou, N. G., Panagiotakos, D. B., Georgiou, A., Zacharias, G. A., Alevra, A. N., … Avgerinos, P. C. (2008). An inverse relationship between cumulating components of the metabolic syndrome and serum magnesium levels. Nutrition Research, 28(10), 659–663. doi:10.1016/j.nutres.2008.07.001

[879] He, K., Song, Y., Belin, R.J. and Chen, Y. (2006), Magnesium Intake and the Metabolic Syndrome: Epidemiologic Evidence to Date. Journal of the CardioMetabolic Syndrome, 1: 351-355. https://doi.org/10.1111/j.1559-4564.2006.05702.x

[880] Moradi et al (2021) 'A pilot study of the effects of chromium picolinate supplementation on serum fetuin-A, metabolic and inflammatory factors in patients with nonalcoholic fatty liver disease: A double-blind, placebo-controlled trial', Journal of Trace Elements in Medicine and Biology, Volume 63, January 2021, 126659.

[881] Coulston (2001) 'CHAPTER 29 - Nutritional Management for Type 2 Diabetes', Nutrition in the Prevention and Treatment of Disease, Pages 441-452.

[882] Costello, R. B., Dwyer, J. T., & Bailey, R. L. (2016). Chromium supplements for glycemic control in type 2 diabetes: limited evidence of effectiveness. Nutrition reviews, 74(7), 455–468. https://doi.org/10.1093/nutrit/nuw011

[883] San Mauro-Martin, I., Ruiz-León, A. M., Camina-Martín, M. A., Garicano-Vilar, E., Collado-Yurrita, L., Mateo-Silleras, B. d., & Redondo Del Río, M. (2016). Nutricion hospitalaria, 33(1), 27. https://doi.org/10.20960/nh.v33i1.27

[884] A scientific review: the role of chromium in insulin resistance. (2004). The Diabetes educator, Suppl, 2–14.

[885] Guerrero-Romero, F., & Rodríguez-Morán, M. (2005). Complementary therapies for diabetes: the case for chromium, magnesium, and antioxidants. Archives of medical research, 36(3), 250–257. https://doi.org/10.1016/j.arcmed.2005.01.004

[886] El-Aal, A. A., El-Ghffar, E., Ghali, A. A., Zughbur, M. R., & Sirdah, M. M. (2018). The effect of vitamin C and/or E supplementations on type 2 diabetic adult males under metformin treatment: A single-blinded randomized controlled clinical trial. Diabetes & metabolic syndrome, 12(4), 483–489. https://doi.org/10.1016/j.dsx.2018.03.013

[887] Chang (2011) Mechanisms Underlying the Abnormal Inositol Metabolisms in Diabetes Mellitus. Thesis, ResearchSpace@Auckland.

[888] Albert I Winegrad; Banting Lecture 1986: Does a Common Mechanism Induce the Diverse Complications of Diabetes?. Diabetes 1 March 1987; 36 (3): 396–406. https://doi.org/10.2337/diab.36.3.396

[889] Asplin et al (1993) 'chiro-Inositol deficiency and insulin resistance: A comparison of the chiro-inositol- and the myo-inositol-containing insulin mediators isolated from urine, hemodialysate, and muscle of control and type II diabetic subjects, Proc. Natl. Acad. Sci. USA, Vol. 90, pp. 5924-5928, July 1993.

[890] Sun, T., Heimark, D. B., Nguygen, T., Nadler, J. L., & Larner, J. (2002). Both myo-inositol to chiro-inositol epimerase activities and chiro-inositol to myo-inositol ratios are decreased in tissues of GK type 2 diabetic rats compared to Wistar controls. Biochemical and Biophysical Research Communications, 293(3), 1092–1098. https://doi.org/10.1016/s0006-291x(02)00313-3

[891] Parthasarathy, L. K., Seelan, R. S., Tobias, C., Casanova, M. F., & Parthasarathy, R. N. (2006). Mammalian inositol 3-phosphate synthase: its role in the biosynthesis of brain inositol and its clinical use as a psychoactive agent. Sub-cellular biochemistry, 39, 293–314. https://doi.org/10.1007/0-387-27600-9_12

892 Bizzarri, M., Fuso, A., Dinicola, S., Cucina, A., & Bevilacqua, A. (2016). Pharmacodynamics and pharmacokinetics of inositol(s) in health and disease. Expert opinion on drug metabolism & toxicology, 12(10), 1181–1196. https://doi.org/10.1080/17425255.2016.1206887

[893] Olgemöller, B., Schwaabe, S., Schleicher, E. D., & Gerbitz, K. D. (1990). Competitive inhibition by glucose of myo-inositol incorporation into cultured porcine aortic endothelial cells. Biochimica et Biophysica Acta (BBA) - Molecular Cell Research, 1052(1), 47–52. https://doi.org/10.1016/0167-4889(90)90056-j

[894] Haneda, M., Kikkawa, R., Arimura, T., Ebata, K., Togawa, M., Maeda, S., Sawada, T., Horide, N., & Shigeta, Y. (1990). Glucose inhibits myo-inositol uptake and reduces myo-inositol content in cultured rat glomerular mesangial cells. Metabolism, 39(1), 40–45. https://doi.org/10.1016/0026-0495(90)90145-3

[895] Yorek, M. A., & Dunlap, J. A. (1989). The effect of elevated glucose levels on myo-inositol metabolism in cultured bovine aortic endothelial cells. Metabolism, 38(1), 16–22. https://doi.org/10.1016/0026-0495(89)90174-1

[896] Greene, D. A., & Lattimer, S. A. (1982). Sodium- and energy-dependent uptake of myo-inositol by rabbit peripheral nerve. Competitive inhibition by glucose and lack of an insulin effect. Journal of Clinical Investigation, 70(5), 1009–1018. https://doi.org/10.1172/jci110688

[897] Kanwar, Y. S., Wada, J., Sun, L., Xie, P., Wallner, E. I., Chen, S., Chugh, S., & Danesh, F. R. (2008). Diabetic nephropathy: mechanisms of renal disease progression. Experimental biology and medicine (Maywood, N.J.), 233(1), 4–11. https://doi.org/10.3181/0705-MR-134

[898] Croze, M. L., & Soulage, C. O. (2013). Potential role and therapeutic interests of myo-inositol in metabolic diseases. Biochimie, 95(10), 1811–1827. https://doi.org/10.1016/j.biochi.2013.05.011

[899] Croze, M. L., & Soulage, C. O. (2013). Potential role and therapeutic interests of myo-inositol in metabolic diseases. Biochimie, 95(10), 1811–1827. https://doi.org/10.1016/j.biochi.2013.05.011

900 Greenwood et al (2001) 'D-PINITOL AUGMENTS WHOLE BODY CREATINE RETENTION IN MAN', Journal of Exercise Physiologyonline, Volume 4 Number 4 November 2001, Accessed Online Sep 15 2021: https://www.asep.org/asep/GreenwoodNOVEMBER2001.pdf

901 Angeloff, L. G., Skoryna, S. C., & Henderson, I. W. (1977). Effects of the hexahydroxyhexane myoinositol on bone uptake of radiocalcium in rats: Effect of inositol and vitamin D2 on bone uptake of 45Ca in rats. Acta pharmacologica et toxicologica, 40(2), 209–215. https://doi.org/10.1111/j.1600-0773.1977.tb02070.x

902 Bevilacqua, A., & Bizzarri, M. (2018). Inositols in Insulin Signaling and Glucose Metabolism. International Journal of Endocrinology, 2018, 1–8. doi:10.1155/2018/1968450

[903] Larner J. (2002). D-chiro-inositol--its functional role in insulin action and its deficit in insulin resistance. International journal of experimental diabetes research, 3(1), 47–60. https://doi.org/10.1080/15604280212528

[904] Gerasimenko, J. V., Flowerdew, S. E., Voronina, S. G., Sukhomlin, T. K., Tepikin, A. V., Petersen, O. H., & Gerasimenko, O. V. (2006). Bile acids induce Ca2+ release from both the endoplasmic reticulum and acidic intracellular calcium stores through activation of inositol trisphosphate receptors and ryanodine receptors. The Journal of biological chemistry, 281(52), 40154–40163. https://doi.org/10.1074/jbc.M606402200

[905] Kukuljan, M., Vergara, L., & Stojilkovic, S. S. (1997). Modulation of the kinetics of inositol 1,4,5-trisphosphate-induced [Ca2+]i oscillations by calcium entry in pituitary gonadotrophs. Biophysical journal, 72(2 Pt 1), 698–707. https://doi.org/10.1016/s0006-3495(97)78706-x

[906] Rapiejko, P. J., Northup, J. K., Evans, T., Brown, J. E., & Malbon, C. C. (1986). G-proteins of fat-cells. Role in hormonal regulation of intracellular inositol 1,4,5-trisphosphate. The Biochemical journal, 240(1), 35–40. https://doi.org/10.1042/bj2400035

[907] Shen, X., Xiao, H., Ranallo, R., Wu, W. H., & Wu, C. (2003). Modulation of ATP-dependent chromatin-remodeling complexes by inositol polyphosphates. Science (New York, N.Y.), 299(5603), 112–114. https://doi.org/10.1126/science.1078068

[908] Steger, D. J., Haswell, E. S., Miller, A. L., Wente, S. R., & O'Shea, E. K. (2003). Regulation of chromatin remodeling by inositol polyphosphates. Science (New York, N.Y.), 299(5603), 114–116. https://doi.org/10.1126/science.1078062

909 Eisenberg, F., & Parthasarathy, R. (1987). Measurement of biosynthesis of myo-inositol from glucose 6-phosphate. Cellular Regulators Part B: Calcium and Lipids, 127–143. doi:10.1016/0076-6879(87)41061-6

[910] A. Santamaria, D. Giordano, F. Corrado, B. Pintaudi, M. L. Interdonato, G. Di Vieste, A. Di Benedetto & R. D'Anna (2012) One-year effects of myo-inositol supplementation in postmenopausal women with metabolic syndrome, Climacteric, 15:5, 490-495, DOI: 10.3109/13697137.2011.631063

[911] D'Anna, R., Scilipoti, A., Giordano, D., Caruso, C., Cannata, M. L., Interdonato, M. L., Corrado, F., & Di Benedetto, A. (2013). myo-Inositol Supplementation and Onset of Gestational Diabetes Mellitus in Pregnant Women With a Family History of Type 2 Diabetes. Diabetes Care, 36(4), 854–857. https://doi.org/10.2337/dc12-1371

[912] Matarrelli, B., Vitacolonna, E., D'angelo, M., Pavone, G., Mattei, P. A., Liberati, M., & Celentano, C. (2013). Effect of dietary myo-inositol supplementation in pregnancy on the incidence of maternal gestational diabetes mellitus and fetal outcomes: a randomized controlled trial. The Journal of Maternal-Fetal & Neonatal Medicine, 26(10), 967–972. https://doi.org/10.3109/14767058.2013.766691

[913] Unfer, V., Carlomagno, G., Dante, G., & Facchinetti, F. (2012). Effects of myo-inositol in women with PCOS: a systematic review of randomized controlled trials. Gynecological Endocrinology, 28(7), 509–515. https://doi.org/10.3109/09513590.2011.650660

[914] Genazzani, A. D., Lanzoni, C., Ricchieri, F., & Jasonni, V. M. (2008). Myo-inositol administration positively affects hyperinsulinemia and hormonal parameters in overweight patients with polycystic ovary syndrome. Gynecological Endocrinology, 24(3), 139–144. https://doi.org/10.1080/09513590801893232

[915] Enrico Papaleo, Vittorio Unfer, Jean-Patrice Baillargeon, Lucia De Santis, Francesco Fusi, Claudio Brigante, Guido Marelli, Ilaria Cino, Anna Redaelli & Augusto Ferrari (2007) Myo-inositol in patients with polycystic ovary syndrome: A novel method for ovulation induction, Gynecological Endocrinology, 23:12, 700-703, DOI: 10.1080/09513590701672405

[916] Emanuela Raffone, Pietro Rizzo & Vincenzo Benedetto (2010) Insulin sensitiser agents alone and in co-treatment with r-FSH for ovulation induction in PCOS women, Gynecological Endocrinology, 26:4, 275-280, DOI: 10.3109/09513590903366996

[917] Artini, P. G., Di Berardino, O. M., Papini, F., Genazzani, A. D., Simi, G., Ruggiero, M., & Cela, V. (2013). Endocrine and clinical effects of myo-inositol administration in polycystic ovary syndrome. A randomized study. Gynecological endocrinology : the official journal of the International Society of Gynecological Endocrinology, 29(4), 375–379. https://doi.org/10.3109/09513590.2012.743020

[918] Giordano, D., Corrado, F., Santamaria, A., Quattrone, S., Pintaudi, B., Di Benedetto, A., & D'Anna, R. (2011). Effects of myo-inositol supplementation in postmenopausal women with metabolic syndrome. Menopause, 18(1), 102–104. https://doi.org/10.1097/gme.0b013e3181e8e1b1

[919] Costantino, D., Minozzi, G., Minozzi, E., & Guaraldi, C. (2009). Metabolic and hormonal effects of myo-inositol in women with polycystic ovary syndrome: a double-blind trial. European review for medical and pharmacological sciences, 13(2), 105–110.

920 Venturella, R., Mocciaro, R., De Trana, E., D'Alessandro, P., Morelli, M., & Zullo, F. (2012). Valutazione delle modificazioni del profilo clinico, endocrino e metabolico di pazienti con sindrome dell'ovaio policistico in trattamento con mio-inositolo [Assessment of the modification of the clinical, endocrinal and metabolical profile of patients with PCOS syndrome treated with myo-inositol]. Minerva ginecologica, 64(3), 239–243.

921 Holub (1986) 'Metabolism and Function of myo-Inositol and Inositol Phospholipids', Annual Review of Nutrition, Vol. 6:563-597.

922 Schlemmer, U., Frølich, W., Prieto, R. M., & Grases, F. (2009). Phytate in foods and significance for humans: Food sources, intake, processing, bioavailability, protective role and analysis. Molecular Nutrition & Food Research, 53(S2), S330–S375. Portico. https://doi.org/10.1002/mnfr.200900099

923 Clements, R. S., Jr, & Darnell, B. (1980). Myo-inositol content of common foods: development of a high-myo-inositol diet. The American journal of clinical nutrition, 33(9), 1954–1967. https://doi.org/10.1093/ajcn/33.9.1954

[924] Corrado, F., D'Anna, R., Di Vieste, G., Giordano, D., Pintaudi, B., Santamaria, A. and Di Benedetto, A. (2011), The effect of myoinositol supplementation on insulin resistance in patients with gestational diabetes. Diabetic Medicine, 28: 972-975. https://doi.org/10.1111/j.1464-5491.2011.03284.x

[925] Taylor, R., & Holman, R. R. (2015). Normal weight individuals who develop type 2 diabetes: the personal fat threshold. Clinical science (London, England : 1979), 128(7), 405–410. https://doi.org/10.1042/CS20140553

[926] Virtue, S., & Vidal-Puig, A. (2010). Adipose tissue expandability, lipotoxicity and the Metabolic Syndrome--an allostatic perspective. Biochimica et biophysica acta, 1801(3), 338–349. https://doi.org/10.1016/j.bbalip.2009.12.006

[927] Ohlson, L. O., Larsson, B., Svärdsudd, K., Welin, L., Eriksson, H., Wilhelmsen, L., Björntorp, P., & Tibblin, G. (1985). The influence of body fat distribution on the incidence of diabetes mellitus. 13.5 years of follow-up of the participants in the study of men born in 1913. Diabetes, 34(10), 1055–1058. https://doi.org/10.2337/diab.34.10.1055

[928] Donahue, R. P., Abbott, R. D., Bloom, E., Reed, D. M., & Yano, K. (1987). Central obesity and coronary heart disease in men. Lancet (London, England), 1(8537), 821–824. https://doi.org/10.1016/s0140-6736(87)91605-9

[929] Ducimetiere and Cambien (1986) 'The pattern of subcutaneous fat distribution in middle-aged men and the risk of coronary heart disease: the Paris Prospective Study.', International Journal of Obesity, 01 Jan 1986, 10(3):229-240.

[930] Lapidus, L., Bengtsson, C., Larsson, B., Pennert, K., Rybo, E., & Sjöström, L. (1984). Distribution of adipose tissue and risk of cardiovascular disease and death: a 12 year follow up of participants in the population study of women in Gothenburg, Sweden. British medical journal (Clinical research ed.), 289(6454), 1257–1261. https://doi.org/10.1136/bmj.289.6454.1257

[931] Larsson et al (1984) 'Abdominal adipose tissue distribution, obesity, and risk of cardiovascular disease and death: 13 year follow up of participants in the study of men born in 1913.', Br Med J (Clin Res Ed) 1984; 288 doi: https://doi.org/10.1136/bmj.288.6428.1401

[932] Pou, K. M., Massaro, J. M., Hoffmann, U., Vasan, R. S., Maurovich-Horvat, P., Larson, M. G., Keaney, J. F., Jr, Meigs, J. B., Lipinska, I., Kathiresan, S., Murabito, J. M., O'Donnell, C. J., Benjamin, E. J., & Fox, C. S. (2007). Visceral and subcutaneous adipose tissue volumes are cross-sectionally related to markers of inflammation and oxidative stress: the Framingham Heart Study. Circulation, 116(11), 1234–1241. https://doi.org/10.1161/CIRCULATIONAHA.107.710509

[933] Pischon, T., Boeing, H., Hoffmann, K., Bergmann, M., Schulze, M. B., Overvad, K., van der Schouw, Y. T., Spencer, E., Moons, K. G., Tjønneland, A., Halkjaer, J., Jensen, M. K., Stegger, J., Clavel-Chapelon, F., Boutron-Ruault, M. C., Chajes, V., Linseisen, J., Kaaks, R., Trichopoulou, A., Trichopoulos, D., … Riboli, E. (2008). General and abdominal adiposity and risk of death in Europe. The New England journal of medicine, 359(20), 2105–2120. https://doi.org/10.1056/NEJMoa0801891

[934] Kern, P. A., Ranganathan, S., Li, C., Wood, L., & Ranganathan, G. (2001). Adipose tissue tumor necrosis factor and interleukin-6 expression in human obesity and insulin resistance. American journal of physiology. Endocrinology and metabolism, 280(5), E745–E751. https://doi.org/10.1152/ajpendo.2001.280.5.E745

[935] Mokdad, A. H., Ford, E. S., Bowman, B. A., Dietz, W. H., Vinicor, F., Bales, V. S., & Marks, J. S. (2003). Prevalence of obesity, diabetes, and obesity-related health risk factors, 2001. JAMA, 289(1), 76–79. https://doi.org/10.1001/jama.289.1.76

[936] Marette A. (2003). Molecular mechanisms of inflammation in obesity-linked insulin resistance. International journal of obesity and related metabolic disorders : journal of the International Association for the Study of Obesity, 27 Suppl 3, S46–S48. https://doi.org/10.1038/sj.ijo.0802500

[937] Montague, C. T., & O'Rahilly, S. (2000). The perils of portliness: causes and consequences of visceral adiposity. Diabetes, 49(6), 883–888. https://doi.org/10.2337/diabetes.49.6.883

[938] Maresky, H. S., Sharfman, Z., Ziv-Baran, T., Gomori, J. M., Copel, L., & Tal, S. (2015). Anthropometric Assessment of Neck Adipose Tissue and Airway Volume Using Multidetector Computed Tomography: An Imaging Approach and Association With Overall Mortality. Medicine, 94(45), e1991. https://doi.org/10.1097/MD.0000000000001991

[939] Batra, A., & Siegmund, B. (2012). The role of visceral fat. Digestive diseases (Basel, Switzerland), 30(1), 70–74. https://doi.org/10.1159/000335722

[940] Ibrahim M. M. (2010). Subcutaneous and visceral adipose tissue: structural and functional differences. Obesity reviews : an official journal of the International Association for the Study of Obesity, 11(1), 11–18. https://doi.org/10.1111/j.1467-789X.2009.00623.x

[941] Price et al (August 2006). "Weight, shape, and mortality risk in older persons: elevated waist-hip ratio, not high body mass index, is associated with a greater risk of death". Am. J. Clin. Nutr. 84 (2): 449–60.

[942] Thomas, E. L., Parkinson, J. R., Frost, G. S., Goldstone, A. P., Doré, C. J., McCarthy, J. P., Collins, A. L., Fitzpatrick, J. A., Durighel, G., Taylor-Robinson, S. D., & Bell, J. D. (2012). The missing risk: MRI and MRS phenotyping of abdominal adiposity and ectopic fat. Obesity (Silver Spring, Md.), 20(1), 76–87. https://doi.org/10.1038/oby.2011.142

[943] Thomas, E. L., Frost, G., Taylor-Robinson, S. D., & Bell, J. D. (2012). Excess body fat in obese and normal-weight subjects. Nutrition research reviews, 25(1), 150–161. https://doi.org/10.1017/S0954422412000054

[944] Thomas, E. L., Parkinson, J. R., Frost, G. S., Goldstone, A. P., Doré, C. J., McCarthy, J. P., Collins, A. L., Fitzpatrick, J. A., Durighel, G., Taylor-Robinson, S. D., & Bell, J. D. (2012). The missing risk: MRI and MRS phenotyping of abdominal adiposity and ectopic fat. Obesity (Silver Spring, Md.), 20(1), 76–87. https://doi.org/10.1038/oby.2011.142

[945] Conus, F., Rabasa-Lhoret, R., & Péronnet, F. (2007). Characteristics of metabolically obese normal-weight (MONW) subjects. Applied physiology, nutrition, and metabolism = Physiologie appliquee, nutrition et metabolisme, 32(1), 4–12. https://doi.org/10.1139/h06-092

[946] Ruderman, N. B., Schneider, S. H., & Berchtold, P. (1981). The "metabolically-obese," normal-weight individual. The American journal of clinical nutrition, 34(8), 1617–1621. https://doi.org/10.1093/ajcn/34.8.1617

[947] Dimitriadis, G., Mitrou, P., Lambadiari, V., Maratou, E., & Raptis, S. A. (2011). Insulin effects in muscle and adipose tissue. Diabetes research and clinical practice, 93 Suppl 1, S52–S59. https://doi.org/10.1016/S0168-8227(11)70014-6

[948] Kuo, L. E., Czarnecka, M., Kitlinska, J. B., Tilan, J. U., Kvetnanský, R., & Zukowska, Z. (2008). Chronic stress, combined with a high-fat/high-sugar diet, shifts sympathetic signaling toward neuropeptide Y and leads to obesity and the metabolic syndrome. Annals of the New York Academy of Sciences, 1148, 232–237. https://doi.org/10.1196/annals.1410.035

[949] Björntorp P. (1996). The regulation of adipose tissue distribution in humans. International journal of obesity and related metabolic disorders : journal of the International Association for the Study of Obesity, 20(4), 291–302.

[950] Mårin, P., Darin, N., Amemiya, T., Andersson, B., Jern, S., & Björntorp, P. (1992). Cortisol secretion in relation to body fat distribution in obese premenopausal women. Metabolism: clinical and experimental, 41(8), 882–886. https://doi.org/10.1016/0026-0495(92)90171-6

[951] Reaven G. M. (2011). The metabolic syndrome: time to get off the merry-go-round?. Journal of internal medicine, 269(2), 127–136. https://doi.org/10.1111/j.1365-2796.2010.02325.x

[952] Rutters, F., Nieuwenhuizen, A. G., Lemmens, S. G., Born, J. M., & Westerterp-Plantenga, M. S. (2010). Hypothalamic-pituitary-adrenal (HPA) axis functioning in relation to body fat distribution. Clinical endocrinology, 72(6), 738–743. https://doi.org/10.1111/j.1365-2265.2009.03712.x

[953] Tchernof, A., & Després, J. P. (2013). Pathophysiology of human visceral obesity: an update. Physiological reviews, 93(1), 359–404. https://doi.org/10.1152/physrev.00033.2011

[954] Chielle, E. O., Feltez, A., & Rossi, E. M. (2017). Influence of obesity on the serum concentration of retinol-binding protein 4 (RBP4) in young adults. Jornal Brasileiro de Patologia e Medicina Laboratorial. https://doi.org/10.5935/1676-2444.20170012

[955] Chang, X., Yan, H., Bian, H., Xia, M., Zhang, L., Gao, J., & Gao, X. (2015). Serum retinol binding protein 4 is associated with visceral fat in human with nonalcoholic fatty liver disease without known diabetes: a cross-sectional study. Lipids in health and disease, 14, 28. https://doi.org/10.1186/s12944-015-0033-2

[956] Patel, P., & Abate, N. (2013). Body fat distribution and insulin resistance. Nutrients, 5(6), 2019–2027. https://doi.org/10.3390/nu5062019

[957] Havel P. J. (2005). Dietary fructose: implications for dysregulation of energy homeostasis and lipid/carbohydrate metabolism. Nutrition reviews, 63(5), 133–157. https://doi.org/10.1301/nr.2005.may.133-157

[958] Lustig R. H. (2010). Fructose: metabolic, hedonic, and societal parallels with ethanol. Journal of the American Dietetic Association, 110(9), 1307–1321. https://doi.org/10.1016/j.jada.2010.06.008

[959] Stanhope, K. L., Schwarz, J. M., Keim, N. L., Griffen, S. C., Bremer, A. A., Graham, J. L., Hatcher, B., Cox, C. L., Dyachenko, A., Zhang, W., McGahan, J. P., Seibert, A., Krauss, R. M., Chiu, S., Schaefer, E. J., Ai, M., Otokozawa, S., Nakajima, K., Nakano, T., Beysen, C., … Havel, P. J. (2009). Consuming fructose-sweetened, not glucose-sweetened, beverages increases visceral adiposity and lipids and decreases insulin sensitivity in overweight/obese humans. The Journal of clinical investigation, 119(5), 1322–1334. https://doi.org/10.1172/JCI37385

[960] Tchernof, A., & Després, J. P. (2013). Pathophysiology of human visceral obesity: an update. Physiological reviews, 93(1), 359–404. https://doi.org/10.1152/physrev.00033.2011

[961] Walker, B. R., & Andrew, R. (2006). Tissue production of cortisol by 11beta-hydroxysteroid dehydrogenase type 1 and metabolic disease. Annals of the New York Academy of Sciences, 1083, 165–184. https://doi.org/10.1196/annals.1367.012

[962] Thieringer, R., Le Grand, C. B., Carbin, L., Cai, T. Q., Wong, B., Wright, S. D., & Hermanowski-Vosatka, A. (2001). 11 Beta-hydroxysteroid dehydrogenase type 1 is induced in human monocytes upon differentiation to macrophages. Journal of immunology (Baltimore, Md. : 1950), 167(1), 30–35. https://doi.org/10.4049/jimmunol.167.1.30

[963] Beck-Nielsen, H., Pedersen, O., & Lindskov, H. O. (1980). Impaired cellular insulin binding and insulin sensitivity induced by high-fructose feeding in normal subjects. The American journal of clinical nutrition, 33(2), 273–278. https://doi.org/10.1093/ajcn/33.2.273

[964] Stanhope, K. L., Schwarz, J. M., Keim, N. L., Griffen, S. C., Bremer, A. A., Graham, J. L., Hatcher, B., Cox, C. L., Dyachenko, A., Zhang, W., McGahan, J. P., Seibert, A., Krauss, R. M., Chiu, S., Schaefer, E. J., Ai, M., Otokozawa, S., Nakajima, K., Nakano, T., Beysen, C., … Havel, P. J. (2009). Consuming fructose-sweetened, not glucose-sweetened, beverages increases visceral adiposity and lipids and decreases insulin sensitivity in overweight/obese humans. The Journal of clinical investigation, 119(5), 1322–1334. https://doi.org/10.1172/JCI37385

[965] Glushakova, O., Kosugi, T., Roncal, C., Mu, W., Heinig, M., Cirillo, P., Sánchez-Lozada, L. G., Johnson, R. J., & Nakagawa, T. (2008). Fructose induces the inflammatory molecule ICAM-1 in endothelial cells. Journal of the American Society of Nephrology : JASN, 19(9), 1712–1720. https://doi.org/10.1681/ASN.2007121304

[966] Basciano, H., Federico, L., & Adeli, K. (2005). Fructose, insulin resistance, and metabolic dyslipidemia. Nutrition & metabolism, 2(1), 5. https://doi.org/10.1186/1743-7075-2-5

[967] DiNicolantonio, J. J., Mehta, V., Onkaramurthy, N., & O'Keefe, J. H. (2018). Fructose-induced inflammation and increased cortisol: A new mechanism for how sugar induces visceral adiposity. Progress in cardiovascular diseases, 61(1), 3–9. https://doi.org/10.1016/j.pcad.2017.12.001

[968] London, E., & Castonguay, T. W. (2011). High fructose diets increase 11β-hydroxysteroid dehydrogenase type 1 in liver and visceral adipose in rats within 24-h exposure. Obesity (Silver Spring, Md.), 19(5), 925–932. https://doi.org/10.1038/oby.2010.284

[969] Vasiljević, A., Bursać, B., Djordjevic, A., Milutinović, D. V., Nikolić, M., Matić, G., & Veličković, N. (2014). Hepatic inflammation induced by high-fructose diet is associated with altered 11βHSD1 expression in the liver of Wistar rats. European journal of nutrition, 53(6), 1393–1402. https://doi.org/10.1007/s00394-013-0641-4

[970] Snel, M., Jonker, J. T., Schoones, J., Lamb, H., de Roos, A., Pijl, H., Smit, J. W., Meinders, A. E., & Jazet, I. M. (2012). Ectopic fat and insulin resistance: pathophysiology and effect of diet and lifestyle interventions. International journal of endocrinology, 2012, 983814. https://doi.org/10.1155/2012/983814

[971] Dekker, M. J., Su, Q., Baker, C., Rutledge, A. C., & Adeli, K. (2010). Fructose: a highly lipogenic nutrient implicated in insulin resistance, hepatic steatosis, and the metabolic syndrome. American Journal of Physiology-Endocrinology and Metabolism, 299(5), E685–E694. https://doi.org/10.1152/ajpendo.00283.2010

[972] Rizkalla S. W. (2010). Health implications of fructose consumption: A review of recent data. Nutrition & metabolism, 7, 82. https://doi.org/10.1186/1743-7075-7-82

[973] Morino, K., Petersen, K. F., & Shulman, G. I. (2006). Molecular mechanisms of insulin resistance in humans and their potential links with mitochondrial dysfunction. Diabetes, 55 Suppl 2(Suppl 2), S9–S15. https://doi.org/10.2337/db06-S002

[974] Sánchez-Lozada, L. G., Le, M., Segal, M., & Johnson, R. J. (2008). How safe is fructose for persons with or without diabetes?. The American journal of clinical nutrition, 88(5), 1189–1190. https://doi.org/10.3945/ajcn.2008.26812

[975] Segal, M. S., Gollub, E., & Johnson, R. J. (2007). Is the fructose index more relevant with regards to cardiovascular disease than the glycemic index?. European journal of nutrition, 46(7), 406–417. https://doi.org/10.1007/s00394-007-0680-9

[976] White J. S. (2013). Challenging the fructose hypothesis: new perspectives on fructose consumption and metabolism. Advances in nutrition (Bethesda, Md.), 4(2), 246–256. https://doi.org/10.3945/an.112.003137

[977] Marriott, B. P., Cole, N., & Lee, E. (2009). National estimates of dietary fructose intake increased from 1977 to 2004 in the United States. The Journal of nutrition, 139(6), 1228S–1235S. https://doi.org/10.3945/jn.108.098277

[978] Bes-Rastrollo, M., Schulze, M. B., Ruiz-Canela, M., & Martinez-Gonzalez, M. A. (2013). Financial conflicts of interest and reporting bias regarding the association between sugar-sweetened beverages and weight gain: a systematic review of systematic reviews. PLoS medicine, 10(12), e1001578. https://doi.org/10.1371/journal.pmed.1001578

[979] Nour, M., Lutze, S. A., Grech, A., & Allman-Farinelli, M. (2018). The Relationship between Vegetable Intake and Weight Outcomes: A Systematic Review of Cohort Studies. Nutrients, 10(11), 1626. https://doi.org/10.3390/nu10111626

[980] Ledoux, T. A., Hingle, M. D., & Baranowski, T. (2011). Relationship of fruit and vegetable intake with adiposity: a systematic review. Obesity reviews : an official journal of the International Association for the Study of Obesity, 12(5), e143–e150. https://doi.org/10.1111/j.1467-789X.2010.00786.x

[981] Merlotti, C., Ceriani, V., Morabito, A., & Pontiroli, A. E. (2017). Subcutaneous fat loss is greater than visceral fat loss with diet and exercise, weight-loss promoting drugs and bariatric surgery: a critical review and meta-analysis. International journal of obesity (2005), 41(5), 672–682. https://doi.org/10.1038/ijo.2017.31

[982] Ross, R., & Rissanen, J. (1994). Mobilization of visceral and subcutaneous adipose tissue in response to energy restriction and exercise. The American journal of clinical nutrition, 60(5), 695–703. https://doi.org/10.1093/ajcn/60.5.695

[983] Hu, F. B., & Malik, V. S. (2010). Sugar-sweetened beverages and risk of obesity and type 2 diabetes: epidemiologic evidence. Physiology & behavior, 100(1), 47–54. https://doi.org/10.1016/j.physbeh.2010.01.036

[984] Stanhope, K. L., Schwarz, J. M., Keim, N. L., Griffen, S. C., Bremer, A. A., Graham, J. L., Hatcher, B., Cox, C. L., Dyachenko, A., Zhang, W., McGahan, J. P., Seibert, A., Krauss, R. M., Chiu, S., Schaefer, E. J., Ai, M., Otokozawa, S., Nakajima, K., Nakano, T., Beysen, C., … Havel, P. J. (2009). Consuming fructose-sweetened, not glucose-sweetened, beverages increases visceral adiposity and lipids and decreases insulin sensitivity in overweight/obese humans. The Journal of clinical investigation, 119(5), 1322–1334. https://doi.org/10.1172/JCI37385

[985] Ma, J., Sloan, M., Fox, C. S., Hoffmann, U., Smith, C. E., Saltzman, E., Rogers, G. T., Jacques, P. F., & McKeown, N. M. (2014). Sugar-sweetened beverage consumption is associated with abdominal fat partitioning in healthy adults. The Journal of nutrition, 144(8), 1283–1290. https://doi.org/10.3945/jn.113.188599

[986] Stanhope, K. L., Griffen, S. C., Bair, B. R., Swarbrick, M. M., Keim, N. L., & Havel, P. J. (2008). Twenty-four-hour endocrine and metabolic profiles following consumption of high-fructose corn syrup-, sucrose-, fructose-, and glucose-sweetened beverages with meals. The American journal of clinical nutrition, 87(5), 1194–1203. https://doi.org/10.1093/ajcn/87.5.1194

[987] Stanhope, K. L., & Havel, P. J. (2008). Endocrine and metabolic effects of consuming beverages sweetened with fructose, glucose, sucrose, or high-fructose corn syrup. The American journal of clinical nutrition, 88(6), 1733S–1737S. https://doi.org/10.3945/ajcn.2008.25825D

[988] Schwarz, J. M., Noworolski, S. M., Erkin-Cakmak, A., Korn, N. J., Wen, M. J., Tai, V. W., Jones, G. M., Palii, S. P., Velasco-Alin, M., Pan, K., Patterson, B. W., Gugliucci, A., Lustig, R. H., & Mulligan, K. (2017). Effects of Dietary Fructose Restriction on Liver Fat, De Novo Lipogenesis, and Insulin Kinetics in Children With Obesity. Gastroenterology, 153(3), 743–752. https://doi.org/10.1053/j.gastro.2017.05.043

[989] Bendsen, N. T., Christensen, R., Bartels, E. M., Kok, F. J., Sierksma, A., Raben, A., & Astrup, A. (2013). Is beer consumption related to measures of abdominal and general obesity? A systematic review and meta-analysis. Nutrition reviews, 71(2), 67–87. https://doi.org/10.1111/j.1753-4887.2012.00548.x

[990] Dorn et al (2003) 'Alcohol Drinking Patterns Differentially Affect Central Adiposity as Measured by Abdominal Height in Women and Men', The Journal of Nutrition, Volume 133, Issue 8, August 2003, Pages 2655–2662, https://doi.org/10.1093/jn/133.8.2655

[991] Kim, K. H., Oh, S. W., Kwon, H., Park, J. H., Choi, H., & Cho, B. (2012). Alcohol consumption and its relation to visceral and subcutaneous adipose tissues in healthy male Koreans. Annals of nutrition & metabolism, 60(1), 52–61. https://doi.org/10.1159/000334710

[992] Cigolini, M., Targher, G., Bergamo Andreis, I. A., Tonoli, M., Filippi, F., Muggeo, M., & De Sandre, G. (1996). Moderate alcohol consumption and its relation to visceral fat and plasma androgens in healthy women. International journal of obesity and related metabolic disorders : journal of the International Association for the Study of Obesity, 20(3), 206–212.

[993] de Souze et al (2015) 'Intake of saturated and trans unsaturated fatty acids and risk of all cause mortality, cardiovascular disease, and type 2 diabetes: systematic review and meta-analysis of observational studies', BMJ 2015; 351 doi: https://doi.org/10.1136/bmj.h3978

[994] Mozaffarian, D., Aro, A., & Willett, W. C. (2009). Health effects of trans-fatty acids: experimental and observational evidence. European journal of clinical nutrition, 63 Suppl 2, S5–S21. https://doi.org/10.1038/sj.ejcn.1602973

[995] Kavanagh, K., Jones, K. L., Sawyer, J., Kelley, K., Carr, J. J., Wagner, J. D., & Rudel, L. L. (2007). Trans fat diet induces abdominal obesity and changes in insulin sensitivity in monkeys. Obesity (Silver Spring, Md.), 15(7), 1675–1684. https://doi.org/10.1038/oby.2007.200

[996] Verheggen, R. J., Maessen, M. F., Green, D. J., Hermus, A. R., Hopman, M. T., & Thijssen, D. H. (2016). A systematic review and meta-analysis on the effects of exercise training versus hypocaloric diet: distinct effects on body weight and visceral adipose tissue. Obesity reviews : an official journal of the International Association for the Study of Obesity, 17(8), 664–690. https://doi.org/10.1111/obr.12406

[997] Ohkawara, K., Tanaka, S., Miyachi, M., Ishikawa-Takata, K., & Tabata, I. (2007). A dose-response relation between aerobic exercise and visceral fat reduction: systematic review of clinical trials. International journal of obesity (2005), 31(12), 1786–1797. https://doi.org/10.1038/sj.ijo.0803683

[998] Coker, R. H., Williams, R. H., Kortebein, P. M., Sullivan, D. H., & Evans, W. J. (2009). Influence of exercise intensity on abdominal fat and adiponectin in elderly adults. Metabolic syndrome and related disorders, 7(4), 363–368. https://doi.org/10.1089/met.2008.0060

[999] Irving, B. A., Davis, C. K., Brock, D. W., Weltman, J. Y., Swift, D., Barrett, E. J., Gaesser, G. A., & Weltman, A. (2008). Effect of exercise training intensity on abdominal visceral fat and body composition. Medicine and science in sports and exercise, 40(11), 1863–1872. https://doi.org/10.1249/MSS.0b013e3181801d40

[1000] Vissers, D., Hens, W., Taeymans, J., Baeyens, J. P., Poortmans, J., & Van Gaal, L. (2013). The effect of exercise on visceral adipose tissue in overweight adults: a systematic review and meta-analysis. PloS one, 8(2), e56415. https://doi.org/10.1371/journal.pone.0056415

[1001] Thomas, E. L., Brynes, A. E., McCarthy, J., Goldstone, A. P., Hajnal, J. V., Saeed, N., Frost, G., & Bell, J. D. (2000). Preferential loss of visceral fat following aerobic exercise, measured by magnetic resonance imaging. Lipids, 35(7), 769–776. https://doi.org/10.1007/s11745-000-0584-0

[1002] Ismail, I., Keating, S. E., Baker, M. K., & Johnson, N. A. (2012). A systematic review and meta-analysis of the effect of aerobic vs. resistance exercise training on visceral fat. Obesity reviews : an official journal of the International Association for the Study of Obesity, 13(1), 68–91. https://doi.org/10.1111/j.1467-789X.2011.00931.x

[1003] Khalafi, M., Malandish, A., Rosenkranz, S. K., & Ravasi, A. A. (2021). Effect of resistance training with and without caloric restriction on visceral fat: A systemic review and meta-analysis. Obesity reviews : an official journal of the International Association for the Study of Obesity, 22(9), e13275. https://doi.org/10.1111/obr.13275

[1004] Hejnová, J., Majercík, M., Polák, J., Richterová, B., Crampes, F., deGlisezinski, I., & Stich, V. (2004). Vliv silove-dynamického tréninku na inzulínovou senzitivitu u inzulínorezistentních mužů [Effect of dynamic strength training on insulin sensitivity in men with insulin resistance]. Casopis lekaru ceskych, 143(11), 762–765.

[1005] Patel, S. R., Malhotra, A., White, D. P., Gottlieb, D. J., & Hu, F. B. (2006). Association between reduced sleep and weight gain in women. American journal of epidemiology, 164(10), 947–954. https://doi.org/10.1093/aje/kwj280

[1006] Hairston, K. G., Bryer-Ash, M., Norris, J. M., Haffner, S., Bowden, D. W., & Wagenknecht, L. E. (2010). Sleep duration and five-year abdominal fat accumulation in a minority cohort: the IRAS family study. Sleep, 33(3), 289–295. https://doi.org/10.1093/sleep/33.3.289

[1007] Beccuti, G., & Pannain, S. (2011). Sleep and obesity. Current opinion in clinical nutrition and metabolic care, 14(4), 402–412. https://doi.org/10.1097/MCO.0b013e3283479109

[1008] Theorell-Haglöw, J., Berne, C., Janson, C., Sahlin, C., & Lindberg, E. (2010). Associations between short sleep duration and central obesity in women. Sleep, 33(5), 593–598.

[1009] Pillar and Shehadeh (2008) 'Abdominal Fat and Sleep Apnea: The chicken or the egg?', Diabetes Care 2008;31(Supplement_2):S303–S309.

[1010] Toyama, Y., Tanizawa, K., Kubo, T., Chihara, Y., Harada, Y., Murase, K., Azuma, M., Hamada, S., Hitomi, T., Handa, T., Oga, T., Chiba, T., Mishima, M., & Chin, K. (2015). Impact of Obstructive Sleep Apnea on Liver Fat Accumulation According to Sex and Visceral Obesity. PLOS ONE, 10(6), e0129513. https://doi.org/10.1371/journal.pone.0129513

[1011] Kim, N. H., Lee, S. K., Eun, C. R., Seo, J. A., Kim, S. G., Choi, K. M., Baik, S. H., Choi, D. S., Yun, C. H., Kim, N. H., & Shin, C. (2013). Short sleep duration combined with obstructive sleep apnea is associated with visceral obesity in Korean adults. Sleep, 36(5), 723–729. https://doi.org/10.5665/sleep.2636

[1012] Chaput, J. P., Bouchard, C., & Tremblay, A. (2014). Change in sleep duration and visceral fat accumulation over 6 years in adults. Obesity (Silver Spring, Md.), 22(5), E9–E12. https://doi.org/10.1002/oby.20701

[1013] Mattson, M. P., Longo, V. D., & Harvie, M. (2017). Impact of intermittent fasting on health and disease processes. Ageing Research Reviews, 39, 46–58. https://doi.org/10.1016/j.arr.2016.10.005

[1014] Arnason, T. G., Bowen, M. W., & Mansell, K. D. (2017). Effects of intermittent fasting on health markers in those with type 2 diabetes: A pilot study. World journal of diabetes, 8(4), 154–164. https://doi.org/10.4239/wjd.v8.i4.154

[1015] Barnosky, A. R., Hoddy, K. K., Unterman, T. G., & Varady, K. A. (2014). Intermittent fasting vs daily calorie restriction for type 2 diabetes prevention: a review of human findings. Translational Research, 164(4), 302–311. https://doi.org/10.1016/j.trsl.2014.05.013

[1016] Volek, J., Sharman, M., Gómez, A., Judelson, D., Rubin, M., Watson, G., Sokmen, B., Silvestre, R., French, D., & Kraemer, W. (2004). Comparison of energy-restricted very low-carbohydrate and low-fat diets on weight loss and body composition in overweight men and women. Nutrition & metabolism, 1(1), 13. https://doi.org/10.1186/1743-7075-1-13

[1017] Gower, B. A., & Goss, A. M. (2015). A lower-carbohydrate, higher-fat diet reduces abdominal and intermuscular fat and increases insulin sensitivity in adults at risk of type 2 diabetes. The Journal of nutrition, 145(1), 177S–83S. https://doi.org/10.3945/jn.114.195065

[1018] Sasakabe, T., Haimoto, H., Umegaki, H., & Wakai, K. (2015). Association of decrease in carbohydrate intake with reduction in abdominal fat during 3-month moderate low-carbohydrate diet among non-obese Japanese patients with type 2 diabetes. Metabolism: clinical and experimental, 64(5), 618–625. https://doi.org/10.1016/j.metabol.2015.01.012

[1019] Goss, A. M., Goree, L. L., Ellis, A. C., Chandler-Laney, P. C., Casazza, K., Lockhart, M. E., & Gower, B. A. (2013). Effects of diet macronutrient composition on body composition and fat distribution during weight maintenance and weight loss. Obesity (Silver Spring, Md.), 21(6), 1139–1142. https://doi.org/10.1002/oby.20191

[1020] Hairston, K. G., Vitolins, M. Z., Norris, J. M., Anderson, A. M., Hanley, A. J., & Wagenknecht, L. E. (2012). Lifestyle factors and 5-year abdominal fat accumulation in a minority cohort: the IRAS Family Study. Obesity (Silver Spring, Md.), 20(2), 421–427. https://doi.org/10.1038/oby.2011.171

[1021] Morrison, D. J., & Preston, T. (2016). Formation of short chain fatty acids by the gut microbiota and their impact on human metabolism. Gut microbes, 7(3), 189–200. https://doi.org/10.1080/19490976.2015.1134082

[1022] Byrne, C. S., Chambers, E. S., Morrison, D. J., & Frost, G. (2015). The role of short chain fatty acids in appetite regulation and energy homeostasis. International journal of obesity (2005), 39(9), 1331–1338. https://doi.org/10.1038/ijo.2015.84

[1023] Tolhurst, G., Heffron, H., Lam, Y. S., Parker, H. E., Habib, A. M., Diakogiannaki, E., Cameron, J., Grosse, J., Reimann, F., & Gribble, F. M. (2012). Short-chain fatty acids stimulate glucagon-like peptide-1 secretion via the G-protein-coupled receptor FFAR2. Diabetes, 61(2), 364–371. https://doi.org/10.2337/db11-1019

1024 Wanders, A. J., van den Borne, J. J., de Graaf, C., Hulshof, T., Jonathan, M. C., Kristensen, M., Mars, M., Schols, H. A., & Feskens, E. J. (2011). Effects of dietary fibre on subjective appetite, energy intake and body weight: a systematic review of randomized controlled trials. Obesity reviews : an official journal of the International Association for the Study of Obesity, 12(9), 724–739. https://doi.org/10.1111/j.1467-789X.2011.00895.x

1025 Clark, M. J., & Slavin, J. L. (2013). The effect of fiber on satiety and food intake: a systematic review. Journal of the American College of Nutrition, 32(3), 200–211. https://doi.org/10.1080/07315724.2013.791194

1026 Burton-Freeman B. (2000). Dietary fiber and energy regulation. The Journal of nutrition, 130(2S Suppl), 272S–275S. https://doi.org/10.1093/jn/130.2.272S

1027 Kristensen, M., Jensen, M. G., Aarestrup, J., Petersen, K. E., Søndergaard, L., Mikkelsen, M. S., & Astrup, A. (2012). Flaxseed dietary fibers lower cholesterol and increase fecal fat excretion, but magnitude of effect depend on food type. Nutrition & metabolism, 9, 8. https://doi.org/10.1186/1743-7075-9-8

1028 Uebelhack, R., Busch, R., Alt, F., Beah, Z. M., & Chong, P. W. (2014). Effects of cactus fiber on the excretion of dietary fat in healthy subjects: a double blind, randomized, placebo-controlled, crossover clinical investigation. Current therapeutic research, clinical and experimental, 76, 39–44. https://doi.org/10.1016/j.curtheres.2014.02.001

[1029] Ogawa, A., Kobayashi, T., Sakai, F., Kadooka, Y., & Kawasaki, Y. (2015). Lactobacillus gasseri SBT2055 suppresses fatty acid release through enlargement of fat emulsion size in vitro and promotes fecal fat excretion in healthy Japanese subjects. Lipids in health and disease, 14, 20. https://doi.org/10.1186/s12944-015-0019-0

[1030] Kadooka, Y., Sato, M., Imaizumi, K., Ogawa, A., Ikuyama, K., Akai, Y., Okano, M., Kagoshima, M., & Tsuchida, T. (2010). Regulation of abdominal adiposity by probiotics (Lactobacillus gasseri SBT2055) in adults with obese tendencies in a randomized controlled trial. European journal of clinical nutrition, 64(6), 636–643. https://doi.org/10.1038/ejcn.2010.19

[1031] Kadooka, Y., Sato, M., Ogawa, A., Miyoshi, M., Uenishi, H., Ogawa, H., Ikuyama, K., Kagoshima, M., & Tsuchida, T. (2013). Effect of Lactobacillus gasseri SBT2055 in fermented milk on abdominal adiposity in adults in a randomised controlled trial. The British journal of nutrition, 110(9), 1696–1703. https://doi.org/10.1017/S0007114513001037

[1032] Pasiakos, S. M., Lieberman, H. R., & Fulgoni, V. L., 3rd (2015). Higher-protein diets are associated with higher HDL cholesterol and lower BMI and waist circumference in US adults. The Journal of nutrition, 145(3), 605–614. https://doi.org/10.3945/jn.114.205203

[1033] Loenneke, J.P., Wilson, J.M., Manninen, A.H. et al. Quality protein intake is inversely related with abdominal fat. Nutr Metab (Lond) 9, 5 (2012). https://doi.org/10.1186/1743-7075-9-5

[1034] Belko, A. Z., Barbieri, T. F., & Wong, E. C. (1986). Effect of energy and protein intake and exercise intensity on the thermic effect of food. The American journal of clinical nutrition, 43(6), 863–869. https://doi.org/10.1093/ajcn/43.6.863

[1035] Fukagawa, N. K., Bandini, L. G., Lim, P. H., Roingeard, F., Lee, M. A., & Young, J. B. (1991). Protein-induced changes in energy expenditure in young and old individuals. The American journal of physiology, 260(3 Pt 1), E345–E352. https://doi.org/10.1152/ajpendo.1991.260.3.E345

[1036] Ahmed, S. H., Guillem, K., & Vandaele, Y. (2013). Sugar addiction: pushing the drug-sugar analogy to the limit. Current opinion in clinical nutrition and metabolic care, 16(4), 434–439. https://doi.org/10.1097/MCO.0b013e328361c8b8

[1037] Lustig R. H. (2010). Fructose: metabolic, hedonic, and societal parallels with ethanol. Journal of the American Dietetic Association, 110(9), 1307–1321. https://doi.org/10.1016/j.jada.2010.06.008

[1038] Toll, B. A., Katulak, N. A., Williams-Piehota, P., & O'Malley, S. (2008). Validation of a scale for the assessment of food cravings among smokers. Appetite, 50(1), 25–32. https://doi.org/10.1016/j.appet.2007.05.001

[1039] Aubin, H. J., Farley, A., Lycett, D., Lahmek, P., & Aveyard, P. (2012). Weight gain in smokers after quitting cigarettes: meta-analysis. BMJ (Clinical research ed.), 345, e4439. https://doi.org/10.1136/bmj.e4439

[1040] West, R., May, S., McEwen, A., McRobbie, H., Hajek, P., & Vangeli, E. (2010). A randomised trial of glucose tablets to aid smoking cessation. Psychopharmacology, 207(4), 631–635. https://doi.org/10.1007/s00213-009-1692-3

[1041] Goldstein, R. Z., Woicik, P. A., Moeller, S. J., Telang, F., Jayne, M., Wong, C., Wang, G. J., Fowler, J. S., & Volkow, N. D. (2010). Liking and wanting of drug and non-drug rewards in active cocaine users: the STRAP-R questionnaire. Journal of psychopharmacology (Oxford, England), 24(2), 257–266. https://doi.org/10.1177/0269881108096982

[1042] Augier, E., Vouillac, C., & Ahmed, S. H. (2012). Diazepam promotes choice of abstinence in cocaine self-administering rats. Addiction biology, 17(2), 378–391. https://doi.org/10.1111/j.1369-1600.2011.00368.x

[1043] Cantin, L., Lenoir, M., Augier, E., Vanhille, N., Dubreucq, S., Serre, F., Vouillac, C., & Ahmed, S. H. (2010). Cocaine is low on the value ladder of rats: possible evidence for resilience to addiction. PloS one, 5(7), e11592. https://doi.org/10.1371/journal.pone.0011592

[1044] Lenoir, M., Serre, F., Cantin, L., & Ahmed, S. H. (2007). Intense sweetness surpasses cocaine reward. PloS one, 2(8), e698. https://doi.org/10.1371/journal.pone.0000698

[1045] Spring, B., Schneider, K., Smith, M., Kendzor, D., Appelhans, B., Hedeker, D., & Pagoto, S. (2008). Abuse potential of carbohydrates for overweight carbohydrate cravers. Psychopharmacology, 197(4), 637–647. https://doi.org/10.1007/s00213-008-1085-z

[1046] Pretlow R. A. (2011). Addiction to highly pleasurable food as a cause of the childhood obesity epidemic: a qualitative Internet study. Eating disorders, 19(4), 295–307. https://doi.org/10.1080/10640266.2011.584803

[1047] Avena, N. M., Rada, P., & Hoebel, B. G. (2008). Evidence for sugar addiction: behavioral and neurochemical effects of intermittent, excessive sugar intake. Neuroscience and biobehavioral reviews, 32(1), 20–39. https://doi.org/10.1016/j.neubiorev.2007.04.019

[1048] Ifland, J. R., Preuss, H. G., Marcus, M. T., Rourke, K. M., Taylor, W. C., Burau, K., Jacobs, W. S., Kadish, W., & Manso, G. (2009). Refined food addiction: a classic substance use disorder. Medical hypotheses, 72(5), 518–526. https://doi.org/10.1016/j.mehy.2008.11.035

[1049] Johnson, R. J., Andrews, P., Benner, S. A., & Oliver, W. (2010). Theodore E. Woodward award. The evolution of obesity: insights from the mid-Miocene. Transactions of the American Clinical and Climatological Association, 121, 295–308.

[1050] Keskitalo, K., Knaapila, A., Kallela, M., Palotie, A., Wessman, M., Sammalisto, S., Peltonen, L., Tuorila, H., & Perola, M. (2007). Sweet taste preferences are partly genetically determined: identification of a trait locus on chromosome 16. The American Journal of Clinical Nutrition, 86(1), 55–63. https://doi.org/10.1093/ajcn/86.1.55

[1051] Steiner J. E. (1979). Human facial expressions in response to taste and smell stimulation. Advances in child development and behavior, 13, 257–295. https://doi.org/10.1016/s0065-2407(08)60349-3

[1052] Berridge, K. C. (1996). Food reward: Brain substrates of wanting and liking. Neuroscience & Biobehavioral Reviews, 20(1), 1–25. https://doi.org/10.1016/0149-7634(95)00033-b

[1053] Drewnowski A. (1997). Taste preferences and food intake. Annual review of nutrition, 17, 237–253. https://doi.org/10.1146/annurev.nutr.17.1.237

[1054] DiNicolantonio JJ, Lucan SC, Season S. It's Everywhere and Addictive: The New York Times, 2014.

[1055] Avena, N. M., Rada, P., & Hoebel, B. G. (2008). Evidence for sugar addiction: behavioral and neurochemical effects of intermittent, excessive sugar intake. Neuroscience and biobehavioral reviews, 32(1), 20–39. https://doi.org/10.1016/j.neubiorev.2007.04.019

[1056] Lieblich, I., Cohen, E., Ganchrow, J. R., Blass, E. M., & Bergmann, F. (1983). Morphine tolerance in genetically selected rats induced by chronically elevated saccharin intake. Science (New York, N.Y.), 221(4613), 871–873. https://doi.org/10.1126/science.6879185

[1057] d'Anci, K. E., Kanarek, R. B., & Marks-Kaufman, R. (1996). Duration of sucrose availability differentially alters morphine-induced analgesia in rats. Pharmacology, biochemistry, and behavior, 54(4), 693–697. https://doi.org/10.1016/0091-3057(96)00016-0

[1058] Levine, A. S., Kotz, C. M., & Gosnell, B. A. (2003). Sugars: hedonic aspects, neuroregulation, and energy balance. The American journal of clinical nutrition, 78(4), 834S–842S. https://doi.org/10.1093/ajcn/78.4.834S

[1059] Volkow, N. D., & Wise, R. A. (2005). How can drug addiction help us understand obesity?. Nature neuroscience, 8(5), 555–560. https://doi.org/10.1038/nn1452

[1060] Kelley, A. E. (2004). Memory and Addiction. Neuron, 44(1), 161–179. https://doi.org/10.1016/j.neuron.2004.09.016!

[1061] Fowler, L., Ivezaj, V., & Saules, K. K. (2014). Problematic intake of high-sugar/low-fat and high glycemic index foods by bariatric patients is associated with development of post-surgical new onset substance use disorders. Eating behaviors, 15(3), 505–508. https://doi.org/10.1016/j.eatbeh.2014.06.009

[1062] Colantuoni, C., Rada, P., McCarthy, J., Patten, C., Avena, N. M., Chadeayne, A., & Hoebel, B. G. (2002). Evidence that intermittent, excessive sugar intake causes endogenous opioid dependence. Obesity research, 10(6), 478–488. https://doi.org/10.1038/oby.2002.66

[1063] DiNicolantonio JJ, et al. Br J Sports Med 2017;0:1–5. doi:10.1136/bjsports-2017-097971

[1064] DiNicolantonio (2017) 'Low-Salt Diets May Be Sensitizing Us to Addiction', VICE, Accessed Online May 6th 2022: https://www.vice.com/amp/en/article/9k5bwe/low-salt-diets-may-be-screwing-with-evolution

[1065] Clark, J. J., & Bernstein, I. L. (2006). A role for D2 but not D1 dopamine receptors in the cross-sensitization between amphetamine and salt appetite. Pharmacology Biochemistry and Behavior, 83(2), 277–284. https://doi.org/10.1016/j.pbb.2006.02.008

[1066] Roitman, M. F., Na, E., Anderson, G., Jones, T. A., & Bernstein, I. L. (2002). Induction of a salt appetite alters dendritic morphology in nucleus accumbens and sensitizes rats to amphetamine. The Journal of neuroscience : the official journal of the Society for Neuroscience, 22(11), RC225. https://doi.org/10.1523/JNEUROSCI.22-11-j0001.2002

[1067] Sakai, R. R., Fine, W. B., Epstein, A. N., & Frankmann, S. P. (1987). Salt appetite is enhanced by one prior episode of sodium depletion in the rat. Behavioral neuroscience, 101(5), 724–731. https://doi.org/10.1037//0735-7044.101.5.724

[1068] Denton, D. A., McKinley, M. J., & Weisinger, R. S. (1996). Hypothalamic integration of body fluid regulation. Proceedings of the National Academy of Sciences of the United States of America, 93(14), 7397–7404. https://doi.org/10.1073/pnas.93.14.7397

[1069] Liedtke, W. B., McKinley, M. J., Walker, L. L., Zhang, H., Pfenning, A. R., Drago, J., Hochendoner, S. J., Hilton, D. L., Lawrence, A. J., & Denton, D. A. (2011). Relation of addiction genes to hypothalamic gene changes subserving genesis and gratification of a classic instinct, sodium appetite. Proceedings of the National Academy of Sciences of the United States of America, 108(30), 12509–12514. https://doi.org/10.1073/pnas.1109199108

[1070] Robinson, T. E., & Berridge, K. C. (1993). The neural basis of drug craving: an incentive-sensitization theory of addiction. Brain research. Brain research reviews, 18(3), 247–291. https://doi.org/10.1016/0165-0173(93)90013-p

[1071] Robinson, T. E., & Kolb, B. (1997). Persistent structural modifications in nucleus accumbens and prefrontal cortex neurons produced by previous experience with amphetamine. The Journal of neuroscience : the official journal of the Society for Neuroscience, 17(21), 8491–8497. https://doi.org/10.1523/JNEUROSCI.17-21-08491.1997

[1072] Clark, J. J., & Bernstein, I. L. (2006). A role for D2 but not D1 dopamine receptors in the cross-sensitization between amphetamine and salt appetite. Pharmacology, biochemistry, and behavior, 83(2), 277–284. https://doi.org/10.1016/j.pbb.2006.02.008

[1073] Konner, M., & Eaton, S. B. (2010). Paleolithic nutrition: twenty-five years later. Nutrition in clinical practice : official publication of the American Society for Parenteral and Enteral Nutrition, 25(6), 594–602. https://doi.org/10.1177/0884533610385702

[1074] Eaton, S. B., & Konner, M. (1985). Paleolithic Nutrition. New England Journal of Medicine, 312(5), 283–289. doi:10.1056/nejm198501313120505

[1075] Heaney R. P. (2015). Making Sense of the Science of Sodium. Nutrition today, 50(2), 63–66. https://doi.org/10.1097/NT.0000000000000084

[1076] Eaton, S. B., & Konner, M. (1985). Paleolithic nutrition. A consideration of its nature and current implications. The New England journal of medicine, 312(5), 283–289. https://doi.org/10.1056/NEJM198501313120505

[1077] Denton D (1982) Hunger for salt, an anthropological, physiological and medical analysis. Springer Berlin, Heidelberg, New York, pp 573–575

[1078] Barlow, R. J., Connell, M. A., Levendig, B. J., Gear, J. S., & Milne, F. J. (1982). A comparative study of urinary sodium and potassium excretion in normotensive urban black and white South African males. South African medical journal = Suid-Afrikaanse tydskrif vir geneeskunde, 62(25), 939–941.

[1079] Grim, C. E., Luft, F. C., Miller, J. Z., Meneely, G. R., Battarbee, H. D., Hames, C. G., & Dahl, L. K. (1980). Racial differences in blood pressure in Evans County, Georgia: relationship to sodium and potassium intake and plasma renin activity. Journal of chronic diseases, 33(2), 87–94. https://doi.org/10.1016/0021-9681(80)90032-6

[1080] Khaw, K. T., & Barrett-Connor, E. (1984). Dietary potassium and blood pressure in a population. The American Journal of Clinical Nutrition, 39(6), 963–968. doi:10.1093/ajcn/39.6.963

[1081] Langford H. G. (1983). Dietary potassium and hypertension: epidemiologic data. Annals of internal medicine, 98(5 Pt 2), 770–772. https://doi.org/10.7326/0003-4819-98-5-770

[1082] FDA (2020) 'Sodium in Your Diet: Use the Nutrition Facts Label and Reduce Your Intake', Nutrition Education Resources & Materials, Accessed Online Dec 30 2020: https://www.fda.gov/food/nutrition-education-resources-materials/sodium-your-diet

[1083] Guinard, J. X., & Brun, P. (1998). Sensory-specific satiety: comparison of taste and texture effects. Appetite, 31(2), 141–157. https://doi.org/10.1006/appe.1998.0159

[1084] Rolls et al (1981) 'Sensory specific satiety in man', Physiology & Behavior, Volume 27, Issue 1, July 1981, Pages 137-142.

[1085] Rolls, B. J., Rowe, E. A., Rolls, E. T., Kingston, B., Megson, A., & Gunary, R. (1981). Variety in a meal enhances food intake in man. Physiology & behavior, 26(2), 215–221. https://doi.org/10.1016/0031-9384(81)90014-7

[1086] Rolls, B. J., Rolls, E. T. & Rowe, E. A. (1982b). The influence of variety on food selection and intake in man. In L. M. Barker (Ed.), Psychobiology of Human Food Selection. Pp. 101–122. Westport, CT: A.V.I. Publishing Co.

[1087] Rolls, B. J., Rowe, E. A., & Rolls, E. T. (1982). How sensory properties of foods affect human feeding behavior. Physiology & behavior, 29(3), 409–417. https://doi.org/10.1016/0031-9384(82)90259-1

[1088] Miller, P. E., & Perez, V. (2014). Low-calorie sweeteners and body weight and composition: a meta-analysis of randomized controlled trials and prospective cohort studies. The American journal of clinical nutrition, 100(3), 765–777. https://doi.org/10.3945/ajcn.113.082826

[1089] Shankar, P., Ahuja, S., & Sriram, K. (2013). Non-nutritive sweeteners: review and update. Nutrition (Burbank, Los Angeles County, Calif.), 29(11-12), 1293–1299. https://doi.org/10.1016/j.nut.2013.03.024

[1090] Rogers, P. J., Hogenkamp, P. S., de Graaf, C., Higgs, S., Lluch, A., Ness, A. R., Penfold, C., Perry, R., Putz, P., Yeomans, M. R., & Mela, D. J. (2016). Does low-energy sweetener consumption affect energy intake and body weight? A systematic review, including meta-analyses, of the evidence from human and animal studies. International journal of obesity (2005), 40(3), 381–394. https://doi.org/10.1038/ijo.2015.177

[1091] Bosetti, C., Gallus, S., Talamini, R., Montella, M., Franceschi, S., Negri, E., & La Vecchia, C. (2009). Artificial Sweeteners and the Risk of Gastric, Pancreatic, and Endometrial Cancers in Italy. Cancer Epidemiology Biomarkers & Prevention, 18(8), 2235–2238. https://doi.org/10.1158/1055-9965.epi-09-0365

[1092] Mishra, A., Ahmed, K., Froghi, S., & Dasgupta, P. (2015). Systematic review of the relationship between artificial sweetener consumption and cancer in humans: analysis of 599,741 participants. International Journal of Clinical Practice, 69(12), 1418–1426. Portico. https://doi.org/10.1111/ijcp.12703

[1093] Rogers, P. J., Hogenkamp, P. S., de Graaf, C., Higgs, S., Lluch, A., Ness, A. R., Penfold, C., Perry, R., Putz, P., Yeomans, M. R., & Mela, D. J. (2016). Does low-energy sweetener consumption affect energy intake and body weight? A systematic review, including meta-analyses, of the evidence from human and animal studies. International journal of obesity (2005), 40(3), 381–394. https://doi.org/10.1038/ijo.2015.177

[1094] Brown, R. J., de Banate, M. A., & Rother, K. I. (2010). Artificial sweeteners: a systematic review of metabolic effects in youth. International journal of pediatric obesity : IJPO : an official journal of the International Association for the Study of Obesity, 5(4), 305–312. https://doi.org/10.3109/17477160903497027

[1095] Bundgaard Anker, C. C., Rafiq, S., & Jeppesen, P. B. (2019). Effect of Steviol Glycosides on Human Health with Emphasis on Type 2 Diabetic Biomarkers: A Systematic Review and Meta-Analysis of Randomized Controlled Trials. Nutrients, 11(9), 1965. https://doi.org/10.3390/nu11091965

[1096] Suez, J., Korem, T., Zeevi, D., Zilberman-Schapira, G., Thaiss, C. A., Maza, O., Israeli, D., Zmora, N., Gilad, S., Weinberger, A., Kuperman, Y., Harmelin, A., Kolodkin-Gal, I., Shapiro, H., Halpern, Z., Segal, E., & Elinav, E. (2014). Artificial sweeteners induce glucose intolerance by altering the gut microbiota. Nature, 514(7521), 181–186. https://doi.org/10.1038/nature13793

[1097] Cinti S. (2005). The adipose organ. Prostaglandins, leukotrienes, and essential fatty acids, 73(1), 9–15. https://doi.org/10.1016/j.plefa.2005.04.010

[1098] Enerbäck S. (2009). The origins of brown adipose tissue. The New England journal of medicine, 360(19), 2021–2023. https://doi.org/10.1056/NEJMcibr0809610

[1099] Kozak, L. P. (2010). Brown Fat and the Myth of Diet-Induced Thermogenesis. Cell Metabolism, 11(4), 263–267. https://doi.org/10.1016/j.cmet.2010.03.009

[1100] Gesta, S., Tseng, Y. H., & Kahn, C. R. (2007). Developmental origin of fat: tracking obesity to its source. Cell, 131(2), 242–256. https://doi.org/10.1016/j.cell.2007.10.004

[1101] Saito, M., Okamatsu-Ogura, Y., Matsushita, M., Watanabe, K., Yoneshiro, T., Nio-Kobayashi, J., Iwanaga, T., Miyagawa, M., Kameya, T., Nakada, K., Kawai, Y., & Tsujisaki, M. (2009). High incidence of metabolically active brown adipose tissue in healthy adult humans: effects of cold exposure and adiposity. Diabetes, 58(7), 1526–1531. https://doi.org/10.2337/db09-0530

[1102] Nedergaard, J., Bengtsson, T., & Cannon, B. (2007). Unexpected evidence for active brown adipose tissue in adult humans. American journal of physiology. Endocrinology and metabolism, 293(2), E444–E452. https://doi.org/10.1152/ajpendo.00691.2006

[1103] Samuelson, I., & Vidal-Puig, A. (2020). Studying Brown Adipose Tissue in a Human in vitro Context. Frontiers in Endocrinology, 11. https://doi.org/10.3389/fendo.2020.00629

[1104] Carrière, A., Jeanson, Y., Cousin, B., Arnaud, E., & Casteilla, L. (2013). Le recrutement et l'activation d'adipocytes bruns et/ou BRITE. Médecine/Sciences, 29(8–9), 729–735. https://doi.org/10.1051/medsci/2013298011

[1105] Liu, X., Zheng, Z., Zhu, X., Meng, M., Li, L., Shen, Y., Chi, Q., Wang, D., Zhang, Z., Li, C., Li, Y., Xue, Y., Speakman, J. R., & Jin, W. (2013). Brown adipose tissue transplantation improves whole-body energy metabolism. Cell research, 23(6), 851–854. https://doi.org/10.1038/cr.2013.64

[1106] Stanford, K. I., Middelbeek, R. J., Townsend, K. L., An, D., Nygaard, E. B., Hitchcox, K. M., Markan, K. R., Nakano, K., Hirshman, M. F., Tseng, Y. H., & Goodyear, L. J. (2013). Brown adipose tissue regulates glucose homeostasis and insulin sensitivity. The Journal of clinical investigation, 123(1), 215–223. https://doi.org/10.1172/JCI62308

[1107] Berbée, J. F., Boon, M. R., Khedoe, P. P., Bartelt, A., Schlein, C., Worthmann, A., Kooijman, S., Hoeke, G., Mol, I. M., John, C., Jung, C., Vazirpanah, N., Brouwers, L. P., Gordts, P. L., Esko, J. D., Hiemstra, P. S., Havekes, L. M., Scheja, L., Heeren, J., & Rensen, P. C. (2015). Brown fat activation reduces hypercholesterolaemia and protects from atherosclerosis development. Nature communications, 6, 6356. https://doi.org/10.1038/ncomms7356

[1108] Bartelt, A., Bruns, O. T., Reimer, R., Hohenberg, H., Ittrich, H., Peldschus, K., Kaul, M. G., Tromsdorf, U. I., Weller, H., Waurisch, C., Eychmüller, A., Gordts, P. L., Rinninger, F., Bruegelmann, K., Freund, B., Nielsen, P., Merkel, M., & Heeren, J. (2011). Brown adipose tissue activity controls triglyceride clearance. Nature medicine, 17(2), 200–205. https://doi.org/10.1038/nm.2297

[1109] Cypess A. M., Lehman, S., Williams, G., Tal, I., Rodman, D., Goldfine, A. B., Kuo, F. C., Palmer, E. L., Tseng, Y. H., Doria, A., Kolodny, G. M., & Kahn, C. R. (2009). Identification and importance of brown adipose tissue in adult humans. The New England journal of medicine, 360(15), 1509–1517. https://doi.org/10.1056/NEJMoa0810780

[1110] Graja, A., & Schulz, T. J. (2014). Mechanisms of Aging-Related Impairment of Brown Adipocyte Development and Function. Gerontology, 61(3), 211–217. Portico. https://doi.org/10.1159/000366557

[1111] Romere, C., Duerrschmid, C., Bournat, J., Constable, P., Jain, M., Xia, F., Saha, P. K., Del Solar, M., Zhu, B., York, B., Sarkar, P., Rendon, D. A., Gaber, M. W., LeMaire, S. A., Coselli, J. S., Milewicz, D. M., Sutton, V. R., Butte, N. F., Moore, D. D., & Chopra, A. R. (2016). Asprosin, a Fasting-Induced Glucogenic Protein Hormone. Cell, 165(3), 566–579. https://doi.org/10.1016/j.cell.2016.02.063

[1112] Martínez-Sánchez N. (2020). There and Back Again: Leptin Actions in White Adipose Tissue. International journal of molecular sciences, 21(17), 6039. https://doi.org/10.3390/ijms21176039

[1113] Alan, M., Gurlek, B., Yilmaz, A., Aksit, M., Aslanipour, B., Gulhan, I., Mehmet, C., & Taner, C. E. (2019). Asprosin: a novel peptide hormone related to insulin resistance in women with polycystic ovary syndrome. Gynecological endocrinology : the official journal of the International Society of Gynecological Endocrinology, 35(3), 220–223. https://doi.org/10.1080/09513590.2018.1512967

[1114] Yuan, M., Li, W., Zhu, Y., Yu, B., & Wu, J. (2020). Asprosin: A Novel Player in Metabolic Diseases. Frontiers in endocrinology, 11, 64. https://doi.org/10.3389/fendo.2020.00064

[1115] Wang, C. Y., Lin, T. A., Liu, K. H., Liao, C. H., Liu, Y. Y., Wu, V. C., Wen, M. S., & Yeh, T. S. (2019). Serum asprosin levels and bariatric surgery outcomes in obese adults. International journal of obesity (2005), 43(5), 1019–1025. https://doi.org/10.1038/s41366-018-0248-1

[1116] Wu, J., Boström, P., Sparks, L. M., Ye, L., Choi, J. H., Giang, A.-H., Khandekar, M., Virtanen, K. A., Nuutila, P., Schaart, G., Huang, K., Tu, H., van Marken Lichtenbelt, W. D., Hoeks, J., Enerbäck, S., Schrauwen, P., & Spiegelman, B. M. (2012). Beige Adipocytes Are a Distinct Type of Thermogenic Fat Cell in Mouse and Human. Cell, 150(2), 366–376. https://doi.org/10.1016/j.cell.2012.05.016

[1117] Miao, Y., Qin, H., Zhong, Y., Huang, K., & Rao, C. (2021). Novel adipokine asprosin modulates browning and adipogenesis in white adipose tissue. The Journal of endocrinology, 249(2), 83–93. https://doi.org/10.1530/JOE-20-0503

[1118] Cedikova, M., Kripnerová, M., Dvorakova, J., Pitule, P., Grundmanova, M., Babuska, V., Mullerova, D., & Kuncova, J. (2016). Mitochondria in White, Brown, and Beige Adipocytes. Stem cells international, 2016, 6067349. https://doi.org/10.1155/2016/6067349

[1119] Lidell, M. E., Betz, M. J., & Enerbäck, S. (2014). Two types of brown adipose tissue in humans. Adipocyte, 3(1), 63–66. https://doi.org/10.4161/adip.26896

[1120] Heaton J. M. (1972). The distribution of brown adipose tissue in the human. Journal of anatomy, 112(Pt 1), 35–39.

[1121] Van Marken Lichtenbelt et al (2009). Cold-Activated Brown Adipose Tissue in Healthy Men. New England Journal of Medicine, 360(15), 1500–1508. doi:10.1056/nejmoa0808718

[1122] Saito, M. (2013). Brown Adipose Tissue as a Regulator of Energy Expenditure and Body Fat in Humans. Diabetes & Metabolism Journal, 37(1), 22. doi:10.4093/dmj.2013.37.1.22

[1123] Nie et al (2015) 'Cold exposure stimulates lipid metabolism, induces inflammatory response in the adipose tissue of mice and promotes the osteogenic differentiation of BMMSCs via the p38 MAPK pathway in vitro', Int J Clin Exp Pathol. 2015; 8(9): 10875–10886.

[1124] Dempersmier et al (2015). Cold-Inducible Zfp516 Activates UCP1 Transcription to Promote Browning of White Fat and Development of Brown Fat. Molecular Cell, 57(2), 235–246. doi:10.1016/j.molcel.2014.12.005

[1125] Hanssen et al (2015). Short-term Cold Acclimation Recruits Brown Adipose Tissue in Obese Humans. Diabetes, 65(5), 1179–1189. doi:10.2337/db15-1372

[1126] Acosta et al (2018). Physiological responses to acute cold exposure in young lean men. PLOS ONE, 13(5), e0196543. doi:10.1371/journal.pone.0196543

[1127] Srámek et al (2000). Human physiological responses to immersion into water of different temperatures. European journal of applied physiology, 81(5), 436–442. https://doi.org/10.1007/s004210050065

[1128] Imbeault, P., Dépault, I., & Haman, F. (2009). Cold exposure increases adiponectin levels in men. Metabolism: clinical and experimental, 58(4), 552–559. https://doi.org/10.1016/j.metabol.2008.11.017

[1129] Schrauwen, P., & van Marken Lichtenbelt, W. D. (2016). Combatting type 2 diabetes by turning up the heat. Diabetologia, 59(11), 2269–2279. doi:10.1007/s00125-016-4068-3

278

[1130] Garritson, J. D., & Boudina, S. (2021). The Effects of Exercise on White and Brown Adipose Tissue Cellularity, Metabolic Activity and Remodeling. Frontiers in physiology, 12, 772894. https://doi.org/10.3389/fphys.2021.772894

[1131] Xu, X., Ying, Z., Cai, M., Xu, Z., Li, Y., Jiang, S. Y., Tzan, K., Wang, A., Parthasarathy, S., He, G., Rajagopalan, S., & Sun, Q. (2011). Exercise ameliorates high-fat diet-induced metabolic and vascular dysfunction, and increases adipocyte progenitor cell population in brown adipose tissue. American journal of physiology. Regulatory, integrative and comparative physiology, 300(5), R1115–R1125. https://doi.org/10.1152/ajpregu.00806.2010

[1132] Fu, P., Zhu, R., Jia, J., Hu, Y., Wu, C., Cieszczyk, P., Holmberg, H. C., & Gong, L. (2021). Aerobic exercise promotes the functions of brown adipose tissue in obese mice via a mechanism involving COX2 in the VEGF signaling pathway. Nutrition & metabolism, 18(1), 56. https://doi.org/10.1186/s12986-021-00581-0

[1133] Loustau, T., Coudiere, E., Karkeni, E., Landrier, J. F., Jover, B., & Riva, C. (2020). Murine double minute-2 mediates exercise-induced angiogenesis in adipose tissue of diet-induced obese mice. Microvascular research, 130, 104003. https://doi.org/10.1016/j.mvr.2020.104003

[1134] Ye J. (2009). Emerging role of adipose tissue hypoxia in obesity and insulin resistance. International journal of obesity (2005), 33(1), 54–66. https://doi.org/10.1038/ijo.2008.229

[1135] Kolahdouzi, S., Talebi-Garakani, E., Hamidian, G., & Safarzade, A. (2019). Exercise training prevents high-fat diet-induced adipose tissue remodeling by promoting capillary density and macrophage polarization. Life sciences, 220, 32–43. https://doi.org/10.1016/j.lfs.2019.01.037

[1136] Wendt (2012) 'Vitamins Come to Dinner', Science History Institute, Accessed Online April 2nd 2022: https://www.sciencehistory.org/distillations/magazine/vitamins-come-to-dinner

[1137] World Health Organization and Food and Agricultural Organization (2016) 'Guidelines on food fortification with micronutrients', Edited by Lindsay Allen, Bruno de Benoist, Omar Dary and Richard Hurrell, Accessed Online Dec 5 2020: https://www.who.int/nutrition/publications/guide_food_fortification_micronutrients.pdf

[1138] McClure R. D. (1935). GOITER PROPHYLAXIS WITH IODIZED SALT. Science (New York, N.Y.), 82(2129), 370–371. https://doi.org/10.1126/science.82.2129.370

[1139] Moline Dispatch & Rock Island Argus (2021) '1933: Milk is enriched with vitamin D', Accessed Online April 11th 2022: https://qconline.com/lifestyles/1933-milk-is-enriched-with-vitamin-d/image_fd832d29-e5c2-5123-a5c5-b68e6b04ed3c.html

[1140] Cannell JJ, Vieth R, Umhau JC, et al. Epidemic influenza and vitamin D. Epidemiol Infect. 2006;134(6):1129-1140. doi:10.1017/S0950268806007175

[1141] Malloy, P. J., & Feldman, D. (2011). The role of vitamin D receptor mutations in the development of alopecia. Molecular and cellular endocrinology, 347(1-2), 90–96. https://doi.org/10.1016/j.mce.2011.05.045

[1142] Bener, A., & Saleh, N. M. (2015). Low vitamin D, and bone mineral density with depressive symptoms burden in menopausal and postmenopausal women. Journal of mid-life health, 6(3), 108–114. https://doi.org/10.4103/0976-7800.165590

[1143] Delange, F., Bürgi, H., Chen, Z. P., & Dunn, J. T. (2002). World status of monitoring iodine deficiency disorders control programs. Thyroid : official journal of the American Thyroid Association, 12(10), 915–924. https://doi.org/10.1089/105072502761016557

[1144] Food and Agricultural Organization of the United Nations 'Micronutrient Fortification of Food: Technology and Quality Control', Accessed Online Dec 5 2020: http://www.fao.org/3/W2840E/w2840e0b.htm

[1145] Harvard Medical School (2014) 'Vitamin and mineral supplements: Do you need them?', Harvard Health Publishing, Accessed Online April 2nd 2022: https://www.health.harvard.edu/newsletter_article/vitamin-and-mineral-supplements-do-you-need-them

[1146] Spedding, S. (2013). Vitamins are more Funky than Casimir thought. Australasian Medical Journal, 6(2), 104–106. https://doi.org/10.4066/amj.2013.1588

[1147] Spedding, S. (2013). Vitamins are more Funky than Casimir thought. Australasian Medical Journal, 6(2), 104–106. https://doi.org/10.4066/amj.2013.1588

[1148] Spedding S. (2013). Vitamins are more Funky than Casimir thought. The Australasian medical journal, 6(2), 104–106. https://doi.org/10.4066/AMJ.2013.1588

[1149] Institute of Medicine (US) Committee on Use of Dietary Reference Intakes in Nutrition Labeling. (2003). Dietary Reference Intakes: Guiding Principles for Nutrition Labeling and Fortification. National Academies Press (US).

[1150] Census (2012) 'Women's History Month: March 2012', Accessed Online April 2nd 2022: https://www.census.gov/newsroom/releases/archives/facts_for_features_special_editions/cb12-ff05.html

[1151] Lehnhardt (2019) '73 Interesting Pregnancy Facts', Fact Retriever, Accessed Online April 2nd 2022: https://www.factretriever.com/interesting-pregnancy-facts

[1152] Amanoel, D. E., Thomas, D. T., Blache, D., Milton, J. T., Wilmot, M. G., Revell, D. K., & Norman, H. C. (2016). Sheep deficient in vitamin E preferentially select for a feed with a higher concentration of vitamin E. Animal : an international journal of animal bioscience, 10(2), 183–191. https://doi.org/10.1017/S1751731115001937

[1153] Amanoel, D. E., Thomas, D. T., Blache, D., Milton, J. T., Wilmot, M. G., Revell, D. K., & Norman, H. C. (2016). Sheep deficient in vitamin E preferentially select for a feed with a higher concentration of vitamin E. Animal : an international journal of animal bioscience, 10(2), 183–191. https://doi.org/10.1017/S1751731115001937

1154 Holt SH et al (1995) 'A satiety index of common foods', Eur J Clin Nutr. 1995 Sep;49(9):675-90.

1155 Hall, K. D., Ayuketah, A., Brychta, R., Cai, H., Cassimatis, T., Chen, K. Y., Chung, S. T., Costa, E., Courville, A., Darcey, V., Fletcher, L. A., Forde, C. G., Gharib, A. M., Guo, J., Howard, R., Joseph, P. V., McGehee, S., Ouwerkerk, R., Raisinger, K., Rozga, I., … Zhou, M. (2019). Ultra-Processed Diets Cause Excess Calorie Intake and Weight Gain: An Inpatient Randomized Controlled Trial of Ad Libitum Food Intake. Cell metabolism, 30(1), 67–77.e3. https://doi.org/10.1016/j.cmet.2019.05.008

[1156] Schatzker (2015) 'More Nutrients, Less Nutrition: The Truth About Fortified Foods', Men's Health, Accessed Online April 2nd 2022: https://www.mensjournal.com/health-fitness/more-nutrients-less-nutrition-the-truth-about-fortified-foods-20151228/

[1157] Schatzker (2015) 'More Nutrients, Less Nutrition: The Truth About Fortified Foods', Men's Health, Accessed Online April 2nd 2022: https://www.mensjournal.com/health-fitness/more-nutrients-less-nutrition-the-truth-about-fortified-foods-20151228/

[1158] PLOS. (2017, November 21). Sugar industry withheld evidence of sucrose's health effects nearly 50 years ago, study suggests. ScienceDaily. Retrieved April 1, 2022 from www.sciencedaily.com/releases/2017/11/171121155819.htm

[1159] Campbell et al (1991) 'NUTRITIONAL CHARACTERISTICS of ORGANIC, FRESHLY STONE-GROUND, SOURDOUGH & -CONVENTIONAL BREADS', EAP Publication - 35, Accessed Online April 2nd 2022: https://eap.mcgill.ca/publications/EAP35.htm

[1160] Campbell et al (1991) 'NUTRITIONAL CHARACTERISTICS of ORGANIC, FRESHLY STONE-GROUND, SOURDOUGH & -CONVENTIONAL BREADS', EAP Publication - 35, Accessed Online April 2nd 2022: https://eap.mcgill.ca/publications/EAP35.htm

[1161] Passwater, Richard; Supernutrition – Mega Vitamin Revolution, NY The Dial Press, 1975.

[1162] Appetite and choice of diet. The ability of the vitamin B deficient rat to discriminate between diets containing and lacking the vitamin. (1933). Proceedings of the Royal Society of London. Series B, Containing Papers of a Biological Character, 113(781), 161–190. https://doi.org/10.1098/rspb.1933.0038

[1163] The National Academies of Sciences Engineering Medicine (2022) 'Summary Report of the Dietary Reference Intakes', Accessed Online April 2nd 2022: https://www.nationalacademies.org/our-work/summary-report-of-the-dietary-reference-intakes

[1164] Schatzker (2015) 'More Nutrients, Less Nutrition: The Truth About Fortified Foods', Men's Health, Accessed Online April 2nd 2022: https://www.mensjournal.com/health-fitness/more-nutrients-less-nutrition-the-truth-about-fortified-foods-20151228/

1165 Martinez-Cordero C et al (2012) 'Testing the Protein Leverage Hypothesis in a free-living human population', Appetite. 2012 Oct;59(2):312-5.

1166 Gannon, M. C., & Nuttall, F. Q. (2011). Effect of a high-protein diet on ghrelin, growth hormone, and insulin-like growth factor-I and binding proteins 1 and 3 in subjects with type 2 diabetes mellitus. Metabolism: clinical and experimental, 60(9), 1300–1311. https://doi.org/10.1016/j.metabol.2011.01.016

1167 Lejeune, M. P., Westerterp, K. R., Adam, T. C., Luscombe-Marsh, N. D., & Westerterp-Plantenga, M. S. (2006). Ghrelin and glucagon-like peptide 1 concentrations, 24-h satiety, and energy and substrate metabolism during a high-protein diet and measured in a respiration chamber. The American journal of clinical nutrition, 83(1), 89–94. https://doi.org/10.1093/ajcn/83.1.89

1168 Halton, T. L., & Hu, F. B. (2004). The effects of high protein diets on thermogenesis, satiety and weight loss: a critical review. Journal of the American College of Nutrition, 23(5), 373–385. https://doi.org/10.1080/07315724.2004.10719381

[1169] Schatzker (2015) 'More Nutrients, Less Nutrition: The Truth About Fortified Foods', Men's Health, Accessed Online April 2nd 2022: https://www.mensjournal.com/health-fitness/more-nutrients-less-nutrition-the-truth-about-fortified-foods-20151228/

[1170] Cook and Reusser (1983) 'Iron Fortification: an Update', Am J Clin Nutr 1983;38:648-659, Accessed Online April 11th 2022: https://pdf.usaid.gov/pdf_docs/PNAAQ794.pdf

[1171] McLean, E., Cogswell, M., Egli, I., Wojdyla, D., & de Benoist, B. (2008). Worldwide prevalence of anaemia, WHO Vitamin and Mineral Nutrition Information System, 1993–2005. Public Health Nutrition, 12(04), 444. doi:10.1017/s1368980008002401

[1172] McClung, J. P., & Karl, J. P. (2009). Iron deficiency and obesity: the contribution of inflammation and diminished iron absorption. Nutrition reviews, 67(2), 100–104. https://doi.org/10.1111/j.1753-4887.2008.00145.x

[1173] Pinhas-Hamiel, O., Newfield, R. S., Koren, I., Agmon, A., Lilos, P., & Phillip, M. (2003). Greater prevalence of iron deficiency in overweight and obese children and adolescents. International Journal of Obesity, 27(3), 416–418. https://doi.org/10.1038/sj.ijo.0802224

[1174] Pinhas-Hamiel, O., Newfield, R. S., Koren, I., Agmon, A., Lilos, P., & Phillip, M. (2003). Greater prevalence of iron deficiency in overweight and obese children and adolescents. International Journal of Obesity, 27(3), 416–418. https://doi.org/10.1038/sj.ijo.0802224

[1175] Aigner, E., Feldman, A., & Datz, C. (2014). Obesity as an emerging risk factor for iron deficiency. Nutrients, 6(9), 3587–3600. https://doi.org/10.3390/nu6093587

[1176] European Commission (2006) 'Questions and Answers on Fortified Foods', MEMO/06/199, Accessed Online April 2nd 2022: https://ec.europa.eu/commission/presscorner/detail/en/MEMO_06_199

[1177] Zimmermann et al (2010) 'The effects of iron fortification on the gut microbiota in African children: a randomized controlled trial in Côte d'Ivoire', The American Journal of Clinical Nutrition, Volume 92, Issue 6, December 2010, Pages 1406–1415, https://doi.org/10.3945/ajcn.110.004564

[1178] Jaeggi, T., Kortman, G. A., Moretti, D., Chassard, C., Holding, P., Dostal, A., Boekhorst, J., Timmerman, H. M., Swinkels, D. W., Tjalsma, H., Njenga, J., Mwangi, A., Kvalsvig, J., Lacroix, C., & Zimmermann, M. B. (2015). Iron fortification adversely affects the gut microbiome, increases pathogen abundance and induces intestinal inflammation in Kenyan infants. Gut, 64(5), 731–742. https://doi.org/10.1136/gutjnl-2014-307720

[1179] Yilmaz, B., & Li, H. (2018). Gut Microbiota and Iron: The Crucial Actors in Health and Disease. Pharmaceuticals, 11(4), 98. https://doi.org/10.3390/ph11040098

[1180] Insel, PM, Turner RE, and Ross D. (2003). Nutrition. 3rd edition. Jones and Bartlett

[1181] Scrimshaw, N. S. (1991). Iron Deficiency. Scientific American, 265(4), 46–53. http://www.jstor.org/stable/24938757

[1182] Zimmermann et al (2010) 'The effects of iron fortification on the gut microbiota in African children : a randomized controlled trial in Côte d'Ivoire', American journal of clinical nutrition, Vol. 92, H. 6. pp. 1406-1415.

[1183] Biemi, F. D., & Ganji, V. (2021). Temporal Relation between Double Fortification of Wheat Flour with Iron and Folic Acid, and Markers and Prevalence of Anemia in Children. Nutrients, 13(6), 2013. https://doi.org/10.3390/nu13062013

[1184] Elvehjem et al (1929) 'IS COPPER A CONSTITUENT OF THE HEMOGLOBIN MOLECULE? THE DISTRIBUTION OF COPPER IN BLOOD', J. Biol. Chem. 1929, 83:21-25.

[1185] Matak P, Zumerle S, Mastrogiannaki M, El Balkhi S, Delga S, Mathieu JRR, et al. (2013) Copper Deficiency Leads to Anemia, Duodenal Hypoxia, Upregulation of HIF-2α and Altered Expression of Iron Absorption Genes in Mice. PLoS ONE 8(3): e59538. https://doi.org/10.1371/journal.pone.0059538

[1186] Istvan Molnar, Dora Il'yasova, Anastasia Ivanova, Mary A. Knovich; The Association between Serum Copper and Anemia in the Adult NHANES II Population.. Blood 2005; 106 (11): 3766. doi: https://doi.org/10.1182/blood.V106.11.3766.3766

[1187] Hart, E. B.; Steenbock, H.; Waddell, J. (1928). "Iron nutrition. VII: Copper is a supplement to iron for hemoglobin building in the rat". The Journal of Biological Chemistry. 77: 797–833.

[1188] BRUBAKER, C., & STURGEON, P. (1956). Copper deficiency in infants; a syndrome characterized by hypocupremia, iron deficiency anemia, and hypoproteinemia. A.M.A. journal of diseases of children, 92(3), 254–265.

[1189] Vulpe, C. D., Kuo, Y. M., Murphy, T. L., Cowley, L., Askwith, C., Libina, N., Gitschier, J., & Anderson, G. J. (1999). Hephaestin, a ceruloplasmin homologue implicated in intestinal iron transport, is defective in the sla mouse. Nature genetics, 21(2), 195–199. https://doi.org/10.1038/5979

[1190] Joseph R. Prohaska, Impact of Copper Limitation on Expression and Function of Multicopper Oxidases (Ferroxidases), Advances in Nutrition, Volume 2, Issue 2, 01 March 2011, Pages 89–95, https://doi.org/10.3945/an.110.000208

[1191] Watts (1989) 'The Nutritional Relationships of Copper', Journal of Orthomolecular Medicine, Vol. 4, No. 2, Accessed Online Nov 4 2020: http://traceelements.com/Docs/The%20Nutritional%20Relationships%20of%20Copper.pdf

[1192] Klevay, L. M. (2001). Iron overload can induce mild copper deficiency. Journal of Trace Elements in Medicine and Biology, 14(4), 237–240. doi:10.1016/s0946-672x(01)80009-2

[1193] LEWIS, M. S. (1931). IRON AND COPPER IN THE TREATMENT OF ANEMIA IN CHILDREN. JAMA: The Journal of the American Medical Association, 96(14), 1135. doi:10.1001/jama.1931.02720400033010

[1194] Chan, L. N., & Mike, L. A. (2014). The science and practice of micronutrient supplementations in nutritional anemia: an evidence-based review. JPEN. Journal of parenteral and enteral nutrition, 38(6), 656–672. https://doi.org/10.1177/0148607114533726

[1195] F. S. Robscheit-Robbins, G. H. Whipple; COPPER AND COBALT RELATED HEMOGLOBIN PRODUCTION IN EXPERIMENTAL ANEMIA . J Exp Med 1 May 1942; 75 (5): 481–487. doi: https://doi.org/10.1084/jem.75.5.481

[1196] G. E. CARTWRIGHT, M. M. WINTROBE, The Question of Copper Deficiency in Man, The American Journal of Clinical Nutrition, Volume 15, Issue 2, August 1964, Pages 94–110, https://doi.org/10.1093/ajcn/15.2.94

[1197] Torti, S. V., & Torti, F. M. (2013). Iron and cancer: more ore to be mined. Nature reviews. Cancer, 13(5), 342–355. https://doi.org/10.1038/nrc3495

[1198] Fleming, R. E., & Ponka, P. (2012). Iron overload in human disease. The New England journal of medicine, 366(4), 348–359. https://doi.org/10.1056/NEJMra1004967

[1199] Höhn, A., Jung, T., Grimm, S., & Grune, T. (2010). Lipofuscin-bound iron is a major intracellular source of oxidants: role in senescent cells. Free radical biology & medicine, 48(8), 1100–1108. https://doi.org/10.1016/j.freeradbiomed.2010.01.030

[1200] Martins (2012) 'Universal iron fortification of foods: the view of a hematologist', Rev. Bras. Hematol. Hemoter. 34 (6), https://doi.org/10.5581/1516-8484.20120113

[1201] Martins (2012) 'Universal iron fortification of foods: the view of a hematologist', Rev. Bras. Hematol. Hemoter. 34 (6), https://doi.org/10.5581/1516-8484.20120113

[1202] Moon (2008) 'Iron: The Most Toxic Metal', George Ohsawa Macrobiotic

[1203] Rossander-Hultén, L., Brune, M., Sandström, B., Lönnerdal, B., & Hallberg, L. (1991). Competitive inhibition of iron absorption by manganese and zinc in humans. The American journal of clinical nutrition, 54(1), 152–156. https://doi.org/10.1093/ajcn/54.1.152

[1204] Oppenheimer, G. M., & Benrubi, I. D. (2014). McGovern's Senate Select Committee on Nutrition and Human Needs Versus the: Meat Industry on the Diet-Heart Question (1976–1977). American Journal of Public Health, 104(1), 59–69. https://doi.org/10.2105/ajph.2013.301464

[1205] Backstrand J. R. (2002). The history and future of food fortification in the United States: a public health perspective. Nutrition reviews, 60(1), 15–26. https://doi.org/10.1301/002966402760240390

[1206] *Moon and Weinberg (2008) 'Iron: The Most Toxic Metal', George Ohsawa Macrobiotic Foundation.*

[1207] Elwood (1977), 'The Enrichment Dabate', Nutrition Today: July-August 1977 - p 18-24..

[1208] Nikoley (2016) 'HOW FOOD ENRICHMENT PROMOTES OBESITY', Medium, Accessed Online April 2nd 2022: https://medium.com/@rnikoley/how-food-enrichment-promotes-obesity-275989cb03b7

[1209] American Bakers Association (2022) https://risetoaction.org/

[1210] Yudkin J. (1979). The avoidance of sucrose by thiamine-deficient rats. International journal for vitamin and nutrition research. Internationale Zeitschrift fur Vitamin- und Ernahrungsforschung. Journal international de vitaminologie et de nutrition, 49(2), 127–135.

[1211] Nosowitz (2015) 'What Exactly Do They Put in Cheetos?', Thrillist, Accessed Online April 2nd 2022: https://www.thrillist.com/health/nation/cheetos-nutrition-what-all-the-ingredients-mean

[1212] Schatzker (2015) 'More Nutrients, Less Nutrition: The Truth About Fortified Foods', Men's Health, Accessed Online April 2nd 2022: https://www.mensjournal.com/health-fitness/more-nutrients-less-nutrition-the-truth-about-fortified-foods-20151228/

[1213] McCarrison (1921) 'Studies in Deficiency Disease', Oxford Medical Publications, Accessed Online April 2nd 2022: https://www.soilandhealth.org/wp-content/uploads/02/0203CAT/020306carison/medtest_mccarrison2.html

[1214] New York State Medical Association (1920) 'New York State Journal Of Medicine, Volume 20', Medical Society of the State of New York.

[1215] Nikoley (2016) 'HOW FOOD ENRICHMENT PROMOTES OBESITY', Medium, Accessed Online April 2nd 2022: https://medium.com/@rnikoley/how-food-enrichment-promotes-obesity-275989cb03b7

[1216] Li, D., Sun, W. P., Zhou, Y. M., Liu, Q. G., Zhou, S. S., Luo, N., Bian, F. N., Zhao, Z. G., & Guo, M. (2010). Chronic niacin overload may be involved in the increased prevalence of obesity in US children. World journal of gastroenterology, 16(19), 2378–2387. https://doi.org/10.3748/wjg.v16.i19.2378

[1217] Zhou, S. S., Li, D., Zhou, Y. M., Sun, W. P., & Liu, Q. G. (2010). B-vitamin consumption and the prevalence of diabetes and obesity among the US adults: population based ecological study. BMC public health, 10, 746. https://doi.org/10.1186/1471-2458-10-746

[1218] Zhou, SS., Zhou, YM., Li, D. et al. Dietary methyl-consuming compounds and metabolic syndrome. Hypertens Res 34, 1239–1245 (2011). https://doi.org/10.1038/hr.2011.133

[1219] Li, D., Tian, Y. J., Guo, J., Sun, W. P., Lun, Y. Z., Guo, M., Luo, N., Cao, Y., Cao, J. M., Gong, X. J., & Zhou, S. S. (2013). Nicotinamide supplementation induces detrimental metabolic and epigenetic changes in developing rats. The British journal of nutrition, 110(12), 2156–2164. https://doi.org/10.1017/S0007114513001815

[1220] Zhou, S.-S. (2014). Excess vitamin intake: An unrecognized risk factor for obesity. World J Diabetes, 5(1), 1. https://doi.org/10.4239/wjd.v5.i1.1

[1221] Zhou, S. S., Li, D., Chen, N. N., & Zhou, Y. (2015). Vitamin paradox in obesity: Deficiency or excess?. World journal of diabetes, 6(10), 1158–1167. https://doi.org/10.4239/wjd.v6.i10.1158

[1222] Zhou, S.-S. (2014). Excess vitamin intake: An unrecognized risk factor for obesity. World J Diabetes, 5(1), 1. https://doi.org/10.4239/wjd.v5.i1.1

[1223] William Reed Ltd (2004) 'Denmark opening up on fortified foods?', Accessed Online April 2nd 2022: https://www.nutraingredients.com/Article/2004/08/17/Denmark-opening-up-on-fortified-foods

[1224] Banting, W (1864) 'Letter on corpulence : addressed to the public', London, 1869, p. 21.

[1225] Galgani, J., & Ravussin, E. (2008). Energy metabolism, fuel selection and body weight regulation. International journal of obesity (2005), 32 Suppl 7(Suppl 7), S109–S119. https://doi.org/10.1038/ijo.2008.246

[1226] CDC (2004) 'Trends in Intake of Energy and Macronutrients --- United States, 1971--2000', Accessed Online April 25th 2022: https://www.cdc.gov/mmwr/preview/mmwrhtml/mm5304a3.htm

[1227] Cercato, C., & Fonseca, F. A. (2019). Cardiovascular risk and obesity. Diabetology & Metabolic Syndrome, 11(1). https://doi.org/10.1186/s13098-019-0468-0

[1228] Liu, A. G., Ford, N. A., Hu, F. B., Zelman, K. M., Mozaffarian, D., & Kris-Etherton, P. M. (2017). A healthy approach to dietary fats: understanding the science and taking action to reduce consumer confusion. Nutrition journal, 16(1), 53. https://doi.org/10.1186/s12937-017-0271-4

[1229] Hiza, HAB and Bente L (2007) 'Nutrient Content of the U.S. Food Supply, 1909-2004, A Summary Report', Center for Nutrition Policy and Promotion, Home Economics Research Report No. 57.

[1230] Guyenet, S. J., & Carlson, S. E. (2015). Increase in Adipose Tissue Linoleic Acid of US Adults in the Last Half Century. Advances in Nutrition, 6(6), 660–664. doi:10.3945/an.115.009944

[1231] Blasbalg, T. L., Hibbeln, J. R., Ramsden, C. E., Majchrzak, S. F., & Rawlings, R. R. (2011). Changes in consumption of omega-3 and omega-6 fatty acids in the United States during the 20th century. The American Journal of Clinical Nutrition, 93(5), 950–962. https://doi.org/10.3945/ajcn.110.006643

[1232] DiNicolantonio, J. J., & O'Keefe, J. H. (2018). Omega-6 vegetable oils as a driver of coronary heart disease: the oxidized linoleic acid hypothesis. Open Heart, 5(2), e000898. doi:10.1136/openhrt-2018-000898

[1233] Blasbalg, T. L., Hibbeln, J. R., Ramsden, C. E., Majchrzak, S. F., & Rawlings, R. R. (2011). Changes in consumption of omega-3 and omega-6 fatty acids in the United States during the 20th century. The American Journal of Clinical Nutrition, 93(5), 950–962. https://doi.org/10.3945/ajcn.110.006643

[1234] Guyenet, S. J., & Carlson, S. E. (2015). Increase in Adipose Tissue Linoleic Acid of US Adults in the Last Half Century. Advances in Nutrition, 6(6), 660–664. https://doi.org/10.3945/an.115.009944

[1235] Flachs, P., Rossmeisl, M., Kuda, O., & Kopecky, J. (2013). Stimulation of mitochondrial oxidative capacity in white fat independent of UCP1: A key to lean phenotype. Biochimica et Biophysica Acta (BBA) - Molecular and Cell Biology of Lipids, 1831(5), 986–1003. doi:10.1016/j.bbalip.2013.02.003

[1236] Flachs, P., Mohamed-Ali, V., Horakova, O., Rossmeisl, M., Hosseinzadeh-Attar, M. J., Hensler, M., … Kopecky, J. (2006). Polyunsaturated fatty acids of marine origin induce adiponectin in mice fed a high-fat diet. Diabetologia, 49(2), 394–397. doi:10.1007/s00125-005-0053-y

[1237] Hensler, M., Bardova, K., Jilkova, Z. M., Wahli, W., Meztger, D., Chambon, P., Kopecky, J., & Flachs, P. (2011). The inhibition of fat cell proliferation by n-3 fatty acids in dietary obese mice. Lipids in health and disease, 10, 128. https://doi.org/10.1186/1476-511X-10-128

[1238] Ruzickova, J., Rossmeisl, M., Prazak, T., Flachs, P., Sponarova, J., Veck, M., Tvrzicka, E., Bryhn, M., & Kopecky, J. (2004). Omega-3 PUFA of marine origin limit diet-induced obesity in mice by reducing cellularity of adipose tissue. Lipids, 39(12), 1177–1185. https://doi.org/10.1007/s11745-004-1345-9

[1239] Alvheim, A. R., Torstensen, B. E., Lin, Y. H., Lillefosse, H. H., Lock, E. J., Madsen, L., Frøyland, L., Hibbeln, J. R., & Malde, M. K. (2014). Dietary linoleic acid elevates the endocannabinoids 2-AG and anandamide and promotes weight gain in mice fed a low fat diet. Lipids, 49(1), 59–69. https://doi.org/10.1007/s11745-013-3842-y

[1240] Hill JO, Peters JC, Lin D, et al. Lipid accumulation and body fat distribution is influenced by type of dietary fat fed to rats. Int J Obes Relat Metab Disord. 1993 Apr;17(4):223-36.

[1241] DiNicolantonio, J. J., & O'Keefe, J. H. (2018). Importance of maintaining a low omega-6/omega-3 ratio for reducing inflammation. Open Heart, 5(2), e000946. doi:10.1136/openhrt-2018-000946

[1242] Lee, T. H., Hoover, R. L., Williams, J. D., Sperling, R. I., Ravalese, J., Spur, B. W., … Austen, K. F. (1985). Effect of Dietary Enrichment with Eicosapentaenoic and Docosahexaenoic Acids on in Vitro Neutrophil and Monocyte Leukotriene Generation and Neutrophil Function. New England Journal of Medicine, 312(19), 1217–1224. doi:10.1056/nejm198505093121903

[1243] Endres, S., Ghorbani, R., Kelley, V. E., Georgilis, K., Lonnemann, G., van der Meer, J. W. M., … Dinarello, C. A. (1989). The Effect of Dietary Supplementation with n—3 Polyunsaturated Fatty Acids on the Synthesis of Interleukin-1 and Tumor Necrosis Factor by Mononuclear Cells. New England Journal of Medicine, 320(5), 265–271. doi:10.1056/nejm198902023200501

[1244] Sperling, R. I., Benincaso, A. I., Knoell, C. T., Larkin, J. K., Austen, K. F., & Robinson, D. R. (1993). Dietary omega-3 polyunsaturated fatty acids inhibit phosphoinositide formation and chemotaxis in neutrophils. Journal of Clinical Investigation, 91(2), 651–660. doi:10.1172/jci116245

[1245] Caughey, G. E., Mantzioris, E., Gibson, R. A., Cleland, L. G., & James, M. J. (1996). The effect on human tumor necrosis factor alpha and interleukin 1 beta production of diets enriched in n-3 fatty acids from vegetable oil or fish oil. The American Journal of Clinical Nutrition, 63(1), 116–122. doi:10.1093/ajcn/63.1.116

[1246] Rees, D., Miles, E. A., Banerjee, T., Wells, S. J., Roynette, C. E., Wahle, K. W., & Calder, P. C. (2006). Dose-related effects of eicosapentaenoic acid on innate immune function in healthy humans: a comparison of young and older men. The American Journal of Clinical Nutrition, 83(2), 331–342. doi:10.1093/ajcn/83.2.331

[1247] Meydani, S. N., Endres, S., Woods, M. M., Goldin, B. R., Soo, C., Morrill-Labrode, A., … Gorbach, S. L. (1991). Oral (n-3) Fatty Acid Supplementation Suppresses Cytokine Production and Lymphocyte Proliferation: Comparison between Young and Older Women. The Journal of Nutrition, 121(4), 547–555. doi:10.1093/jn/121.4.547

[1248] von Schacky, C., Kiefl, R., Jendraschak, E., & Kaminski, W. E. (1993). n-3 fatty acids and cysteinyl-leukotriene formation in humans in vitro, ex vivo, and in vivo. The Journal of laboratory and clinical medicine, 121(2), 302–309.

[1249] Simopoulos, A. P., & DiNicolantonio, J. J. (2016). The importance of a balanced ω-6 to ω-3 ratio in the prevention and management of obesity. Open Heart, 3(2), e000385. doi:10.1136/openhrt-2015-000385

[1250] DiNicolantonio, J. J., & O'Keefe, J. H. (2018). Omega-6 vegetable oils as a driver of coronary heart disease: the oxidized linoleic acid hypothesis. Open Heart, 5(2), e000898. doi:10.1136/openhrt-2018-000898

[1251] DiNicolantonio, J. J., & O'Keefe, J. H. (2018). Importance of maintaining a low omega-6/omega-3 ratio for reducing inflammation. Open Heart, 5(2), e000946. doi:10.1136/openhrt-2018-000946

[1252] PM Kris-Etherton, Denise Shaffer Taylor, Shaomei Yu-Poth, Peter Huth, Kristin Moriarty, Valerie Fishell, Rebecca L Hargrove, Guixiang Zhao, Terry D Etherton; Polyunsaturated fatty acids in the food chain in the United States, The American Journal of Clinical Nutrition, Volume 71, Issue 1, 1 January 2000, Pages 179S–188S.

[1253] Russo GL (2009) 'Dietary n-6 and n-3 polyunsaturated fatty acids: from biochemistry to clinical implications in cardiovascular prevention', Biochem Pharmacol. 2009 Mar 15;77(6):937-46.

[1254] Simopoulos (1999) 'Essential fatty acids in health and chronic disease 1,2', American Journal of Clinical Nutrition 70(3 Suppl):560S-569S

[1255] Calder, P. C. (2009). Polyunsaturated fatty acids and inflammatory processes: New twists in an old tale. Biochimie, 91(6), 791–795. doi:10.1016/j.biochi.2009.01.008

1256 Gutiérrez, S., Svahn, S. L., & Johansson, M. E. (2019). Effects of Omega-3 Fatty Acids on Immune Cells. International Journal of Molecular Sciences, 20(20), 5028. doi:10.3390/ijms20205028

1257 Harvard T.H. Chan, The Nutrition Source, 'Omega-3 Fatty Acids: An Essential Contribution', Accessed Online: https://www.hsph.harvard.edu/nutritionsource/what-should-you-eat/fats-and-cholesterol/types-of-fat/omega-3-fats/

[1258] Gago-Dominguez, M., Jiang, X., & Castelao, J. E. (2007). Lipid peroxidation, oxidative stress genes and dietary factors in breast cancer protection: a hypothesis. Breast cancer research : BCR, 9(1), 201. https://doi.org/10.1186/bcr1628

[1259] Tsimikas S, Philis-Tsimikas A, Alexopoulos S, et al. LDL isolated from Greek subjects on a typical diet or from American subjects on an oleate-supplemented diet induces less monocyte chemotaxis and adhesion when exposed to oxidative stress. Arteriosclerosis, thrombosis, and vascular biology 1999;19:122-30.

[1260] Aviram, M., & Eias, K. (1993). Dietary olive oil reduces low-density lipoprotein uptake by macrophages and decreases the susceptibility of the lipoprotein to undergo lipid peroxidation. Annals of nutrition & metabolism, 37(2), 75–84. https://doi.org/10.1159/000177753

[1261] Reaven, P., Parthasarathy, S., Grasse, B. J., Miller, E., Steinberg, D., & Witztum, J. L. (1993). Effects of oleate-rich and linoleate-rich diets on the susceptibility of low density lipoprotein to oxidative modification in mildly hypercholesterolemic subjects. The Journal of clinical investigation, 91(2), 668–676. https://doi.org/10.1172/JCI116247

[1262] Reaven, P. D., Grasse, B. J., & Tribble, D. L. (1994). Effects of linoleate-enriched and oleate-enriched diets in combination with alpha-tocopherol on the susceptibility of LDL and LDL subfractions to oxidative modification in humans. Arteriosclerosis and thrombosis : a journal of vascular biology, 14(4), 557–566. https://doi.org/10.1161/01.atv.14.4.557

[1263] Berry, E. M., Eisenberg, S., Haratz, D., Friedlander, Y., Norman, Y., Kaufmann, N. A., & Stein, Y. (1991). Effects of diets rich in monounsaturated fatty acids on plasma lipoproteins--the Jerusalem Nutrition Study: high MUFAs vs high PUFAs. The American journal of clinical nutrition, 53(4), 899–907. https://doi.org/10.1093/ajcn/53.4.899

1264 Salonen, J. T., Korpela, H., Salonen, R., Nyyssonen, K., Yla-Herttuala, S., Yamamoto, R., … Witztum, J. L. (1992). Autoantibody against oxidised LDL and progression of carotid atherosclerosis. The Lancet, 339(8798), 883–887. doi:10.1016/0140-6736(92)90926-t

1265 Holvoet, P., Stassen, J.-M., Van Cleemput, J., Collen, D., & Vanhaecke, J. (1998). Oxidized Low Density Lipoproteins in Patients With Transplant-Associated Coronary Artery Disease. Arteriosclerosis, Thrombosis, and Vascular Biology, 18(1), 100–107. doi:10.1161/01.atv.18.1.100

1266 Holvoet, P., Vanhaecke, J., Janssens, S., Van de Werf, F., & Collen, D. (1998). Oxidized LDL and Malondialdehyde-Modified LDL in Patients With Acute Coronary Syndromes and Stable Coronary Artery Disease. Circulation, 98(15), 1487–1494. doi:10.1161/01.cir.98.15.1487

1267 Parthasarathy S et al (2012) 'Oxidized Low-Density Lipoprotein', Methods Mol Biol. 2010; 610: 403–417.

1268 Silaste, M.-L., Rantala, M., Alfthan, G., Aro, A., Witztum, J. L., Kesäniemi, Y. A., & Hörkkö, S. (2004). Changes in Dietary Fat Intake Alter Plasma Levels of Oxidized Low-Density Lipoprotein and Lipoprotein(a). Arteriosclerosis, Thrombosis, and Vascular Biology, 24(3), 498–503. doi:10.1161/01.atv.0000118012.64932.f4

[1269] Salonen, J. T., Korpela, H., Salonen, R., Nyyssonen, K., Yla-Herttuala, S., Yamamoto, R., … Witztum, J. L. (1992). Autoantibody against oxidised LDL and progression of carotid atherosclerosis. The Lancet, 339(8798), 883–887. doi:10.1016/0140-6736(92)90926-t

[1270] Holvoet, P., Stassen, J.-M., Van Cleemput, J., Collen, D., & Vanhaecke, J. (1998). Oxidized Low Density Lipoproteins in Patients With Transplant-Associated Coronary Artery Disease. Arteriosclerosis, Thrombosis, and Vascular Biology, 18(1), 100–107. doi:10.1161/01.atv.18.1.100

[1271] Holvoet, P., Vanhaecke, J., Janssens, S., Van de Werf, F., & Collen, D. (1998). Oxidized LDL and Malondialdehyde-Modified LDL in Patients With Acute Coronary Syndromes and Stable Coronary Artery Disease. Circulation, 98(15), 1487–1494. doi:10.1161/01.cir.98.15.1487

[1272] Jira, W., Spiteller, G., Carson, W., & Schramm, A. (1998). Strong increase in hydroxy fatty acids derived from linoleic acid in human low density lipoproteins of atherosclerotic patients. Chemistry and Physics of Lipids, 91(1), 1–11. doi:10.1016/s0009-3084(97)00095-9

[1273] Haberland, M. E., Fogelman, A. M., & Edwards, P. A. (1982). Specificity of receptor-mediated recognition of malondialdehyde-modified low density lipoproteins. Proceedings of the National Academy of Sciences, 79(6), 1712–1716. doi:10.1073/pnas.79.6.1712

[1274] Haberland ME , Olch CL , Folgelman AM . Role of lysines in mediating interaction of modified low density lipoproteins with the scavenger receptor of human monocyte macrophages. J Biol Chem 1984;259:11305–11.

[1275] Francis, G. A. (2000). High density lipoprotein oxidation: in vitro susceptibility and potential in vivo consequences. Biochimica et Biophysica Acta (BBA) - Molecular and Cell Biology of Lipids, 1483(2), 217–235. doi:10.1016/s1388-1981(99)00181-x

[1276] Reaven, P., Parthasarathy, S., Grasse, B. J., Miller, E., Steinberg, D., & Witztum, J. L. (1993). Effects of oleate-rich and linoleate-rich diets on the susceptibility of low density lipoprotein to oxidative modification in mildly hypercholesterolemic subjects. Journal of Clinical Investigation, 91(2), 668–676. doi:10.1172/jci116247

[1277] Belkner, J., Wiesner, R., Kühn, H., & Lankin, V. Z. (1991). The oxygenation of cholesterol esters by the reticulocyte lipoxygenase. FEBS Letters, 279(1), 110–114. doi:10.1016/0014-5793(91)80263-3

[1278] Burdge, G. C., & Wootton, S. A. (2002). Conversion of alpha-linolenic acid to eicosapentaenoic, docosapentaenoic and docosahexaenoic acids in young women. The British journal of nutrition, 88(4), 411–420. https://doi.org/10.1079/BJN2002689

[1279] Rodriguez-Leyva, D., Dupasquier, C. M., McCullough, R., & Pierce, G. N. (2010). The cardiovascular effects of flaxseed and its omega-3 fatty acid, alpha-linolenic acid. The Canadian journal of cardiology, 26(9), 489–496. https://doi.org/10.1016/s0828-282x(10)70455-4

[1280] Okuyama, H., Kobayashi, T., & Watanabe, S. (1996). Dietary fatty acids--the N-6/N-3 balance and chronic elderly diseases. Excess linoleic acid and relative N-3 deficiency syndrome seen in Japan. Progress in lipid research, 35(4), 409–457. https://doi.org/10.1016/s0163-7827(96)00012-4

[1281] Dias, C. B., Garg, R., Wood, L. G., & Garg, M. L. (2014). Saturated fat consumption may not be the main cause of increased blood lipid levels. Medical Hypotheses, 82(2), 187–195. doi:10.1016/j.mehy.2013.11.036

[1282] Bowe, W. P., & Logan, A. C. (2010). Clinical implications of lipid peroxidation in acne vulgaris: old wine in new bottles. Lipids in Health and Disease, 9(1), 141. doi:10.1186/1476-511x-9-141

[1283] Mandal and Chatterjee (1980) 'Ultraviolet- and Sunlight-Induced Lipid Peroxidation in Liposomal Membrane', Radiation Research, Vol. 83, No. 2 (Aug., 1980), pp. 290-302.

[1284] Qi, M., Chen, D., Liu, K., & Auborn, K. J. (2002). n-6 Polyunsaturated fatty acids increase skin but not cervical cancer in human papillomavirus 16 transgenic mice. Cancer research, 62(2), 433–436.

[1285] Black, H. S., & Rhodes, L. E. (2016). Potential Benefits of Omega-3 Fatty Acids in Non-Melanoma Skin Cancer. Journal of clinical medicine, 5(2), 23. https://doi.org/10.3390/jcm5020023

[1286] Park, M. K., Li, W. Q., Qureshi, A. A., & Cho, E. (2018). Fat Intake and Risk of Skin Cancer in U.S. Adults. Cancer epidemiology, biomarkers & prevention : a publication of the American Association for Cancer Research, cosponsored by the American Society of Preventive Oncology, 27(7), 776–782. https://doi.org/10.1158/1055-9965.EPI-17-0782

[1287] Fischer, M.A., & Black, H.S. (1991). MODIFICATION OF MEMBRANE COMPOSITION, EICOSANOID METABOLISM, AND IMMUNORESPONSIVENESS BY DIETARY OMEGA-3 AND OMEGA-6 FATTY ACID SOURCES, MODULATORS OF ULTRAVIOLET-CARCINOGENESIS. Photochemistry and Photobiology, 54.

[1288] Black, H. S., Thornby, J. I., Gerguis, J., & Lenger, W. (1992). Influence of dietary omega-6, -3 fatty acid sources on the initiation and promotion stages of photocarcinogenesis. Photochemistry and photobiology, 56(2), 195–199. https://doi.org/10.1111/j.1751-1097.1992.tb02147.x

[1289] Cowing, B. E., & Saker, K. E. (2001). Polyunsaturated fatty acids and epidermal growth factor receptor/mitogen-activated protein kinase signaling in mammary cancer. The Journal of nutrition, 131(4), 1125–1128. https://doi.org/10.1093/jn/131.4.1125

[1290] Black, H. S., Thornby, J. I., Wolf, J. E., Goldberg, L. H., Herd, J. A., Rosen, T., Bruce, S., Tschen, J. A., Scott, L. W., Jaax, S., Foreyt, J. P., & Reusser, B. (1995). Evidence that a low-fat diet reduces the occurrence of non-melanoma skin cancer. International Journal of Cancer, 62(2), 165–169. https://doi.org/10.1002/ijc.2910620210

[1291] Cope, R. B., Bosnic, M., Boehm-Wilcox, C., Mohr, D., & Reeve, V. E. (1996). Dietary butter protects against ultraviolet radiation-induced suppression of contact hypersensitivity in Skh:HR-1 hairless mice. The Journal of nutrition, 126(3), 681–692. https://doi.org/10.1093/jn/126.3.681

[1292] Urbańska, M., Nowak, G., & Florek, E. (2012). Wpływ palenia tytoniu na starzenie sie skóry [Cigarette smoking and its influence on skin aging]. Przeglad lekarski, 69(10), 1111–1114.

[1293] Elias, P. M., Brown, B. E., & Ziboh, V. A. (1980). The permeability barrier in essential fatty acid deficiency: evidence for a direct role for linoleic acid in barrier function. The Journal of investigative dermatology, 74(4), 230–233. https://doi.org/10.1111/1523-1747.ep12541775

[1294] ORENGO, I.F., BLACK, H.S., KETTLER, A.H. and WOLF, J.E., JR. (1989), INFLUENCE OF DIETARY MENHADEN OIL UPON CARCINOGENESIS AND VARIOUS CUTANEOUS REspONSES TO ULTRAVIOLET RADIATION. Photochemistry and Photobiology, 49: 71-77. https://doi.org/10.1111/j.1751-1097.1989.tb04080.x

[1295] Brain, S., Camp, R., Dowd, P., Black, A. K., & Greaves, M. (1984). The release of leukotriene B4-like material in biologically active amounts from the lesional skin of patients with psoriasis. The Journal of investigative dermatology, 83(1), 70–73. https://doi.org/10.1111/1523-1747.ep12261712

[1296] Ziboh, V. A., Miller, C. C., & Cho, Y. (2000). Metabolism of polyunsaturated fatty acids by skin epidermal enzymes: generation of antiinflammatory and antiproliferative metabolites. The American Journal of Clinical Nutrition, 71(1), 361s–366s. https://doi.org/10.1093/ajcn/71.1.361s

[1297] Duell, E. A., Ellis, C. N., & Voorhees, J. J. (1988). Determination of 5,12, and 15-lipoxygenase products in keratomed biopsies of normal and psoriatic skin. The Journal of investigative dermatology, 91(5), 446–450. https://doi.org/10.1111/1523-1747.ep12476562

[1298] Ip C. (1987). Fat and essential fatty acid in mammary carcinogenesis. The American journal of clinical nutrition, 45(1 Suppl), 218–224. https://doi.org/10.1093/ajcn/45.1.218

[1299] Hammarström, S., Hamberg, M., Samuelsson, B., Duell, E. A., Stawiski, M., & Voorhees, J. J. (1975). Increased concentrations of nonesterified arachidonic acid, 12L-hydroxy-5,8,10,14-eicosatetraenoic acid, prostaglandin E2, and prostaglandin F2alpha in epidermis of psoriasis. Proceedings of the National Academy of Sciences of the United States of America, 72(12), 5130–5134. https://doi.org/10.1073/pnas.72.12.5130

[1300] Pearce, M. L., & Dayton, S. (1971). Incidence of cancer in men on a diet high in polyunsaturated fat. Lancet (London, England), 1(7697), 464–467. https://doi.org/10.1016/s0140-6736(71)91086-5

[1301] Black, H. S., Lenger, W., Phelps, A. W., & Thornby, J. I. (1984). Influence of dietary lipid upon ultraviolet light-carcinogenesis. Journal of environmental pathology, toxicology and oncology : official organ of the International Society for Environmental Toxicology and Cancer, 5(4-5), 271–282.

[1302] Black, H. S. (2015). The role of nutritional lipids and antioxidants in UV-induced skin cancer. Frontiers in Bioscience, 7(1), 30–39. https://doi.org/10.2741/s422

[1303] Denisenko, Y. K., Kytikova, O. Y., Novgorodtseva, T. P., Antonyuk, M. V., Gvozdenko, T. A., & Kantur, T. A. (2020). Lipid-Induced Mechanisms of Metabolic Syndrome. Journal of obesity, 2020, 5762395. https://doi.org/10.1155/2020/5762395

[1304] Sarbijani, H. M., Khoshnia, M., & Marjani, A. (2016). The association between Metabolic Syndrome and serum levels of lipid peroxidation and interleukin-6 in Gorgan. Diabetes & metabolic syndrome, 10(1 Suppl 1), S86–S89. https://doi.org/10.1016/j.dsx.2015.09.024

[1305] Li, M., Zhao, Y., Dai, Q., Milne, G., Long, J., Cai, Q., Chen, Q., Zhang, X., Lan, Q., Rothman, N., Gao, Y. T., Shu, X. O., Zheng, W., & Yang, G. (2022). Lipid peroxidation biomarkers associated with height and obesity measures in the opposite direction in women. Obesity (Silver Spring, Md.), 10.1002/oby.23408. Advance online publication. https://doi.org/10.1002/oby.23408

[1306] Schooneveldt, Y. L., Paul, S., Calkin, A. C., & Meikle, P. J. (2022). Ether Lipids in Obesity: From Cells to Population Studies. Frontiers in physiology, 13, 841278. https://doi.org/10.3389/fphys.2022.841278

[1307] Sohet, F. M., Neyrinck, A. M., Dewulf, E. M., Bindels, L. B., Portois, L., Malaisse, W. J., Carpentier, Y. A., Cani, P. D., & Delzenne, N. M. (2009). Lipid peroxidation is not a prerequisite for the development of obesity and diabetes in high-fat-fed mice. The British journal of nutrition, 102(3), 462–469. https://doi.org/10.1017/S0007114508191243

[1308] Yesilbursa, D., Serdar, Z., Serdar, A., Sarac, M., Coskun, S., & Jale, C. (2005). Lipid peroxides in obese patients and effects of weight loss with orlistat on lipid peroxides levels. International journal of obesity (2005), 29(1), 142–145. https://doi.org/10.1038/sj.ijo.0802794

[1309] Ginter, E., & Simko, V. (2016). New data on harmful effects of trans-fatty acids. Bratislavske lekarske listy, 117(5), 251–253. https://doi.org/10.4149/bll_2016_048

[1310] Bendsen, N. T., Chabanova, E., Thomsen, H. S., Larsen, T. M., Newman, J. W., Stender, S., Dyerberg, J., Haugaard, S. B., & Astrup, A. (2011). Effect of trans fatty acid intake on abdominal and liver fat deposition and blood lipids: a randomized trial in overweight postmenopausal women. Nutrition & diabetes, 1(1), e4. https://doi.org/10.1038/nutd.2010.4

[1311] Wanders, A. J., Zock, P. L., & Brouwer, I. A. (2017). Trans Fat Intake and Its Dietary Sources in General Populations Worldwide: A Systematic Review. Nutrients, 9(8), 840. https://doi.org/10.3390/nu9080840

[1312] Hyseni, L., Bromley, H., Kypridemos, C., O'Flaherty, M., Lloyd-Williams, F., Guzman-Castillo, M., Pearson-Stuttard, J., & Capewell, S. (2017). Systematic review of dietary trans-fat reduction interventions. Bulletin of the World Health Organization, 95(12), 821–830G. https://doi.org/10.2471/BLT.16.189795

[1313] Iqbal M. P. (2014). Trans fatty acids - A risk factor for cardiovascular disease. Pakistan journal of medical sciences, 30(1), 194–197. https://doi.org/10.12669/pjms.301.4525

[1314] Barnard N et al (2014) 'Saturated and trans fats and dementia: a systematic review', Neurobiology of Aging, Volume 35, Supplement 2, September 2014, Pages S65-S73.

[1315] Pase CS et al (2013) 'Influence of perinatal trans fat on behavioral responses and brain oxidative status of adolescent rats acutely exposed to stress', Neuroscience. 2013 Sep 5;247:242-52.

[1316] LEE, K. W., LEE, H. J., CHO, H. Y., & KIM, Y. J. (2005). Role of the Conjugated Linoleic Acid in the Prevention of Cancer. Critical Reviews in Food Science and Nutrition, 45(2), 135–144. doi:10.1080/10408690490911800

[1317] Wang, Y., Jacome-Sosa, M. M., Ruth, M. R., Goruk, S. D., Reaney, M. J., Glimm, D. R., ... Proctor, S. D. (2009). Trans-11 Vaccenic Acid Reduces Hepatic Lipogenesis and Chylomicron Secretion in JCR:LA-cp Rats. The Journal of Nutrition, 139(11), 2049–2054. doi:10.3945/jn.109.109488

[1318] Consumerlab.com (2018) 'Fish Oil and Omega-3 and -7 Supplements Review (Including Krill, Algae, Calamari, and Sea Buckthorn)', Product Reviews, Accessed Online: https://www.consumerlab.com/reviews/fish_oil_supplements_review/omega3/

[1319] Aviram, M., & Eias, K. (1993). Dietary Olive Oil Reduces Low-Density Lipoprotein Uptake by Macrophages and Decreases the Susceptibility of the Lipoprotein to Undergo Lipid Peroxidation. Annals of Nutrition and Metabolism, 37(2), 75–84. doi:10.1159/000177753

[1320] Loffredo, L., Perri, L., Di Castelnuovo, A., Iacoviello, L., De Gaetano, G., & Violi, F. (2015). Supplementation with vitamin E alone is associated with reduced myocardial infarction: A meta-analysis. Nutrition, Metabolism and Cardiovascular Diseases, 25(4), 354–363. doi:10.1016/j.numecd.2015.01.008

[1321] Huang et al (2002) 'Effects of vitamin C and vitamin E on in vivo lipid peroxidation: results of a randomized controlled trial', The American Journal of Clinical Nutrition, Volume 76, Issue 3, September 2002, Pages 549–555, https://doi.org/10.1093/ajcn/76.3.549

[1322] DiNicolantonio, J. J., Mangan, D., & O'Keefe, J. H. (2018). Copper deficiency may be a leading cause of ischaemic heart disease. Open Heart, 5(2), e000784. doi:10.1136/openhrt-2018-000784

[1323] Jaarin, K., & Kamisah, Y. (2012). Repeatedly Heated Vegetable Oils and Lipid Peroxidation. Lipid Peroxidation. doi:10.5772/46076

[1324] Doll, S. and Conrad, M. (2017), Iron and ferroptosis: A still ill-defined liaison. IUBMB Life, 69: 423-434. doi:10.1002/iub.1616

[1325] DiNicolantonio, J. J., Mangan, D., & O'Keefe, J. H. (2018). Copper deficiency may be a leading cause of ischaemic heart disease. Open Heart, 5(2), e000784. doi:10.1136/openhrt-2018-000784

[1326] Chisté et al (2014) 'Carotenoids inhibit lipid peroxidation and hemoglobin oxidation, but not the depletion of glutathione induced by ROS in human erythrocytes', Life Sciences, Volume 99, Issues 1–2, 18 March 2014, Pages 52-60.

[1327] Zhang et al (1991). Carotenoids enhance gap junctional communication and inhibit lipid peroxidation in C3H/10T1/2 cells: relationship to their cancer chemopreventive action. Carcinogenesis, 12(11), 2109–2114. https://doi.org/10.1093/carcin/12.11.2109

[1328] Lu et al (2006). Preventive effects of Spirulina platensis on skeletal muscle damage under exercise-induced oxidative stress. European journal of applied physiology, 98(2), 220–226. https://doi.org/10.1007/s00421-006-0263-0

[1329] Ould Amara-Leffad, L., Ramdane, H., Nekhoul, K., Ouznadji, A., & Koceir, E. A. (2018). Spirulina effect on modulation of toxins provided by food, impact on hepatic and renal functions. Archives of Physiology and Biochemistry, 125(2), 184–194. doi:10.1080/13813455.2018.1444059

[1330] Jabbari et al (2005). Comparison between swallowing and chewing of garlic on levels of serum lipids, cyclosporine, creatinine and lipid peroxidation in Renal Transplant Recipients, Lipids in Health and Disease, 4(1), 11. doi:10.1186/1476-511x-4-11

[1331] Reddy, A. C., & Lokesh, B. R. (1994). Effect of dietary turmeric (Curcuma longa) on iron-induced lipid peroxidation in the rat liver. Food and chemical toxicology : an international journal published for the British Industrial Biological Research Association, 32(3), 279–283. https://doi.org/10.1016/0278-6915(94)90201-1

[1332] Ji Z. (2010). Targeting DNA damage and repair by curcumin. Breast cancer : basic and clinical research, 4, 1–3.

[1333] Spasov, A. A., Zheltova, A. A., & Kharitonov, M. V. (2012). Rossiiskii fiziologicheskii zhurnal imeni I.M. Sechenova, 98(7), 915–923.

[1334] Kumar, B. P., & Shivakumar, K. (1997). Depressed antioxidant defense in rat heart in experimental magnesium deficiency implications for the pathogenesis of myocardial lesions. Biological Trace Element Research, 60(1-2), 139–144. doi:10.1007/bf02783317

[1335] Wiles, M. E., Wagner, T. L., & Weglicki, W. B. (1996). Effect of acute magnesium deficiency (MgD) on aortic endothelial cell (EC) oxidant production. Life Sciences, 60(3), 221–236. doi:10.1016/s0024-3205(96)00619-4

[1336] Zheltova, A. A., Kharitonova, M. V., Iezhitsa, I. N., & Spasov, A. A. (2016). Magnesium deficiency and oxidative stress: an update. BioMedicine, 6(4). doi:10.7603/s40681-016-0020-6

[1337] Kanner, J., Selhub, J., Shpaizer, A., Rabkin, B., Shacham, I., & Tirosh, O. (2017). Redox homeostasis in stomach medium by foods: The Postprandial Oxidative Stress Index (POSI) for balancing nutrition and human health. Redox Biology, 12, 929–936. doi:10.1016/j.redox.2017.04.029

[1338] Li, Z., Henning, S. M., Zhang, Y., Rahnama, N., Zerlin, A., Thames, G., ... Heber, D. (2013). Decrease of postprandial endothelial dysfunction by spice mix added to high-fat hamburger meat in men with Type 2 diabetes mellitus. Diabetic Medicine, 30(5), 590–595. doi:10.1111/dme.12120

[1339] Kanner, J. (2007). Dietary advanced lipid oxidation endproducts are risk factors to human health. Molecular Nutrition & Food Research, 51(9), 1094–1101. doi:10.1002/mnfr.200600303

[1340] Skulas-Ray, A. C., Kris-Etherton, P. M., Teeter, D. L., Chen, C.-Y. O., Vanden Heuvel, J. P., & West, S. G. (2011). A High Antioxidant Spice Blend Attenuates Postprandial Insulin and Triglyceride Responses and Increases Some Plasma Measures of Antioxidant Activity in Healthy, Overweight Men. The Journal of Nutrition, 141(8), 1451–1457. doi:10.3945/jn.111.138966

[1341] Li, Z., Henning, S. M., Zhang, Y., Zerlin, A., Li, L., Gao, K., ... Heber, D. (2010). Antioxidant-rich spice added to hamburger meat during cooking results in reduced meat, plasma, and urine malondialdehyde concentrations. The American Journal of Clinical Nutrition, 91(5), 1180–1184. doi:10.3945/ajcn.2009.28526

[1342] Zhang, H., Zhang, H., Troise, A. D., & Fogliano, V. (2019). Melanoidins from Coffee, Cocoa, and Bread Are Able to Scavenge α-Dicarbonyl Compounds under Simulated Physiological Conditions. Journal of Agricultural and Food Chemistry, 67(39), 10921–10929. doi:10.1021/acs.jafc.9b03744

[1343] Sirota et al (2013) 'Coffee polyphenols protect human plasma from postprandial carbonyl modifications', Molecular Nutrition & Food Research 57(5).

[1344] Urquiaga, I., Troncoso, D., Mackenna, M., Urzúa, C., Pérez, D., Dicenta, S., ... Rigotti, A. (2018). The Consumption of Beef Burgers Prepared with Wine Grape Pomace Flour Improves Fasting Glucose, Plasma Antioxidant Levels, and Oxidative Damage Markers in Humans: A Controlled Trial. Nutrients, 10(10), 1388. doi:10.3390/nu10101388

1345 McCarty et al (2019) 'Activated Glycine Receptors May Decrease Endosomal NADPH Oxidase Activity by Opposing ClC-3-Mediated Efflux of Chloride from Endosomes', Medical Hypotheses 123, DOI: 10.1016/j.mehy.2019.01.012

1346 Bloomer, R. J., Tschume, L. C., & Smith, W. A. (2009). Glycine Propionyl-L-carnitine Modulates Lipid Peroxidation and Nitric Oxide in Human Subjects. International Journal for Vitamin and Nutrition Research, 79(3), 131–141. doi:10.1024/0300-9831.79.3.131

[1347] Gannon et al (2002) 'The metabolic response to ingested glycine', The American Journal of Clinical Nutrition, Volume 76, Issue 6, December 2002, Pages 1302–1307, https://doi.org/10.1093/ajcn/76.6.1302

[1348] Self Nutrition Data (2018) 'Oil, olive, salad or cooking', Accessed Online May 4th 2022: https://nutritiondata.self.com/facts/fats-and-oils/509/2

[1349] Abdullah, M. M., Jew, S., & Jones, P. J. (2017). Health benefits and evaluation of healthcare cost savings if oils rich in monounsaturated fatty acids were substituted for conventional dietary oils in the United States. Nutrition reviews, 75(3), 163–174. https://doi.org/10.1093/nutrit/nuw062

[1350] Bastida, S., & Sánchez-Muniz, F. J. (2001). Thermal Oxidation of Olive Oil, Sunflower Oil and a Mix of Both Oils during Forty Discontinuous Domestic Fryings of Different Foods. Food Science and Technology International, 7(1), 15–21. https://doi.org/10.1106/1898-PLW3-6Y6H-8K22

[1351] Casal, S., Malheiro, R., Sendas, A., Oliveira, B. P., & Pereira, J. A. (2010). Olive oil stability under deep-frying conditions. Food and chemical toxicology : an international journal published for the British Industrial Biological Research Association, 48(10), 2972–2979. https://doi.org/10.1016/j.fct.2010.07.036

[1352] Qian, F., Korat, A. A., Malik, V., & Hu, F. B. (2016). Metabolic Effects of Monounsaturated Fatty Acid-Enriched Diets Compared With Carbohydrate or Polyunsaturated Fatty Acid-Enriched Diets in Patients With Type 2 Diabetes: A Systematic Review and Meta-analysis of Randomized Controlled Trials. Diabetes care, 39(8), 1448–1457. https://doi.org/10.2337/dc16-0513

[1353] Joris, P. J., & Mensink, R. P. (2016). Role of cis-Monounsaturated Fatty Acids in the Prevention of Coronary Heart Disease. Current atherosclerosis reports, 18(7), 38. https://doi.org/10.1007/s11883-016-0597-y

[1354] Guasch-Ferré, M., Zong, G., Willett, W. C., Zock, P. L., Wanders, A. J., Hu, F. B., & Sun, Q. (2019). Associations of Monounsaturated Fatty Acids From Plant and Animal Sources With Total and Cause-Specific Mortality in Two US Prospective Cohort Studies. Circulation research, 124(8), 1266–1275. https://doi.org/10.1161/CIRCRESAHA.118.313996

[1355] Guasch-Ferré, M., Hu, F. B., Martínez-González, M. A., Fitó, M., Bulló, M., Estruch, R., Ros, E., Corella, D., Recondo, J., Gómez-Gracia, E., Fiol, M., Lapetra, J., Serra-Majem, L., Muñoz, M. A., Pintó, X., Lamuela-Raventós, R. M., Basora, J., Buil-Cosiales, P., Sorlí, J. V., Ruiz-Gutiérrez, V., … Salas-Salvadó, J. (2014). Olive oil intake and risk of cardiovascular disease and mortality in the PREDIMED Study. BMC medicine, 12, 78. https://doi.org/10.1186/1741-7015-12-78

[1356] Schwingshackl, L., & Hoffmann, G. (2014). Monounsaturated fatty acids, olive oil and health status: a systematic review and meta-analysis of cohort studies. Lipids in health and disease, 13, 154. https://doi.org/10.1186/1476-511X-13-154

[1357] Mennella, I., Savarese, M., Ferracane, R., Sacchi, R., & Vitaglione, P. (2015). Oleic acid content of a meal promotes oleoylethanolamide response and reduces subsequent energy intake in humans. Food & function, 6(1), 204–210. https://doi.org/10.1039/c4fo00697f

[1358] Wansink, B., & Linder, L. R. (2003). Interactions between forms of fat consumption and restaurant bread consumption. International journal of obesity and related metabolic disorders : journal of the International Association for the Study of Obesity, 27(7), 866–868. https://doi.org/10.1038/sj.ijo.0802291

[1359] DiNicolantonio and Mercola (2018) 'Superfuel', Hay House Inc.

[1360] Singh, R. B., DeMeester, F., & Wilczynska, A. (2010). The Tsim Tsoum Approaches for Prevention of Cardiovascular Disease. Cardiology Research and Practice, 2010, 1–18. doi:10.4061/2010/824938

[1361] Sanders, T. A., Lewis, F. J., Goff, L. M., Chowienczyk, P. J., & RISCK Study Group (2013). SFAs do not impair endothelial function and arterial stiffness. The American journal of clinical nutrition, 98(3), 677–683. https://doi.org/10.3945/ajcn.113.063644

[1362] Pimpin, L., Wu, J. H., Haskelberg, H., Del Gobbo, L., & Mozaffarian, D. (2016). Is Butter Back? A Systematic Review and Meta-Analysis of Butter Consumption and Risk of Cardiovascular Disease, Diabetes, and Total Mortality. PloS one, 11(6), e0158118. https://doi.org/10.1371/journal.pone.0158118

[1363] AHA (2021) 'Saturated Fat', Accessed Online May 1st 2022: https://www.heart.org/en/healthy-living/healthy-eating/eat-smart/fats/saturated-fats

[1364] DiNicolantonio and Mercola (2018) 'Superfuel', Hay House Inc.

[1365] Kuipers, R. S., Luxwolda, M. F., Janneke Dijck-Brouwer, D. A., Eaton, S. B., Crawford, M. A., Cordain, L., & Muskiet, F. A. J. (2010). Estimated macronutrient and fatty acid intakes from an East African Paleolithic diet. British Journal of Nutrition, 104(11), 1666–1687. doi:10.1017/s0007114510002679

[1366] Eaton, S. B., Eaton III, S. B., Sinclair, A. J., Cordain, L., & Mann, N. J. (1998). Dietary Intake of Long-Chain Polyunsaturated Fatty Acids during the Paleolithic. The Return of W3 Fatty Acids into the Food Supply, 12–23. doi:10.1159/000059672

[1367] DeFilippis, A. P., & Sperling, L. S. (2006). Understanding omega-3's. American Heart Journal, 151(3), 564–570. doi:10.1016/j.ahj.2005.03.051

[1368] Wells, HF, Buzby JC. Dietary assessment of major trends in U.S. food consumption, 1970-2005. ERS Report Summary. 2008 Mar.

[1369] Hite, A. H., Feinman, R. D., Guzman, G. E., Satin, M., Schoenfeld, P. A., & Wood, R. J. (2010). In the face of contradictory evidence: Report of the Dietary Guidelines for Americans Committee. Nutrition, 26(10), 915–924. doi:10.1016/j.nut.2010.08.012

[1370] Food and Drug Administration, HHS (2003). Food labeling: trans fatty acids in nutrition labeling, nutrient content claims, and health claims. Final rule. Federal register, 68(133), 41433–41506.

1371 Hunt SM, Groff JL, Gropper SA (1995). Advanced Nutrition and Human Metabolism. Belmont, California: West Pub. Co. p. 98.

1372 Brody, Tom (1999). Nutritional Biochemistry (2nd ed.). Academic Press. p. 320.

1373 Wong et al (2006). "Colonic health: Fermentation and short chain fatty acids". Journal of Clinical Gastroenterology. 40 (3): 235–43.

1374 Mueller, N. T., Zhang, M., Juraschek, S. P., Miller, E. R., & Appel, L. J. (2020). Effects of high-fiber diets enriched with carbohydrate, protein, or unsaturated fat on circulating short chain fatty acids: results from the OmniHeart randomized trial. The American journal of clinical nutrition, 111(3), 545–554. https://doi.org/10.1093/ajcn/nqz322

1375 Byrne, C. S., Chambers, E. S., Morrison, D. J., & Frost, G. (2015). The role of short chain fatty acids in appetite regulation and energy homeostasis. International journal of obesity (2005), 39(9), 1331–1338. https://doi.org/10.1038/ijo.2015.84

[1376] Nagao, K., & Yanagita, T. (2010). Medium-chain fatty acids: functional lipids for the prevention and treatment of the metabolic syndrome. Pharmacological research, 61(3), 208–212. https://doi.org/10.1016/j.phrs.2009.11.007

1377 St-Onge, M. P., & Jones, P. J. (2002). Physiological effects of medium-chain triglycerides: potential agents in the prevention of obesity. The Journal of nutrition, 132(3), 329–332. https://doi.org/10.1093/jn/132.3.329

1378 St-Onge, M.-P., & Jones, P. J. H. (2003). Greater rise in fat oxidation with medium-chain triglyceride consumption relative to long-chain triglyceride is associated with lower initial body weight and greater loss of subcutaneous adipose tissue. International Journal of Obesity, 27(12), 1565–1571. doi:10.1038/sj.ijo.0802467

[1379] Maher, T., Sampson, A., Goslawska, M., Pangua-Irigaray, C., Shafat, A., & Clegg, M. E. (2019). Food Intake and Satiety Response after Medium-Chain Triglycerides Ingested as Solid or Liquid. Nutrients, 11(7), 1638. https://doi.org/10.3390/nu11071638

1380 Maher, T., & Clegg, M. E. (2021). A systematic review and meta-analysis of medium-chain triglycerides effects on acute satiety and food intake. Critical reviews in food science and nutrition, 61(4), 636–648. https://doi.org/10.1080/10408398.2020.1742654

1381 Breckenridge, W. C., & Kuksis, A. (1967). Molecular weight distributions of milk fat triglycerides from seven species. Journal of lipid research, 8(5), 473–478.

[1382] Leonard, W. R., Snodgrass, J. J., & Robertson, M. L. (2010). Evolutionary Perspectives on Fat Ingestion and Metabolism in Humans. In J. P. Montmayeur (Eds.) et. al., Fat Detection: Taste, Texture, and Post Ingestive Effects. CRC Press/Taylor & Francis.

[1383] Lindseth, G., & Petros, T. (2016). Neurobehavioral Effects of Consuming Dietary Fatty Acids. Biological research for nursing, 18(5), 573–581. https://doi.org/10.1177/1099800416657638

[1384] Haro, D., Marrero, P. F., & Relat, J. (2019). Nutritional Regulation of Gene Expression: Carbohydrate-, Fat- and Amino Acid-Dependent Modulation of Transcriptional Activity. International journal of molecular sciences, 20(6), 1386. https://doi.org/10.3390/ijms20061386

1385 Subramaniam, S., Fahy, E., Gupta, S., Sud, M., Byrnes, R. W., Cotter, D., Dinasarapu, A. R., & Maurya, M. R. (2011). Bioinformatics and systems biology of the lipidome. Chemical reviews, 111(10), 6452–6490. https://doi.org/10.1021/cr200295k

1386 Fahy, E., Subramaniam, S., Murphy, R. C., Nishijima, M., Raetz, C. R., Shimizu, T., Spener, F., van Meer, G., Wakelam, M. J., & Dennis, E. A. (2009). Update of the LIPID MAPS comprehensive classification system for lipids. Journal of lipid research, 50 Suppl(Suppl), S9–S14. https://doi.org/10.1194/jlr.R800095-JLR200

1387 Hellerstein, M. K., Christiansen, M., Kaempfer, S., Kletke, C., Wu, K., Reid, J. S., Mulligan, K., Hellerstein, N. S., & Shackleton, C. H. (1991). Measurement of de novo hepatic lipogenesis in humans using stable isotopes. The Journal of clinical investigation, 87(5), 1841–1852. https://doi.org/10.1172/JCI115206

1388 Fats and oils in human nutrition. Report of a joint expert consultation. Food and Agriculture Organization of the United Nations and the World Health Organization. (1994). FAO food and nutrition paper, 57, i–147.

1389 Sanders, T. A. (2010), The role of fat in the diet – quantity, quality and sustainability. Nutrition Bulletin, 35: 138-146.

1390 Hämäläinen, E., Adlercreutz, H., Puska, P., & Pietinen, P. (1984). Diet and serum sex hormones in healthy men. Journal of steroid biochemistry, 20(1), 459–464. https://doi.org/10.1016/0022-4731(84)90254-1

1391 Burdge, G. C., & Wootton, S. A. (2002). Conversion of α-linolenic acid to eicosapentaenoic, docosapentaenoic and docosahexaenoic acids in young women. British Journal of Nutrition, 88(4), 411–420. doi:10.1079/bjn2002689

1392 EFSA Panel on Dietetic Products, Nutrition and Allergies (NDA); Scientific Opinion related to the Tolerable Upper Intake Level of eicosapentaenoic acid (EPA), docosahexaenoic acid (DHA) and docosapentaenoic acid (DPA). EFSA Journal 2012;10(7):2815.

1393 Mickleborough T. D. (2013). Omega-3 polyunsaturated fatty acids in physical performance optimization. International journal of sport nutrition and exercise metabolism, 23(1), 83–96. https://doi.org/10.1123/ijsnem.23.1.83

1394 Jouris, K. B., McDaniel, J. L., & Weiss, E. P. (2011). The Effect of Omega-3 Fatty Acid Supplementation on the Inflammatory Response to eccentric strength exercise. Journal of sports science & medicine, 10(3), 432–438.

1395 Bloomer, R. J., Larson, D. E., Fisher-Wellman, K. H., Galpin, A. J., & Schilling, B. K. (2009). Effect of eicosapentaenoic and docosahexaenoic acid on resting and exercise-induced inflammatory and oxidative stress biomarkers: a randomized, placebo controlled, cross-over study. Lipids in health and disease, 8, 36. https://doi.org/10.1186/1476-511X-8-36

1396 da Silva, E. P., Jr, Nachbar, R. T., Levada-Pires, A. C., Hirabara, S. M., & Lambertucci, R. H. (2016). Omega-3 fatty acids differentially modulate enzymatic anti-oxidant systems in skeletal muscle cells. Cell stress & chaperones, 21(1), 87–95. https://doi.org/10.1007/s12192-015-0642-8

1397 Jakeman, J. R., Lambrick, D. M., Wooley, B., Babraj, J. A., & Faulkner, J. A. (2017). Effect of an acute dose of omega-3 fish oil following exercise-induced muscle damage. European journal of applied physiology, 117(3), 575–582. https://doi.org/10.1007/s00421-017-3543-y

1398 Da Boit, M., Hunter, A. M., & Gray, S. R. (2017). Fit with good fat? The role of n-3 polyunsaturated fatty acids on exercise performance. Metabolism: clinical and experimental, 66, 45–54. https://doi.org/10.1016/j.metabol.2016.10.007

1399 Lewis, E. J., Radonic, P. W., Wolever, T. M., & Wells, G. D. (2015). 21 days of mammalian omega-3 fatty acid supplementation improves aspects of neuromuscular function and performance in male athletes compared to olive oil placebo. Journal of the International Society of Sports Nutrition, 12, 28. https://doi.org/10.1186/s12970-015-0089-4

[1400] Kromhout et al (1985). The inverse relation between fish consumption and 20-year mortality from coronary heart disease. The New England journal of medicine, 312(19), 1205–1209. https://doi.org/10.1056/NEJM198505093121901

[1401] Oomen et al (2000). Fish consumption and coronary heart disease mortality in Finland, Italy, and The Netherlands. American journal of epidemiology, 151(10), 999–1006. https://doi.org/10.1093/oxfordjournals.aje.a010144

[1402] Keli, S. O., Feskens, E. J., & Kromhout, D. (1994). Fish consumption and risk of stroke. The Zutphen Study. Stroke, 25(2), 328–332. https://doi.org/10.1161/01.str.25.2.328

[1403] Burr, M. L., Gilbert, J. F., Holliday, R. M., Elwood, P. C., Fehily, A. M., Rogers, S., … Deadman, N. M. (1989). EFFECTS OF CHANGES IN FAT, FISH, AND FIBRE INTAKES ON DEATH AND MYOCARDIAL REINFARCTION: DIET AND REINFARCTION TRIAL (DART). The Lancet, 334(8666), 757–761. doi:10.1016/s0140-6736(89)90828-3

[1404] De Lorgeril, M., Salen, P., Defaye, P., & Rabaeus, M. (2013). Recent findings on the health effects of omega-3 fatty acids and statins, and their interactions: do statins inhibit omega-3? BMC Medicine, 11(1). doi:10.1186/1741-7015-11-5

[1405] Einvik, G., Klemsdal, T. O., Sandvik, L., & Hjerkinn, E. M. (2010). A randomized clinical trial on n-3 polyunsaturated fatty acids supplementation and all-cause mortality in elderly men at high cardiovascular risk. European journal of cardiovascular prevention and rehabilitation : official journal of the European Society of Cardiology, Working Groups on Epidemiology & Prevention and Cardiac Rehabilitation and Exercise Physiology, 17(5), 588–592. https://doi.org/10.1097/HJR.0b013e328339cc70

[1406] Burr, M. L., Sweetham, P. M., & Fehily, A. M. (1994). Diet and reinfarction. European heart journal, 15(8), 1152–1153. https://doi.org/10.1093/oxfordjournals.eurheartj.a060645

[1407] Marchioli, R., Barzi, F., Bomba, E., Chieffo, C., Di Gregorio, D., Di Mascio, R., … Valagussa, F. (2002). Early Protection Against Sudden Death by n-3 Polyunsaturated Fatty Acids After Myocardial Infarction. Circulation, 105(16), 1897–1903. doi:10.1161/01.cir.0000014682.14181.f2

[1408] Dietary supplementation with n-3 polyunsaturated fatty acids and vitamin E after myocardial infarction: results of the GISSI-Prevenzione trial. Gruppo Italiano per lo Studio della Sopravvivenza nell'Infarto miocardico. (1999). Lancet (London, England), 354(9177), 447–455.

[1409] GISSI-HF investigators. (2008). Effect of n-3 polyunsaturated fatty acids in patients with chronic heart failure (the GISSI-HF trial): a randomised, double-blind, placebo-controlled trial. The Lancet, 372(9645), 1223–1230. doi:10.1016/s0140-6736(08)61239-8

[1410] Hooper et al (2006). Risks and benefits of omega 3 fats for mortality, cardiovascular disease, and cancer: systematic review. BMJ (Clinical research ed.), 332(7544), 752–760. https://doi.org/10.1136/bmj.38755.366331.2F

[1411] Norwegian Scientific Committee for Food Safety (2011) 'Description of the processes in the value chain and risk assessment of decomposition substances and oxidation products in fish oils', Opinion of Steering Committee of the Norwegian Scientific Committee for Food Safety, 08-504-4-final, Accessed Online: https://web.archive.org/web/20160909213119/http://english.vkm.no/dav/0fd42c8b08.pdf

[1412] Consumerlab.com (2018) 'Fish Oil and Omega-3 and -7 Supplements Review (Including Krill, Algae, Calamari, and Sea Buckthorn)', Product Reviews, Accessed Online: https://www.consumerlab.com/reviews/fish_oil_supplements_review/omega3/

[1413] Ulven et al (2010). Metabolic Effects of Krill Oil are Essentially Similar to Those of Fish Oil but at Lower Dose of EPA and DHA, in Healthy Volunteers. Lipids, 46(1), 37–46. doi:10.1007/s11745-010-3490-4

[1414] Martin et al (2010). Intestinal digestion of fish oils and ω-3 concentrates under in vitro conditions. European Journal of Lipid Science and Technology, 112(12), 1315–1322. doi:10.1002/ejlt.201000329

[1415] DiNicolantonio and Mercola (2018) 'Superfuel', Hay House Inc.

[1416] Simopoulos, A. P., Leaf, A., & Salem, N., Jr (1999). Essentiality of and recommended dietary intakes for omega-6 and omega-3 fatty acids. Annals of nutrition & metabolism, 43(2), 127–130. https://doi.org/10.1159/000012777

[1417] Harris, W. S., & von Schacky, C. (2004). The Omega-3 Index: a new risk factor for death from coronary heart disease? Preventive Medicine, 39(1), 212–220. doi:10.1016/j.ypmed.2004.02.030

[1418] Bhandari, P., & Sapra, A. (2022). Low Fat Diet. In StatPearls. StatPearls Publishing.

[1419] Briggs, M. A., Petersen, K. S., & Kris-Etherton, P. M. (2017). Saturated Fatty Acids and Cardiovascular Disease: Replacements for Saturated Fat to Reduce Cardiovascular Risk. Healthcare (Basel, Switzerland), 5(2), 29. https://doi.org/10.3390/healthcare5020029

[1420] Upadhyay R. K. (2015). Emerging risk biomarkers in cardiovascular diseases and disorders. Journal of lipids, 2015, 971453. https://doi.org/10.1155/2015/971453

[1421] Cromwell, W. C., Otvos, J. D., Keyes, M. J., Pencina, M. J., Sullivan, L., Vasan, R. S., Wilson, P. W., & D'Agostino, R. B. (2007). LDL Particle Number and Risk of Future Cardiovascular Disease in the Framingham Offspring Study - Implications for LDL Management. Journal of clinical lipidology, 1(6), 583–592. https://doi.org/10.1016/j.jacl.2007.10.001

[1422] Siri-Tarino, P. W., Chiu, S., Bergeron, N., & Krauss, R. M. (2015). Saturated Fats Versus Polyunsaturated Fats Versus Carbohydrates for Cardiovascular Disease Prevention and Treatment. Annual review of nutrition, 35, 517–543. https://doi.org/10.1146/annurev-nutr-071714-034449

[1423] Berglund, L., Lefevre, M., Ginsberg, H. N., Kris-Etherton, P. M., Elmer, P. J., Stewart, P. W., Ershow, A., Pearson, T. A., Dennis, B. H., Roheim, P. S., Ramakrishnan, R., Reed, R., Stewart, K., Phillips, K. M., & DELTA Investigators (2007). Comparison of monounsaturated fat with carbohydrates as a replacement for saturated fat in subjects with a high metabolic risk profile: studies in the fasting and postprandial states. The American journal of clinical nutrition, 86(6), 1611–1620. https://doi.org/10.1093/ajcn/86.5.1611

[1424] Sacks, F. M., Lichtenstein, A. H., Wu, J., Appel, L. J., Creager, M. A., Kris-Etherton, P. M., Miller, M., Rimm, E. B., Rudel, L. L., Robinson, J. G., Stone, N. J., Van Horn, L. V., & American Heart Association (2017). Dietary Fats and Cardiovascular Disease: A Presidential Advisory From the American Heart Association. Circulation, 136(3), e1–e23. https://doi.org/10.1161/CIR.0000000000000510

[1425] Siri-Tarino, P. W., Sun, Q., Hu, F. B., & Krauss, R. M. (2010). Saturated fat, carbohydrate, and cardiovascular disease. The American journal of clinical nutrition, 91(3), 502–509. https://doi.org/10.3945/ajcn.2008.26285

[1426] Mensink, R. P., & Katan, M. B. (1992). Effect of dietary fatty acids on serum lipids and lipoproteins. A meta-analysis of 27 trials. Arteriosclerosis and thrombosis : a journal of vascular biology, 12(8), 911–919. https://doi.org/10.1161/01.atv.12.8.911

[1427] Ginsberg, H. N., Kris-Etherton, P., Dennis, B., Elmer, P. J., Ershow, A., Lefevre, M., Pearson, T., Roheim, P., Ramakrishnan, R., Reed, R., Stewart, K., Stewart, P., Phillips, K., & Anderson, N. (1998). Effects of reducing dietary saturated fatty acids on plasma lipids and lipoproteins in healthy subjects: the DELTA Study, protocol 1. Arteriosclerosis, thrombosis, and vascular biology, 18(3), 441–449. https://doi.org/10.1161/01.atv.18.3.441

[1428] Andraski, A. B., Singh, S. A., Lee, L. H., Higashi, H., Smith, N., Zhang, B., Aikawa, M., & Sacks, F. M. (2019). Effects of Replacing Dietary Monounsaturated Fat With Carbohydrate on HDL (High-Density Lipoprotein) Protein Metabolism and Proteome Composition in Humans. Arteriosclerosis, thrombosis, and vascular biology, 39(11), 2411–2430. https://doi.org/10.1161/ATVBAHA.119.312889

[1429] Estruch, R., Ros, E., Salas-Salvadó, J., Covas, M.-I., Corella, D., Arós, F., Gómez-Gracia, E., Ruiz-Gutiérrez, V., Fiol, M., Lapetra, J., Lamuela-Raventos, R. M., Serra-Majem, L., Pintó, X., Basora, J., Muñoz, M. A., Sorlí, J. V., Martínez, J. A., & Martínez-González, M. A. (2013). Primary Prevention of Cardiovascular Disease with a Mediterranean Diet. New England Journal of Medicine, 368(14), 1279–1290. https://doi.org/10.1056/nejmoa1200303

[1430] Bendall, C. L., Mayr, H. L., Opie, R. S., Bes-Rastrollo, M., Itsiopoulos, C., & Thomas, C. J. (2018). Central obesity and the Mediterranean diet: A systematic review of intervention trials. Critical reviews in food science and nutrition, 58(18), 3070–3084. https://doi.org/10.1080/10408398.2017.1351917

[1431] D'Innocenzo, S., Biagi, C., & Lanari, M. (2019). Obesity and the Mediterranean Diet: A Review of Evidence of the Role and Sustainability of the Mediterranean Diet. Nutrients, 11(6), 1306. https://doi.org/10.3390/nu11061306

[1432] Jimenez-Torres, J., Alcalá-Diaz, J. F., Torres-Peña, J. D., Gutierrez-Mariscal, F. M., Leon-Acuña, A., Gómez-Luna, P., Fernández-Gandara, C., Quintana-Navarro, G. M., Fernandez-Garcia, J. C., Perez-Martinez, P., Ordovas, J. M., Delgado-Lista, J., Yubero-Serrano, E. M., & Lopez-Miranda, J. (2021). Mediterranean Diet Reduces Atherosclerosis Progression in Coronary Heart Disease: An Analysis of the CORDIOPREV Randomized Controlled Trial. Stroke, 52(11), 3440–3449. https://doi.org/10.1161/STROKEAHA.120.033214

[1433] Dontas, A. S., Zerefos, N. S., Panagiotakos, D. B., Vlachou, C., & Valis, D. A. (2007). Mediterranean diet and prevention of coronary heart disease in the elderly. Clinical interventions in aging, 2(1), 109–115. https://doi.org/10.2147/ciia.2007.2.1.109

[1434] Montserrat et al (2007) 'Effect of a Traditional Mediterranean Diet on Lipoprotein Oxidation: A Randomized Controlled Trial', Arch Intern Med. 2007;167(11):1195-1203. doi:10.1001/archinte.167.11.1195

[1435] Volek, J. S., Sharman, M. J., Love, D. M., Avery, N. G., Gómez, A. L., Scheett, T. P., & Kraemer, W. J. (2002). Body composition and hormonal responses to a carbohydrate-restricted diet. Metabolism: clinical and experimental, 51(7), 864–870. https://doi.org/10.1053/meta.2002.32037

[1436] Jeong, E. A., Jeon, B. T., Shin, H. J., Kim, N., Lee, D. H., Kim, H. J., Kang, S. S., Cho, G. J., Choi, W. S., & Roh, G. S. (2011). Ketogenic diet-induced peroxisome proliferator-activated receptor-γ activation decreases neuroinflammation in the mouse hippocampus after kainic acid-induced seizures. Experimental neurology, 232(2), 195–202. https://doi.org/10.1016/j.expneurol.2011.09.001

[1437] Haces et al (2008). Antioxidant capacity contributes to protection of ketone bodies against oxidative damage induced during hypoglycemic conditions. Experimental neurology, 211(1), 85–96. https://doi.org/10.1016/j.expneurol.2007.12.029

[1438] Shimazu et al (2013). Suppression of oxidative stress by β-hydroxybutyrate, an endogenous histone deacetylase inhibitor. Science (New York, N.Y.), 339(6116), 211–214. https://doi.org/10.1126/science.1227166

[1439] Milder, J. B., Liang, L. P., & Patel, M. (2010). Acute oxidative stress and systemic Nrf2 activation by the ketogenic diet. Neurobiology of disease, 40(1), 238–244. https://doi.org/10.1016/j.nbd.2010.05.030

[1440] Jarrett, S. G., Milder, J. B., Liang, L. P., & Patel, M. (2008). The ketogenic diet increases mitochondrial glutathione levels. Journal of neurochemistry, 106(3), 1044–1051. https://doi.org/10.1111/j.1471-4159.2008.05460.x

[1441] Masuda, R., Monahan, J. W., & Kashiwaya, Y. (2005). D-beta-hydroxybutyrate is neuroprotective against hypoxia in serum-free hippocampal primary cultures. Journal of neuroscience research, 80(4), 501–509. https://doi.org/10.1002/jnr.20464

[1442] Gibson, A. A., Seimon, R. V., Lee, C. M., Ayre, J., Franklin, J., Markovic, T. P., Caterson, I. D., & Sainsbury, A. (2015). Do ketogenic diets really suppress appetite? A systematic review and meta-analysis. Obesity reviews : an official journal of the International Association for the Study of Obesity, 16(1), 64–76. https://doi.org/10.1111/obr.12230

[1443] Sumithran, P., Prendergast, L., Delbridge, E. et al. Ketosis and appetite-mediating nutrients and hormones after weight loss. Eur J Clin Nutr 67, 759–764 (2013). https://doi.org/10.1038/ejcn.2013.90

[1444] Martin et al (2011). Change in food cravings, food preferences, and appetite during a low-carbohydrate and low-fat diet. Obesity (Silver Spring, Md.), 19(10), 1963–1970. https://doi.org/10.1038/oby.2011.62

[1445] Westman et al (2008). The effect of a low-carbohydrate, ketogenic diet versus a low-glycemic index diet on glycemic control in type 2 diabetes mellitus. Nutrition & metabolism, 5, 36. https://doi.org/10.1186/1743-7075-5-36

[1446] Volek and Phinney (2012) 'The Art and Science of Low Carbohydrate Performance', Beyond Obesity LLC

[1447] Rezaei, S., Abdurahman, A. A., Saghazadeh, A., Badv, R. S., & Mahmoudi, M. (2019). Short-term and long-term efficacy of classical ketogenic diet and modified Atkins diet in children and adolescents with epilepsy: A systematic review and meta-analysis. Nutritional neuroscience, 22(5), 317–334. https://doi.org/10.1080/1028415X.2017.1387721

[1448] Wilder R. (1921). The effect of ketonemia on the course of epilepsy. Mayo Clin. Proc. 2 307–308.

[1449] Meira et al (2019). Ketogenic Diet and Epilepsy: What We Know So Far. Frontiers in Neuroscience, 13. doi:10.3389/fnins.2019.00005

[1450] Dashti, H. M., Mathew, T. C., Hussein, T., Asfar, S. K., Behbahani, A., Khoursheed, M. A., Al-Sayer, H. M., Bo-Abbas, Y. Y., & Al-Zaid, N. S. (2004). Long-term effects of a ketogenic diet in obese patients. Experimental and clinical cardiology, 9(3), 200–205.

[1451] Sharman, M. J., Kraemer, W. J., Love, D. M., Avery, N. G., Gómez, A. L., Scheett, T. P., & Volek, J. S. (2002). A ketogenic diet favorably affects serum biomarkers for cardiovascular disease in normal-weight men. The Journal of nutrition, 132(7), 1879–1885. https://doi.org/10.1093/jn/132.7.1879

[1452] Kinzig, K. P., Honors, M. A., & Hargrave, S. L. (2010). Insulin sensitivity and glucose tolerance are altered by maintenance on a ketogenic diet. Endocrinology, 151(7), 3105–3114. https://doi.org/10.1210/en.2010-0175

[1453] Kinzig, K. P., Honors, M. A., & Hargrave, S. L. (2010). Insulin sensitivity and glucose tolerance are altered by maintenance on a ketogenic diet. Endocrinology, 151(7), 3105–3114. https://doi.org/10.1210/en.2010-0175

[1454] Webster, C. C., van Boom, K. M., Armino, N., Larmuth, K., Noakes, T. D., Smith, J. A., & Kohn, T. A. (2020). Reduced Glucose Tolerance and Skeletal Muscle GLUT4 and IRS1 Content in Cyclists Habituated to a Long-Term Low-Carbohydrate, High-Fat Diet. International Journal of Sport Nutrition and Exercise Metabolism, 30(3), 210–217. https://doi.org/10.1123/ijsnem.2019-0359

[1455] Berry, M. N., Phillips, J. W., Henly, D. C., & Clark, D. G. (1993). Effects of fatty acid oxidation on glucose utilization by isolated hepatocytes. FEBS letters, 319(1-2), 26–30. https://doi.org/10.1016/0014-5793(93)80030-x

1456 Fothergill, E., Guo, J., Howard, L., Kerns, J.C., Knuth, N.D., Brychta, R., Chen, K.Y., Skarulis, M.C., Walter, M., Walter, P.J. and Hall, K.D. (2016), Persistent metabolic adaptation 6 years after "The Biggest Loser" competition. Obesity, 24: 1612-1619. https://doi.org/10.1002/oby.21538

1457 Hall K. D. (2013). Diet versus exercise in "the biggest loser" weight loss competition. Obesity (Silver Spring, Md.), 21(5), 957–959. https://doi.org/10.1002/oby.20065

1458 Garthe, I., Raastad, T., Refsnes, P. E., Koivisto, A., & Sundgot-Borgen, J. (2011). Effect of two different weight-loss rates on body composition and strength and power-related performance in elite athletes. International journal of sport nutrition and exercise metabolism, 21(2), 97–104. https://doi.org/10.1123/ijsnem.21.2.97

1459 Chaston, T. B., Dixon, J. B., & O'Brien, P. E. (2007). Changes in fat-free mass during significant weight loss: a systematic review. International journal of obesity (2005), 31(5), 743–750. https://doi.org/10.1038/sj.ijo.0803483

1460 Trexler, E. T., Smith-Ryan, A. E., & Norton, L. E. (2014). Metabolic adaptation to weight loss: implications for the athlete. Journal of the International Society of Sports Nutrition, 11(1), 7. https://doi.org/10.1186/1550-2783-11-7

1461 Leibel, R. L., Rosenbaum, M., & Hirsch, J. (1995). Changes in energy expenditure resulting from altered body weight. The New England journal of medicine, 332(10), 621–628. https://doi.org/10.1056/NEJM199503093321001

1462 Ravussin, E., Burnand, B., Schutz, Y., & Jéquier, E. (1985). Energy expenditure before and during energy restriction in obese patients. The American Journal of Clinical Nutrition, 41(4), 753–759. doi:10.1093/ajcn/41.4.753

1463 Doucet, E., Imbeault, P., St-Pierre, S., Alméras, N., Mauriège, P., Després, J. P., Bouchard, C., & Tremblay, A. (2003). Greater than predicted decrease in energy expenditure during exercise after body weight loss in obese men. Clinical science (London, England : 1979), 105(1), 89–95. https://doi.org/10.1042/CS20020252

1464 Rosenbaum, M. (2005). Low-dose leptin reverses skeletal muscle, autonomic, and neuroendocrine adaptations to maintenance of reduced weight. Journal of Clinical Investigation, 115(12), 3579–3586. doi:10.1172/jci25977

1465 Sumithran, P., Prendergast, L. A., Delbridge, E., Purcell, K., Shulkes, A., Kriketos, A., & Proietto, J. (2011). Long-term persistence of hormonal adaptations to weight loss. The New England journal of medicine, 365(17), 1597–1604. https://doi.org/10.1056/NEJMoa1105816

1466 Doucet, E., St-Pierre, S., Alméras, N., Després, J. P., Bouchard, C., & Tremblay, A. (2001). Evidence for the existence of adaptive thermogenesis during weight loss. The British journal of nutrition, 85(6), 715–723. https://doi.org/10.1079/bjn2001348

1467 Dulloo, A. G., & Jacquet, J. (1998). Adaptive reduction in basal metabolic rate in response to food deprivation in humans: a role for feedback signals from fat stores. The American Journal of Clinical Nutrition, 68(3), 599–606. doi:10.1093/ajcn/68.3.599

1468 Bevilacqua, L., Ramsey, J. J., Hagopian, K., Weindruch, R., & Harper, M.-E. (2004). Effects of short- and medium-term calorie restriction on muscle mitochondrial proton leak and reactive oxygen species production. American Journal of Physiology-Endocrinology and Metabolism, 286(5), E852–E861. doi:10.1152/ajpendo.00367.2003

1469 Esterbauer, H., Oberkofler, H., Dallinger, G., Breban, D., Hell, E., Krempler, F., & Patsch, W. (1999). Uncoupling protein-3 gene expression: reduced skeletal muscle mRNA in obese humans during pronounced weight loss. Diabetologia, 42(3), 302–309. doi:10.1007/s001250051155

1470 Rosenbaum, M., Hirsch, J., Gallagher, D. A., & Leibel, R. L. (2008). Long-term persistence of adaptive thermogenesis in subjects who have maintained a reduced body weight. The American journal of clinical nutrition, 88(4), 906–912. https://doi.org/10.1093/ajcn/88.4.906

1471 Weigle, D. S., & Brunzell, J. D. (1990). Assessment of energy expenditure in ambulatory reduced-obese subjects by the techniques of weight stabilization and exogenous weight replacement. International journal of obesity, 14 Suppl 1, 69–81.

1472 Weigle D. S. (1988). Contribution of decreased body mass to diminished thermic effect of exercise in reduced-obese men. International journal of obesity, 12(6), 567–578.

1473 von Loeffelholz, C., & Birkenfeld, A. (2018). The Role of Non-exercise Activity Thermogenesis in Human Obesity. In K. R. Feingold (Eds.) et. al., Endotext. MDText.com, Inc.

1474 Mäestu, J., Jürimäe, J., Valter, I., & Jürimäe, T. (2008). Increases in ghrelin and decreases in leptin without altering adiponectin during extreme weight loss in male competitive bodybuilders. Metabolism, 57(2), 221–225. doi:10.1016/j.metabol.2007.09.004

1475 Kim B. (2008). Thyroid hormone as a determinant of energy expenditure and the basal metabolic rate. Thyroid : official journal of the American Thyroid Association, 18(2), 141–144. https://doi.org/10.1089/thy.2007.0266

1476 Chin-Chance, C., Polonsky, K. S., & Schoeller, D. A. (2000). Twenty-four-hour leptin levels respond to cumulative short-term energy imbalance and predict subsequent intake. The Journal of clinical endocrinology and metabolism, 85(8), 2685–2691. https://doi.org/10.1210/jcem.85.8.6755

1477 Dirlewanger, M., di Vetta, V., Guenat, E., Battilana, P., Seematter, G., Schneiter, P., Jéquier, E., & Tappy, L. (2000). Effects of short-term carbohydrate or fat overfeeding on energy expenditure and plasma leptin concentrations in healthy female subjects. International journal of obesity and related metabolic disorders : journal of the International Association for the Study of Obesity, 24(11), 1413–1418. https://doi.org/10.1038/sj.ijo.0801395

1478 Spaulding, S. W., Chopra, I. J., Sherwin, R. S., & Lyall, S. S. (1976). EFFECT OF CALORIC RESTRICTION AND DIETARY COMPOSITION ON SERUM T3AND REVERSE T3IN MAN. The Journal of Clinical Endocrinology & Metabolism, 42(1), 197–200. doi:10.1210/jcem-42-1-197

1479 Jenkins, A. B., Markovic, T. P., Fleury, A., & Campbell, L. V. (1997). Carbohydrate intake and short-term regulation of leptin in humans. Diabetologia, 40(3), 348–351. https://doi.org/10.1007/s001250050686

1480 Levine, J. A., Eberhardt, N. L., & Jensen, M. D. (1999). Role of nonexercise activity thermogenesis in resistance to fat gain in humans. Science (New York, N.Y.), 283(5399), 212–214. https://doi.org/10.1126/science.283.5399.212

1481 Byrne, N. M., Sainsbury, A., King, N. A., Hills, A. P., & Wood, R. E. (2017). Intermittent energy restriction improves weight loss efficiency in obese men: the MATADOR study. International Journal of Obesity, 42(2), 129–138. doi:10.1038/ijo.2017.206

1482 Müller, M. J., Bosy-Westphal, A., & Heymsfield, S. B. (2010). Is there evidence for a set point that regulates human body weight?. F1000 medicine reports, 2, 59. https://doi.org/10.3410/M2-59

1483 Harris R. B. (1990). Role of set-point theory in regulation of body weight. FASEB journal : official publication of the Federation of American Societies for Experimental Biology, 4(15), 3310–3318. https://doi.org/10.1096/fasebj.4.15.2253845

1484 Harvard T.H. Chan (2021) 'Genes Are Not Destiny', Accessed Online Aug 17 2021: https://www.hsph.harvard.edu/obesity-prevention-source/obesity-causes/genes-and-obesity/

[1485] Byrne, N. M., Sainsbury, A., King, N. A., Hills, A. P., & Wood, R. E. (2017). Intermittent energy restriction improves weight loss efficiency in obese men: the MATADOR study. International Journal of Obesity, 42(2), 129–138. https://doi.org/10.1038/ijo.2017.206

[1486] Nindl, BC. et al (2000), 'Regional body composition changes in women after 6 months of periodized physical training', J Appl Physiol (1985), Vol 88(6), p 2251-9.

[1487] Demling, RH. and DeSanti, L. (2000) 'Effect of a hypocaloric diet, increased protein intake and resistance training on lean mass gains and fat mass loss in overweight police officers', Ann Nutr Metab, Vol 44(1), p 21-9.

[1488] Mark (2021) 'The Surprising Number Of Calories The Average American Eats Every Day', Health Digest, Accessed Online April 27th 2022: https://www.healthdigest.com/244223/the-surprising-number-of-calories-the-average-american-eats-every-day/

1489 Kerns, J. C., Guo, J., Fothergill, E., Howard, L., Knuth, N. D., Brychta, R., Chen, K. Y., Skarulis, M. C., Walter, P. J., & Hall, K. D. (2017). Increased Physical Activity Associated with Less Weight Regain Six Years After "The Biggest Loser" Competition. Obesity (Silver Spring, Md.), 25(11), 1838–1843. https://doi.org/10.1002/oby.21986

1490 Hill, J. O., Wyatt, H. R., & Peters, J. C. (2012). Energy balance and obesity. Circulation, 126(1), 126–132. https://doi.org/10.1161/CIRCULATIONAHA.111.087213

1491 Krajmalnik-Brown, R., Ilhan, Z. E., Kang, D. W., & DiBaise, J. K. (2012). Effects of gut microbes on nutrient absorption and energy regulation. Nutrition in clinical practice : official publication of the American Society for Parenteral and Enteral Nutrition, 27(2), 201–214. https://doi.org/10.1177/0884533611436116

1492 Sivieri, K., Morales, M. L., Adorno, M. A., Sakamoto, I. K., Saad, S. M., & Rossi, E. A. (2013). Lactobacillus acidophilus CRL 1014 improved "gut health" in the SHIME reactor. BMC gastroenterology, 13, 100. https://doi.org/10.1186/1471-230X-13-100

1493 Hall K. D. (2008). What is the required energy deficit per unit weight loss?. International journal of obesity (2005), 32(3), 573–576. https://doi.org/10.1038/sj.ijo.0803720

1494 Forbes G. B. (2000). Body fat content influences the body composition response to nutrition and exercise. Annals of the New York Academy of Sciences, 904, 359–365. https://doi.org/10.1111/j.1749-6632.2000.tb06482.x

1495 Forbes G. B. (1987). Lean body mass-body fat interrelationships in humans. Nutrition reviews, 45(8), 225–231. https://doi.org/10.1111/j.1753-4887.1987.tb02684.x

1496 Martin, A. D., Daniel, M. Z., Drinkwater, D. T., & Clarys, J. P. (1994). Adipose tissue density, estimated adipose lipid fraction and whole body adiposity in male cadavers. International journal of obesity and related metabolic disorders : journal of the International Association for the Study of Obesity, 18(2), 79–83.

1497 ENTENMAN, C., GOLDWATER, W. H., AYRES, N. S., & BEHNKE, A. R., Jr (1958). Analysis of adipose tissue in relation to body weight loss in man. Journal of applied physiology, 13(1), 129–134. https://doi.org/10.1152/jappl.1958.13.1.129

1498 Dulloo, A. G., Jacquet, J., & Montani, J. P. (2012). How dieting makes some fatter: from a perspective of human body composition autoregulation. The Proceedings of the Nutrition Society, 71(3), 379–389. https://doi.org/10.1017/S0029665112000225

1499 Forbes G. B. (1999). Longitudinal changes in adult fat-free mass: influence of body weight. The American journal of clinical nutrition, 70(6), 1025–1031. https://doi.org/10.1093/ajcn/70.6.1025

1500 Vogels, N., & Westerterp-Plantenga, M. S. (2007). Successful Long-term Weight Maintenance: A 2-year Follow-up*. Obesity, 15(5), 1258–1266. doi:10.1038/oby.2007.147

1501 Muller, M. J., Bosy-Westphal, A., Kutzner, D., & Heller, M. (2002). Metabolically active components of fat-free mass and resting energy expenditure in humans: recent lessons from imaging technologies. Obesity Reviews, 3(2), 113–122. doi:10.1046/j.1467-789x.2002.00057.x

1502 Ravussin, E., Lillioja, S., Knowler, W. C., Christin, L., Freymond, D., Abbott, W. G., Boyce, V., Howard, B. V., & Bogardus, C. (1988). Reduced rate of energy expenditure as a risk factor for body-weight gain. The New England journal of medicine, 318(8), 467–472. https://doi.org/10.1056/NEJM198802253180802

1503 Rice, B., Janssen, I., Hudson, R., & Ross, R. (1999). Effects of aerobic or resistance exercise and/or diet on glucose tolerance and plasma insulin levels in obese men. Diabetes Care, 22(5), 684–691. doi:10.2337/diacare.22.5.684

1504 Janssen, I., Fortier, A., Hudson, R., & Ross, R. (2002). Effects of an Energy-Restrictive Diet With or Without Exercise on Abdominal Fat, Intermuscular Fat, and Metabolic Risk Factors in Obese Women. Diabetes Care, 25(3), 431–438. doi:10.2337/diacare.25.3.431

1505 Janssen, I., & Ross, R. (1999). Effects of sex on the change in visceral, subcutaneous adipose tissue and skeletal muscle in response to weight loss. International Journal of Obesity, 23(10), 1035–1046. doi:10.1038/sj.ijo.0801038

1506 Chomentowski, P., Dubé, J. J., Amati, F., Stefanovic-Racic, M., Zhu, S., Toledo, F. G., & Goodpaster, B. H. (2009). Moderate exercise attenuates the loss of skeletal muscle mass that occurs with intentional caloric restriction-induced weight loss in older, overweight to obese adults. The journals of gerontology. Series A, Biological sciences and medical sciences, 64(5), 575–580. https://doi.org/10.1093/gerona/glp007

1507 Miller, W. C., Koceja, D. M., & Hamilton, E. J. (1997). A meta-analysis of the past 25 years of weight loss research using diet, exercise or diet plus exercise intervention. International journal of obesity and related metabolic disorders : journal of the International Association for the Study of Obesity, 21(10), 941–947. https://doi.org/10.1038/sj.ijo.0800499

1508 Hansen, D., Dendale, P., Berger, J., van Loon, L. J., & Meeusen, R. (2007). The effects of exercise training on fat-mass loss in obese patients during energy intake restriction. Sports medicine (Auckland, N.Z.), 37(1), 31–46. https://doi.org/10.2165/00007256-200737010-00003

1509 Stiegler, P., & Cunliffe, A. (2006). The role of diet and exercise for the maintenance of fat-free mass and resting metabolic rate during weight loss. Sports medicine (Auckland, N.Z.), 36(3), 239–262. https://doi.org/10.2165/00007256-200636030-00005

1510 Layman, D. K., Evans, E., Baum, J. I., Seyler, J., Erickson, D. J., & Boileau, R. A. (2005). Dietary protein and exercise have additive effects on body composition during weight loss in adult women. The Journal of nutrition, 135(8), 1903–1910. https://doi.org/10.1093/jn/135.8.1903

1511 Sardeli, A. V., Komatsu, T. R., Mori, M. A., Gáspari, A. F., & Chacon-Mikahil, M. (2018). Resistance Training Prevents Muscle Loss Induced by Caloric Restriction in Obese Elderly Individuals: A Systematic Review and Meta-Analysis. Nutrients, 10(4), 423. https://doi.org/10.3390/nu10040423

1512 Bryner, R. W., Ullrich, I. H., Sauers, J., Donley, D., Hornsby, G., Kolar, M., & Yeater, R. (1999). Effects of resistance vs. aerobic training combined with an 800 calorie liquid diet on lean body mass and resting metabolic rate. Journal of the American College of Nutrition, 18(2), 115–121. https://doi.org/10.1080/07315724.1999.10718838

1513 Vechetti, I. J., Peck, B. D., Wen, Y., Walton, R. G., Valentino, T. R., Alimov, A. P., ... McCarthy, J. J. (2021). Mechanical overload-induced muscle-derived extracellular vesicles promote adipose tissue lipolysis. The FASEB Journal, 35(6). doi:10.1096/fj.202100242r

1514 Hejnová, J., Majercík, M., Polák, J., Richterová, B., Crampes, F., deGlisezinski, I., & Stich, V. (2004). Vliv silove-dynamického tréninku na inzulínovou senzitivitu u inzulínorezistentních mužů [Effect of dynamic strength training on insulin sensitivity in men with insulin resistance]. Casopis lekaru ceskych, 143(11), 762–765.

1515 Burns, R. D., Fu, Y., & Zhang, P. (2019). Resistance Training and Insulin Sensitivity in Youth: A Meta-analysis. American journal of health behavior, 43(2), 228–242. https://doi.org/10.5993/AJHB.43.2.1

1516 Hansen, E., Landstad, B. J., Gundersen, K. T., Torjesen, P. A., & Svebak, S. (2012). Insulin sensitivity after maximal and endurance resistance training. Journal of strength and conditioning research, 26(2), 327–334. https://doi.org/10.1519/JSC.0b013e318220e70f

1517 Shaibi, G. Q., Cruz, M. L., Ball, G. D., Weigensberg, M. J., Salem, G. J., Crespo, N. C., & Goran, M. I. (2006). Effects of resistance training on insulin sensitivity in overweight Latino adolescent males. Medicine and science in sports and exercise, 38(7), 1208–1215. https://doi.org/10.1249/01.mss.0000227304.88406.0f

1518 Heilbronn, L., Smith, S. R., & Ravussin, E. (2004). Failure of fat cell proliferation, mitochondrial function and fat oxidation results in ectopic fat storage, insulin resistance and type II diabetes mellitus. International Journal of Obesity, 28(S4), S12–S21. doi:10.1038/sj.ijo.0802853

1519 Kullmann, S., Valenta, V., Wagner, R., Tschritter, O., Machann, J., Häring, H.-U., ... Heni, M. (2020). Brain insulin sensitivity is linked to adiposity and body fat distribution. Nature Communications, 11(1). doi:10.1038/s41467-020-15686-y

1520 Caro, J. F., Dohm, L. G., Pories, W. J., & Sinha, M. K. (1989). Cellular alterations in liver, skeletal muscle, and adipose tissue responsible for insulin resistance in obesity and type II diabetes. Diabetes/metabolism reviews, 5(8), 665–689. https://doi.org/10.1002/dmr.5610050804

1521 Holten, M. K., Zacho, M., Gaster, M., Juel, C., Wojtaszewski, J. F. P., & Dela, F. (2004). Strength Training Increases Insulin-Mediated Glucose Uptake, GLUT4 Content, and Insulin Signaling in Skeletal Muscle in Patients With Type 2 Diabetes. Diabetes, 53(2), 294–305. doi:10.2337/diabetes.53.2.294

1522 METTLER, S., MITCHELL, N., & TIPTON, K. D. (2010). Increased Protein Intake Reduces Lean Body Mass Loss during Weight Loss in Athletes. Medicine & Science in Sports & Exercise, 42(2), 326–337. doi:10.1249/mss.0b013e3181b2ef8e

1523 Longland, T. M., Oikawa, S. Y., Mitchell, C. J., Devries, M. C., & Phillips, S. M. (2016). Higher compared with lower dietary protein during an energy deficit combined with intense exercise promotes greater lean mass gain and fat mass loss: a randomized trial. The American Journal of Clinical Nutrition, 103(3), 738–746. doi:10.3945/ajcn.115.119339

1524 Calbet, J. A. L., Ponce-González, J. G., Calle-Herrero, J. de L., Perez-Suarez, I., Martin-Rincon, M., Santana, A., ... Holmberg, H.-C. (2017). Exercise Preserves Lean Mass and Performance during Severe Energy Deficit: The Role of Exercise Volume and Dietary Protein Content. Frontiers in Physiology, 8. doi:10.3389/fphys.2017.00483

1525 Bhasin, S., Storer, T. W., Berman, N., Callegari, C., Clevenger, B., Phillips, J., ... Casaburi, R. (1996). The Effects of Supraphysiologic Doses of Testosterone on Muscle Size and Strength in Normal Men. New England Journal of Medicine, 335(1), 1–7. doi:10.1056/nejm199607043350101

1526 Apró, W., & Blomstrand, E. (2010). Influence of supplementation with branched-chain amino acids in combination with resistance exercise on p70S6 kinase phosphorylation in resting and exercising human skeletal muscle. Acta Physiologica, no–no. doi:10.1111/j.1748-1716.2010.02151.x

1527 Krug, A. L. O., Macedo, A. G., Zago, A. S., Rush, J. W. E., Santos, C. F., & Amaral, S. L. (2016). High-intensity resistance training attenuates dexamethasone-induced muscle atrophy. Muscle & Nerve, 53(5), 779–788. doi:10.1002/mus.24906

1528 Crowley, M. A., & Matt, K. S. (1996). Hormonal regulation of skeletal muscle hypertrophy in rats: the testosterone to cortisol ratio. European Journal of Applied Physiology and Occupational Physiology, 73(1-2), 66–72. doi:10.1007/bf00262811

1529 Watson, P., Shirreffs, S. M., & Maughan, R. J. (2004). The effect of acute branched-chain amino acid supplementation on prolonged exercise capacity in a warm environment. European journal of applied physiology, 93(3), 306–314. https://doi.org/10.1007/s00421-004-1206-2

1530 Arroyo-Cerezo, A., Cerrillo, I., Ortega, Á., & FernÁndez-PachÓn, M. S. (2021). Intake of branched chain amino acids favors post-exercise muscle recovery and may improve muscle function: optimal dosage regimens and consumption conditions. The Journal of sports medicine and physical fitness, 10.23736/S0022-4707.21.11843-2. Advance online publication. https://doi.org/10.23736/S0022-4707.21.11843-2

1531 Khemtong, C., Kuo, C. H., Chen, C. Y., Jaime, S. J., & Condello, G. (2021). Does Branched-Chain Amino Acids (BCAAs) Supplementation Attenuate Muscle Damage Markers and Soreness after Resistance Exercise in Trained Males? A Meta-Analysis of Randomized Controlled Trials. Nutrients, 13(6), 1880. https://doi.org/10.3390/nu13061880

1532 Pasiakos, S. M., & McClung, J. P. (2011). Supplemental dietary leucine and the skeletal muscle anabolic response to essential amino acids. Nutrition reviews, 69(9), 550–557. https://doi.org/10.1111/j.1753-4887.2011.00420.x

1533 Volpi, E., Kobayashi, H., Sheffield-Moore, M., Mittendorfer, B., & Wolfe, R. R. (2003). Essential amino acids are primarily responsible for the amino acid stimulation of muscle protein anabolism in healthy elderly adults. The American journal of clinical nutrition, 78(2), 250–258. https://doi.org/10.1093/ajcn/78.2.250

1534 Børsheim, E., Tipton, K. D., Wolf, S. E., & Wolfe, R. R. (2002). Essential amino acids and muscle protein recovery from resistance exercise. American journal of physiology. Endocrinology and metabolism, 283(4), E648–E657. https://doi.org/10.1152/ajpendo.00466.2001

1535 Wilkinson, D. J., Hossain, T., Hill, D. S., Phillips, B. E., Crossland, H., Williams, J., Loughna, P., Churchward-Venne, T. A., Breen, L., Phillips, S. M., Etheridge, T., Rathmacher, J. A., Smith, K., Szewczyk, N. J., & Atherton, P. J. (2013). Effects of leucine and its metabolite β-hydroxy-β-methylbutyrate on human skeletal muscle protein metabolism. The Journal of physiology, 591(11), 2911–2923. https://doi.org/10.1113/jphysiol.2013.253203

1536 Norton, L. E., & Layman, D. K. (2006). Leucine regulates translation initiation of protein synthesis in skeletal muscle after exercise. The Journal of nutrition, 136(2), 533S–537S. https://doi.org/10.1093/jn/136.2.533S

1537 Blomstrand, E., Eliasson, J., Karlsson, H. K. R., & Köhnke, R. (2006). Branched-Chain Amino Acids Activate Key Enzymes in Protein Synthesis after Physical Exercise. The Journal of Nutrition, 136(1), 269S–273S. doi:10.1093/jn/136.1.269s

1538 Kohlmeier M (May 2015). "Leucine". Nutrient Metabolism: Structures, Functions, and Genes (2nd ed.). Academic Press. pp. 385–388.

1539 Nair, K. S., Schwartz, R. G., & Welle, S. (1992). Leucine as a regulator of whole body and skeletal muscle protein metabolism in humans. The American journal of physiology, 263(5 Pt 1), E928–E934. https://doi.org/10.1152/ajpendo.1992.263.5.E928

1540 van Loon L. J. (2012). Leucine as a pharmaconutrient in health and disease. Current opinion in clinical nutrition and metabolic care, 15(1), 71–77. https://doi.org/10.1097/MCO.0b013e32834d617a

1541 Panton, L. B., Rathmacher, J. A., Baier, S., & Nissen, S. (2000). Nutritional supplementation of the leucine metabolite beta-hydroxy-beta-methylbutyrate (hmb) during resistance training. Nutrition (Burbank, Los Angeles County, Calif.), 16(9), 734–739. https://doi.org/10.1016/s0899-9007(00)00376-2

1542 Slater, G. J., & Jenkins, D. (2000). Beta-hydroxy-beta-methylbutyrate (HMB) supplementation and the promotion of muscle growth and strength. Sports medicine (Auckland, N.Z.), 30(2), 105–116. https://doi.org/10.2165/00007256-200030020-00004

1543 Vukovich, M. D., Stubbs, N. B., & Bohlken, R. M. (2001). Body composition in 70-year-old adults responds to dietary beta-hydroxy-beta-methylbutyrate similar to that of young adults. The Journal of nutrition, 131(7), 2049–2052. https://doi.org/10.1093/jn/131.7.2049

1544 Wilson, G. J., Wilson, J. M., & Manninen, A. H. (2008). Effects of beta-hydroxy-beta-methylbutyrate (HMB) on exercise performance and body composition across varying levels of age, sex, and training experience: A review. Nutrition & Metabolism, 5(1). doi:10.1186/1743-7075-5-1

1545 Rahimi, M. H., Mohammadi, H., Eshaghi, H., Askari, G., & Miraghajani, M. (2018). The Effects of Beta-Hydroxy-Beta-Methylbutyrate Supplementation on Recovery Following Exercise-Induced Muscle Damage: A Systematic Review and Meta-Analysis. Journal of the American College of Nutrition, 37(7), 640–649. https://doi.org/10.1080/07315724.2018.1451789

1546 Silva, V. R., Belozo, F. L., Micheletti, T. O., Conrado, M., Stout, J. R., Pimentel, G. D., & Gonzalez, A. M. (2017). β-hydroxy-β-methylbutyrate free acid supplementation may improve recovery and muscle adaptations after resistance training: a systematic review. Nutrition Research, 45, 1–9. doi:10.1016/j.nutres.2017.07.008

1547 Knitter, A. E., Panton, L., Rathmacher, J. A., Petersen, A., & Sharp, R. (2000). Effects of beta-hydroxy-beta-methylbutyrate on muscle damage after a prolonged run. Journal of applied physiology (Bethesda, Md. : 1985), 89(4), 1340–1344. https://doi.org/10.1152/jappl.2000.89.4.1340

1548 Smith, H. J., Wyke, S. M., & Tisdale, M. J. (2004). Mechanism of the attenuation of proteolysis-inducing factor stimulated protein degradation in muscle by beta-hydroxy-beta-methylbutyrate. Cancer research, 64(23), 8731–8735. https://doi.org/10.1158/0008-5472.CAN-04-1760

1549 Wilson JM and Lowery RP et al (2013) 'β-Hydroxy-β-methylbutyrate free acid reduces markers of exercise-induced muscle damage and improves recovery in resistance-trained men', Br J Nutr. 2013 Aug 28;110(3):538-44.

1550 Wilson, J. M., Fitschen, P. J., Campbell, B., Wilson, G. J., Zanchi, N., Taylor, L., Wilborn, C., Kalman, D. S., Stout, J. R., Hoffman, J. R., Ziegenfuss, T. N., Lopez, H. L., Kreider, R. B., Smith-Ryan, A. E., & Antonio, J. (2013). International Society of Sports Nutrition Position Stand: beta-hydroxy-beta-methylbutyrate (HMB). Journal of the International Society of Sports Nutrition, 10(1), 6. https://doi.org/10.1186/1550-2783-10-6

1551 Sanchez-Martinez, J., Santos-Lozano, A., Garcia-Hermoso, A., Sadarangani, K. P., & Cristi-Montero, C. (2018). Effects of beta-hydroxy-beta-methylbutyrate supplementation on strength and body composition in trained and competitive athletes: A meta-analysis of randomized controlled trials. Journal of science and medicine in sport, 21(7), 727–735. https://doi.org/10.1016/j.jsams.2017.11.003

1552 Kreider, R. B., Ferreira, M., Wilson, M., & Almada, A. L. (1999). Effects of calcium beta-hydroxy-beta-methylbutyrate (HMB) supplementation during resistance-training on markers of catabolism, body composition and strength. International journal of sports medicine, 20(8), 503–509. https://doi.org/10.1055/s-1999-8835

1553 Ransone, J., Neighbors, K., Lefavi, R., & Chromiak, J. (2003). The effect of beta-hydroxy beta-methylbutyrate on muscular strength and body composition in collegiate football players. Journal of strength and conditioning research, 17(1), 34–39. https://doi.org/10.1519/1533-4287(2003)017<0034:teohmo>2.0.co;2

1554 Slater, G., Jenkins, D., Logan, P., Lee, H., Vukovich, M., Rathmacher, J. A., & Hahn, A. G. (2001). Beta-hydroxy-beta-methylbutyrate (HMB) supplementation does not affect changes in strength or body composition during resistance training in trained men. International journal of sport nutrition and exercise metabolism, 11(3), 384–396. https://doi.org/10.1123/ijsnem.11.3.384

1555 Holeček M. (2017). Beta-hydroxy-beta-methylbutyrate supplementation and skeletal muscle in healthy and muscle-wasting conditions. Journal of cachexia, sarcopenia and muscle, 8(4), 529–541. https://doi.org/10.1002/jcsm.12208

1556 Rossi, A. P., D'Introno, A., Rubele, S., Caliari, C., Gattazzo, S., Zoico, E., Mazzali, G., Fantin, F., & Zamboni, M. (2017). The Potential of β-Hydroxy-β-Methylbutyrate as a New Strategy for the Management of Sarcopenia and Sarcopenic Obesity. Drugs & aging, 34(11), 833–840. https://doi.org/10.1007/s40266-017-0496-0

1557 Wilson, J. M., Lowery, R. P., Joy, J. M., Walters, J. A., Baier, S. M., Fuller, J. C., Jr, Stout, J. R., Norton, L. E., Sikorski, E. M., Wilson, S. M., Duncan, N. M., Zanchi, N. E., & Rathmacher, J. (2013). β-Hydroxy-β-methylbutyrate free acid reduces markers of exercise-induced muscle damage and improves recovery in resistance-trained men. The British journal of nutrition, 110(3), 538–544. https://doi.org/10.1017/S0007114512005387

1558 Molfino, A., Gioia, G., Rossi Fanelli, F., & Muscaritoli, M. (2013). Beta-hydroxy-beta-methylbutyrate supplementation in health and disease: a systematic review of randomized trials. Amino acids, 45(6), 1273–1292. https://doi.org/10.1007/s00726-013-1592-z

1559 Gallagher, P. M., Carrithers, J. A., Godard, M. P., Schulze, K. E., & Trappe, S. W. (2000). Beta-hydroxy-beta-methylbutyrate ingestion, Part I: effects on strength and fat free mass. Medicine and science in sports and exercise, 32(12), 2109–2115. https://doi.org/10.1097/00005768-200012000-00022

1560 Wilson, G. J., Wilson, J. M., & Manninen, A. H. (2008). Effects of beta-hydroxy-beta-methylbutyrate (HMB) on exercise performance and body composition across varying levels of age, sex, and training experience: A review. Nutrition & metabolism, 5, 1. https://doi.org/10.1186/1743-7075-5-1

1561 Rathmacher, J. A., Nissen, S., Panton, L., Clark, R. H., Eubanks May, P., Barber, A. E., D'Olimpio, J., & Abumrad, N. N. (2004). Supplementation with a combination of beta-hydroxy-beta-methylbutyrate (HMB), arginine, and glutamine is safe and could improve hematological parameters. JPEN. Journal of parenteral and enteral nutrition, 28(2), 65–75. https://doi.org/10.1177/014860710402800265

1562 Borack, M. S., & Volpi, E. (2016). Efficacy and Safety of Leucine Supplementation in the Elderly. The Journal of nutrition, 146(12), 2625S–2629S. https://doi.org/10.3945/jn.116.230771

1563 Nissen, S., Sharp, R. L., Panton, L., Vukovich, M., Trappe, S., & Fuller, J. C., Jr (2000). beta-hydroxy-beta-methylbutyrate (HMB) supplementation in humans is safe and may decrease cardiovascular risk factors. The Journal of nutrition, 130(8), 1937–1945. https://doi.org/10.1093/jn/130.8.1937

1564 Kaats, G. R., Blum, K., Pullin, D., Keith, S. C., & Wood, R. (1998). A randomized, double-masked, placebo-controlled study of the effects of chromium picolinate supplementation on body composition: A replication and extension of a previous study. Current Therapeutic Research, 59(6), 379–388. doi:10.1016/s0011-393x(98)85040-6

1565 Willoughby, D., Hewlings, S., & Kalman, D. (2018). Body Composition Changes in Weight Loss: Strategies and Supplementation for Maintaining Lean Body Mass, a Brief Review. Nutrients, 10(12), 1876. https://doi.org/10.3390/nu10121876

1566 Bahadori, B., Wallner, S., Schneider, H., Wascher, T. C., & Toplak, H. (1997). Effekt von Chromhefe und Chrompicolinat auf die Körperzusammensetzung bei übergewichtigen, nichtdiabetischen Patienten während und nach einer Formula-Diät [Effect of chromium yeast and chromium picolinate on body composition of obese, non-diabetic patients during and after a formula diet]. Acta medica Austriaca, 24(5), 185–187.

1567 Moradi, F., Kooshki, F., Nokhostin, F., Khoshbaten, M., Bazyar, H., & Pourghassem Gargari, B. (2021). A pilot study of the effects of chromium picolinate supplementation on serum fetuin-A, metabolic and inflammatory factors in patients with nonalcoholic fatty liver disease: A double-blind, placebo-controlled trial. Journal of Trace Elements in Medicine and Biology, 63, 126659. doi:10.1016/j.jtemb.2020.126659

1568 Anderson, R. A., Cheng, N., Bryden, N. A., Polansky, M. M., Cheng, N., Chi, J., & Feng, J. (1997). Elevated intakes of supplemental chromium improve glucose and insulin variables in individuals with type 2 diabetes. Diabetes, 46(11), 1786–1791. https://doi.org/10.2337/diab.46.11.1786

1569 Pittler, M. H., Stevinson, C., & Ernst, E. (2003). Chromium picolinate for reducing body weight: meta-analysis of randomized trials. International journal of obesity and related metabolic disorders : journal of the International Association for the Study of Obesity, 27(4), 522–529. https://doi.org/10.1038/sj.ijo.0802262

1570 Onakpoya, I., Posadzki, P., & Ernst, E. (2013). Chromium supplementation in overweight and obesity: a systematic review and meta-analysis of randomized clinical trials. Obesity reviews : an official journal of the International Association for the Study of Obesity, 14(6), 496–507. https://doi.org/10.1111/obr.12026

1571 Willoughby, D., Hewlings, S., & Kalman, D. (2018). Body Composition Changes in Weight Loss: Strategies and Supplementation for Maintaining Lean Body Mass, a Brief Review. Nutrients, 10(12), 1876. https://doi.org/10.3390/nu10121876

1572 Doisy et al (1976) 'Chromium Metabolism in Man and Biochemical Effects', in Trace Elements in Human Health and Disease, Volume II: Essential and Toxic Elements, Academic Press, New York, pp 79-80.

1573 Tsang, C., Taghizadeh, M., Aghabagheri, E., Asemi, Z., & Jafarnejad, S. (2019). A meta-analysis of the effect of chromium supplementation on anthropometric indices of subjects with overweight or obesity. Clinical obesity, 9(4), e12313. https://doi.org/10.1111/cob.12313

1574 Costello, R. B., Dwyer, J. T., & Bailey, R. L. (2016). Chromium supplements for glycemic control in type 2 diabetes: limited evidence of effectiveness. Nutrition reviews, 74(7), 455–468. https://doi.org/10.1093/nutrit/nuw011

1575 Amato, P., Morales, A. J., & Yen, S. S. C. (2000). Effects of Chromium Picolinate Supplementation on Insulin Sensitivity, Serum Lipids, and Body Composition in Healthy, Nonobese, Older Men and Women. The Journals of Gerontology Series A: Biological Sciences and Medical Sciences, 55(5), M260–M263. doi:10.1093/gerona/55.5.m260

1576 Wilson, B. E., & Gondy, A. (1995). Effects of chromium supplementation on fasting insulin levels and lipid parameters in healthy, non-obese young subjects. Diabetes research and clinical practice, 28(3), 179–184. https://doi.org/10.1016/0168-8227(95)01097-w

1577 Bulbulian et al (1996) 'CHROMIUM PICOLINATE SUPPLEMENTATION IN MALE AND FEMALE SWIMMERS 664', Medicine & Science in Sports & Exercise: May 1996 - Volume 28 - Issue 5 - p 111.

1578 Evans GW. The effect of chromium picolinate on insulin controlled parameters in humans. Int J Biosocial Med Res 1989; 11: 163–80.

1579 Lefavi, R. G., Anderson, R. A., Keith, R. E., Wilson, G. D., McMillan, J. L., & Stone, M. H. (1992). Efficacy of chromium supplementation in athletes: emphasis on anabolism. International journal of sport nutrition, 2(2), 111–122. https://doi.org/10.1123/ijsn.2.2.111

1580 Bunker, V. W., Lawson, M. S., Delves, H. T., & Clayton, B. E. (1984). The uptake and excretion of chromium by the elderly. The American Journal of Clinical Nutrition, 39(5), 797–802. doi:10.1093/ajcn/39.5.797

1581 NIH (2020) 'Chromium: Fact Sheet for Health Professionals', Dietary Supplement Fact Sheets, Accessed Online Jan 18 2021: https://ods.od.nih.gov/factsheets/Chromium-HealthProfessional/

1582 Saraymen et al (2004) 'Sweat Copper, Zinc, Iron, Magnesium and Chromium Levels in National Wrestler', İnönü Üniversitesi Tıp Fakültesi Dergisi 11(1) 7-10.

1583 CONSOLAZIO, C. F., NELSON, R. A., MATOUSH, L. O., HUGHES, R. C., & URONE, P. (1964). THE TRACE MINERAL LOSSES IN SWEAT. REP NO. 284. Report. U.S. Army Medical Research and Nutrition Laboratory, 1–14.

1584 European Food Safety Authority NDA Panel. Scientific Opinion on Dietary Reference Values for chromium. EFSA Journal 2014;12(10):3845.

1585 Chaston, T. B., Dixon, J. B., & O'Brien, P. E. (2006). Changes in fat-free mass during significant weight loss: a systematic review. International Journal of Obesity, 31(5), 743–750. doi:10.1038/sj.ijo.0803483

1586 Hoie, L. H., Bruusgaard, D., & Thom, E. (1993). Reduction of body mass and change in body composition on a very low calorie diet. International journal of obesity and related metabolic disorders : journal of the International Association for the Study of Obesity, 17(1), 17–20.

1587 Cahill, G. F. (2006). Fuel Metabolism in Starvation. Annual Review of Nutrition, 26(1), 1–22. doi:10.1146/annurev.nutr.26.061505.111258

1588 Brandt (1999) 'Endocrine Regulation of Glucose Metabolism', Endocrine Core Notes, Accessed Online Aug 16 2021: https://www.rose-hulman.edu/~brandt/Chem330/EndocrineNotes/Chapter_5_Glucose.pdf

1589 Watford M, Goodridge AG. Regulation of fuel utilization. In: Stipanuk MH, editor. Biochemical and Physiological Aspects of Human Nutrition. Philadelphia, PA: W.B. Saunders Company; 2000. pp. 384–407.

1590 Jensen, N. J., Wodschow, H. Z., Nilsson, M., & Rungby, J. (2020). Effects of Ketone Bodies on Brain Metabolism and Function in Neurodegenerative Diseases. International journal of molecular sciences, 21(22), 8767. https://doi.org/10.3390/ijms21228767

1591 Owen, O. E., Morgan, A. P., Kemp, H. G., Sullivan, J. M., Herrera, M. G., & Cahill, G. F., Jr (1967). Brain metabolism during fasting. The Journal of clinical investigation, 46(10), 1589–1595. https://doi.org/10.1172/JCI105650

1592 Baba, H., Zhang, X. J., & Wolfe, R. R. (1995). Glycerol gluconeogenesis in fasting humans. Nutrition (Burbank, Los Angeles County, Calif.), 11(2), 149–153.

1593 Wyss, M. T., Jolivet, R., Buck, A., Magistretti, P. J., & Weber, B. (2011). In Vivo Evidence for Lactate as a Neuronal Energy Source. Journal of Neuroscience, 31(20), 7477–7485. doi:10.1523/jneurosci.0415-11.2011

1594 Koutnik, A. P., Poff, A. M., Ward, N. P., DeBlasi, J. M., Soliven, M. A., Romero, M. A., ... D'Agostino, D. P. (2020). Ketone Bodies Attenuate Wasting in Models of Atrophy. Journal of Cachexia, Sarcopenia and Muscle, 11(4), 973–996. doi:10.1002/jcsm.12554

1595 Thomsen, H. H., Rittig, N., Johannsen, M., Møller, A. B., Jørgensen, J. O., Jessen, N., & Møller, N. (2018). Effects of 3-hydroxybutyrate and free fatty acids on muscle protein kinetics and signaling during LPS-induced inflammation in humans: anticatabolic impact of ketone bodies. The American Journal of Clinical Nutrition, 108(4), 857–867. doi:10.1093/ajcn/nqy170

1596 Yang, D., & Wan, Y. (2019). NR Supplementation During Lactation: Benefiting Mother and Child. Trends in Endocrinology & Metabolism, 30(4), 225–227. doi:10.1016/j.tem.2019.02.004

1597 Hall, K. D., Chen, K. Y., Guo, J., Lam, Y. Y., Leibel, R. L., Mayer, L. E., Reitman, M. L., Rosenbaum, M., Smith, S. R., Walsh, B. T., & Ravussin, E. (2016). Energy expenditure and body composition changes after an isocaloric ketogenic diet in overweight and obese men. The American journal of clinical nutrition, 104(2), 324–333. https://doi.org/10.3945/ajcn.116.133561

1598 Frisch, S., Zittermann, A., Berthold, H. K., Götting, C., Kuhn, J., Kleesiek, K., Stehle, P., & Körtke, H. (2009). A randomized controlled trial on the efficacy of carbohydrate-reduced or fat-reduced diets in patients attending a telemedically guided weight loss program. Cardiovascular diabetology, 8, 36. https://doi.org/10.1186/1475-2840-8-36

1599 Napoleão, A., Fernandes, L., Miranda, C., & Marum, A. P. (2021). Effects of Calorie Restriction on Health Span and Insulin Resistance: Classic Calorie Restriction Diet vs. Ketosis-Inducing Diet. Nutrients, 13(4), 1302. https://doi.org/10.3390/nu13041302

1600 Tinsley, G. M., & Willoughby, D. S. (2016). Fat-Free Mass Changes During Ketogenic Diets and the Potential Role of Resistance Training. International journal of sport nutrition and exercise metabolism, 26(1), 78–92. https://doi.org/10.1123/ijsnem.2015-0070

1601 Gomez-Arbelaez, D., Bellido, D., Castro, A. I., Ordoñez-Mayan, L., Carreira, J., Galban, C., Martinez-Olmos, M. A., Crujeiras, A. B., Sajoux, I., & Casanueva, F. F. (2017). Body Composition Changes After Very-Low-Calorie Ketogenic Diet in Obesity Evaluated by 3 Standardized Methods. The Journal of clinical endocrinology and metabolism, 102(2), 488–498. https://doi.org/10.1210/jc.2016-2385

1602 Hall, K. D., Bemis, T., Brychta, R., Chen, K. Y., Courville, A., Crayner, E. J., Goodwin, S., Guo, J., Howard, L., Knuth, N. D., Miller, B. V., 3rd, Prado, C. M., Siervo, M., Skarulis, M. C., Walter, M., Walter, P. J., & Yannai, L. (2015). Calorie for Calorie, Dietary Fat Restriction Results in More Body Fat Loss than Carbohydrate Restriction in People with Obesity. Cell metabolism, 22(3), 427–436. https://doi.org/10.1016/j.cmet.2015.07.021

1603 Bradley, U., Spence, M., Courtney, C. H., McKinley, M. C., Ennis, C. N., McCance, D. R., McEneny, J., Bell, P. M., Young, I. S., & Hunter, S. J. (2009). Low-fat versus low-carbohydrate weight reduction diets: effects on weight loss, insulin resistance, and cardiovascular risk: a randomized control trial. Diabetes, 58(12), 2741–2748. https://doi.org/10.2337/db09-0098

1604 Hu, T., Mills, K. T., Yao, L., Demanelis, K., Eloustaz, M., Yancy, W. S., Jr, Kelly, T. N., He, J., & Bazzano, L. A. (2012). Effects of low-carbohydrate diets versus low-fat diets on metabolic risk factors: a meta-analysis of randomized controlled clinical trials. American journal of epidemiology, 176 Suppl 7(Suppl 7), S44–S54. https://doi.org/10.1093/aje/kws264

1605 Nordmann, A. J., Nordmann, A., Briel, M., Keller, U., Yancy, W. S., Jr, Brehm, B. J., & Bucher, H. C. (2006). Effects of low-carbohydrate vs low-fat diets on weight loss and cardiovascular risk factors: a meta-analysis of randomized controlled trials. Archives of internal medicine, 166(3), 285–293. https://doi.org/10.1001/archinte.166.3.285

1606 Manninen A. H. (2004). Is a calorie really a calorie? Metabolic advantage of low-carbohydrate diets. Journal of the International Society of Sports Nutrition, 1(2), 21–26. https://doi.org/10.1186/1550-2783-1-2-21

1607 Brehm, B. J., Spang, S. E., Lattin, B. L., Seeley, R. J., Daniels, S. R., & D'Alessio, D. A. (2005). The role of energy expenditure in the differential weight loss in obese women on low-fat and low-carbohydrate diets. The Journal of clinical endocrinology and metabolism, 90(3), 1475–1482. https://doi.org/10.1210/jc.2004-1540

1608 Hendrickson, S., & Mattes, R. (2007). Financial incentive for diet recall accuracy does not affect reported energy intake or number of underreporters in a sample of overweight females. Journal of the American Dietetic Association, 107(1), 118–121. https://doi.org/10.1016/j.jada.2006.10.003

1609 Champagne, C. M., Bray, G. A., Kurtz, A. A., Monteiro, J. B., Tucker, E., Volaufova, J., & Delany, J. P. (2002). Energy intake and energy expenditure: a controlled study comparing dietitians and non-dietitians. Journal of the American Dietetic Association, 102(10), 1428–1432. https://doi.org/10.1016/s0002-8223(02)90316-0

1610 Schoeller, D. A., Thomas, D., Archer, E., Heymsfield, S. B., Blair, S. N., Goran, M. I., Hill, J. O., Atkinson, R. L., Corkey, B. E., Foreyt, J., Dhurandhar, N. V., Kral, J. G., Hall, K. D., Hansen, B. C., Heitmann, B. L., Ravussin, E., & Allison, D. B. (2013). Self-report-based estimates of energy intake offer an inadequate basis for scientific conclusions. The American journal of clinical nutrition, 97(6), 1413–1415. https://doi.org/10.3945/ajcn.113.062125

1611 Layman, D. K., Boileau, R. A., Erickson, D. J., Painter, J. E., Shiue, H., Sather, C., & Christou, D. D. (2003). A reduced ratio of dietary carbohydrate to protein improves body composition and blood lipid profiles during weight loss in adult women. The Journal of nutrition, 133(2), 411–417. https://doi.org/10.1093/jn/133.2.411

1612 Hall, K. D., Guyenet, S. J., & Leibel, R. L. (2018). The Carbohydrate-Insulin Model of Obesity Is Difficult to Reconcile With Current Evidence. JAMA internal medicine, 178(8), 1103–1105. https://doi.org/10.1001/jamainternmed.2018.2920

1613 Gardner, C. D., Trepanowski, J. F., Del Gobbo, L. C., Hauser, M. E., Rigdon, J., Ioannidis, J. P. A., ... King, A. C. (2018). Effect of Low-Fat vs Low-Carbohydrate Diet on 12-Month Weight Loss in Overweight Adults and the Association With Genotype Pattern or Insulin Secretion. JAMA, 319(7), 667. doi:10.1001/jama.2018.0245

1614 Schoeller, D. A., & Buchholz, A. C. (2005). Energetics of obesity and weight control: does diet composition matter?. Journal of the American Dietetic Association, 105(5 Suppl 1), S24–S28. https://doi.org/10.1016/j.jada.2005.02.025

1615 Howell, S., & Kones, R. (2017). "Calories in, calories out" and macronutrient intake: the hope, hype, and science of calories. American journal of physiology. Endocrinology and metabolism, 313(5), E608–E612. https://doi.org/10.1152/ajpendo.00156.2017

1616 Wanders, A. J., van den Borne, J. J., de Graaf, C., Hulshof, T., Jonathan, M. C., Kristensen, M., Mars, M., Schols, H. A., & Feskens, E. J. (2011). Effects of dietary fibre on subjective appetite, energy intake and body weight: a systematic review of randomized controlled trials. Obesity reviews : an official journal of the International Association for the Study of Obesity, 12(9), 724–739. https://doi.org/10.1111/j.1467-789X.2011.00895.x

1617 Clark, M. J., & Slavin, J. L. (2013). The effect of fiber on satiety and food intake: a systematic review. Journal of the American College of Nutrition, 32(3), 200–211. https://doi.org/10.1080/07315724.2013.791194

1618 Burton-Freeman B. (2000). Dietary fiber and energy regulation. The Journal of nutrition, 130(2S Suppl), 272S–275S. https://doi.org/10.1093/jn/130.2.272S

1619 Kristensen, M., Jensen, M. G., Aarestrup, J., Petersen, K. E., Søndergaard, L., Mikkelsen, M. S., & Astrup, A. (2012). Flaxseed dietary fibers lower cholesterol and increase fecal fat excretion, but magnitude of effect depend on food type. Nutrition & metabolism, 9, 8. https://doi.org/10.1186/1743-7075-9-8

1620 Uebelhack, R., Busch, R., Alt, F., Beah, Z. M., & Chong, P. W. (2014). Effects of cactus fiber on the excretion of dietary fat in healthy subjects: a double blind, randomized, placebo-controlled, crossover clinical investigation. Current therapeutic research, clinical and experimental, 76, 39–44. https://doi.org/10.1016/j.curtheres.2014.02.001

1621 Hall, K. D., Guo, J., Courville, A. B., Boring, J., Brychta, R., Chen, K. Y., Darcey, V., Forde, C. G., Gharib, A. M., Gallagher, I., Howard, R., Joseph, P. V., Milley, L., Ouwerkerk, R., Raisinger, K., Rozga, I., Schick, A., Stagliano, M., Torres, S., Walter, M., ... Chung, S. T. (2021). Effect of a plant-based, low-fat diet versus an animal-based, ketogenic diet on ad libitum energy intake. Nature medicine, 27(2), 344–353. https://doi.org/10.1038/s41591-020-01209-1

1622 BLOOM, W. L., & AZAR, G. J. (1963). SIMILARITIES OF CARBOHYDRATE DEFICIENCY AND FASTING. I. WEIGHT LOSS, ELECTROLYTE EXCRETION, AND FATIGUE. Archives of internal medicine, 112, 333–337. https://doi.org/10.1001/archinte.1963.03860030087006

1623 BLOOM, W. L., & AZAR, G. J. (1963). SIMILARITIES OF CARBOHYDRATE DEFICIENCY AND FASTING. I. WEIGHT LOSS, ELECTROLYTE EXCRETION, AND FATIGUE. Archives of internal medicine, 112, 333–337. https://doi.org/10.1001/archinte.1963.03860030087006

1624 Consolazio, C. F., Matoush, L. O., Johnson, H. L., Krzywicki, H. J., Isaac, G. J., & Witt, N. F. (1968). Metabolic aspects of calorie restriction: nitrogen and mineral balances and vitamin excretion. The American journal of clinical nutrition, 21(8), 803–812. https://doi.org/10.1093/ajcn/21.8.803

1625 Woodie, L. N., Luo, Y., Wayne, M. J., Graff, E. C., Ahmed, B., O'Neill, A. M., & Greene, M. W. (2018). Restricted feeding for 9h in the active period partially abrogates the detrimental metabolic effects of a Western diet with liquid sugar consumption in mice. Metabolism: clinical and experimental, 82, 1–13. https://doi.org/10.1016/j.metabol.2017.12.004

1626 Delahaye, L. B., Bloomer, R. J., Butawan, M. B., Wyman, J. M., Hill, J. L., Lee, H. W., Liu, A. C., McAllan, L., Han, J. C., & van der Merwe, M. (2018). Time-restricted feeding of a high-fat diet in male C57BL/6 mice reduces adiposity but does not protect against increased systemic inflammation. Applied physiology, nutrition, and metabolism = Physiologie appliquee, nutrition et metabolisme, 43(10), 1033–1042. https://doi.org/10.1139/apnm-2017-0706

1627 Olsen, M. K., Choi, M. H., Kulseng, B., Zhao, C. M., & Chen, D. (2017). Time-restricted feeding on weekdays restricts weight gain: A study using rat models of high-fat diet-induced obesity. Physiology & behavior, 173, 298–304. https://doi.org/10.1016/j.physbeh.2017.02.032

1628 Villanueva, J. E., Livelo, C., Trujillo, A. S., Chandran, S., Woodworth, B., Andrade, L., Le, H. D., Manor, U., Panda, S., & Melkani, G. C. (2019). Time-restricted feeding restores muscle function in Drosophila models of obesity and circadian-rhythm disruption. Nature communications, 10(1), 2700. https://doi.org/10.1038/s41467-019-10563-9

1629 Hatori, M., Vollmers, C., Zarrinpar, A., DiTacchio, L., Bushong, E. A., Gill, S., Leblanc, M., Chaix, A., Joens, M., Fitzpatrick, J. A., Ellisman, M. H., & Panda, S. (2012). Time-restricted feeding without reducing caloric intake prevents metabolic diseases in mice fed a high-fat diet. Cell metabolism, 15(6), 848–860. https://doi.org/10.1016/j.cmet.2012.04.019

1630 Chaix, A., Zarrinpar, A., Miu, P., & Panda, S. (2014). Time-restricted feeding is a preventative and therapeutic intervention against diverse nutritional challenges. Cell metabolism, 20(6), 991–1005. https://doi.org/10.1016/j.cmet.2014.11.001

1631 Jamshed, H., Beyl, R. A., Della Manna, D. L., Yang, E. S., Ravussin, E., & Peterson, C. M. (2019). Early Time-Restricted Feeding Improves 24-Hour Glucose Levels and Affects Markers of the Circadian Clock, Aging, and Autophagy in Humans. Nutrients, 11(6), 1234. https://doi.org/10.3390/nu11061234

1632 Panda S. (2016). Circadian physiology of metabolism. Science (New York, N.Y.), 354(6315), 1008–1015. https://doi.org/10.1126/science.aah4967

1633 de Cabo et al (2018) 'A time to fast', Science, Vol. 362, Issue 6416, pp. 770-775.

1634 Longo, V. D., & Mattson, M. P. (2014). Fasting: Molecular Mechanisms and Clinical Applications. Cell Metabolism, 19(2), 181–192. doi:10.1016/j.cmet.2013.12.008

1635 Varady, K. A., Bhutani, S., Church, E. C., & Klempel, M. C. (2009). Short-term modified alternate-day fasting: a novel dietary strategy for weight loss and cardioprotection in obese adults. The American journal of clinical nutrition, 90(5), 1138–1143. https://doi.org/10.3945/ajcn.2009.28380

1636 Barnosky, A. R., Hoddy, K. K., Unterman, T. G., & Varady, K. A. (2014). Intermittent fasting vs daily calorie restriction for type 2 diabetes prevention: a review of human findings. Translational Research, 164(4), 302–311. doi:10.1016/j.trsl.2014.05.013

[1637] Stote, K. S., Baer, D. J., Spears, K., Paul, D. R., Harris, G. K., Rumpler, W. V., Strycula, P., Najjar, S. S., Ferrucci, L., Ingram, D. K., Longo, D. L., & Mattson, M. P. (2007). A controlled trial of reduced meal frequency without caloric restriction in healthy, normal-weight, middle-aged adults. The American journal of clinical nutrition, 85(4), 981–988. https://doi.org/10.1093/ajcn/85.4.981

[1638] Chow, L. S., Manoogian, E., Alvear, A., Fleischer, J. G., Thor, H., Dietsche, K., Wang, Q., Hodges, J. S., Esch, N., Malaeb, S., Harindhanavudhi, T., Nair, K. S., Panda, S., & Mashek, D. G. (2020). Time-Restricted Eating Effects on Body Composition and Metabolic Measures in Humans who are Overweight: A Feasibility Study. Obesity (Silver Spring, Md.), 28(5), 860–869. https://doi.org/10.1002/oby.22756

[1639] Anton, S. D., Lee, S. A., Donahoo, W. T., McLaren, C., Manini, T., Leeuwenburgh, C., & Pahor, M. (2019). The Effects of Time Restricted Feeding on Overweight, Older Adults: A Pilot Study. Nutrients, 11(7), 1500. https://doi.org/10.3390/nu11071500

[1640] Moro, T., Tinsley, G., Bianco, A., Marcolin, G., Pacelli, Q. F., Battaglia, G., Palma, A., Gentil, P., Neri, M., & Paoli, A. (2016). Effects of eight weeks of time-restricted feeding (16/8) on basal metabolism, maximal strength, body composition, inflammation, and cardiovascular risk factors in resistance-trained males. Journal of translational medicine, 14(1), 290. https://doi.org/10.1186/s12967-016-1044-0

[1641] Gabel, K., Marcell, J., Cares, K., Kalam, F., Cienfuegos, S., Ezpeleta, M., & Varady, K. A. (2020). Effect of time restricted feeding on the gut microbiome in adults with obesity: A pilot study. Nutrition and Health, 26(2), 79–85. doi:10.1177/0260106020910907

[1642] LeCheminant, J. D., Christenson, E., Bailey, B. W., & Tucker, L. A. (2013). Restricting night-time eating reduces daily energy intake in healthy young men: a short-term cross-over study. The British journal of nutrition, 110(11), 2108–2113. https://doi.org/10.1017/S0007114513001359

[1643] Liu, D., Huang, Y., Huang, C., Yang, S., Wei, X., Zhang, P., Guo, D., Lin, J., Xu, B., Li, C., He, H., He, J., Liu, S., Shi, L., Xue, Y., & Zhang, H. (2022). Calorie Restriction with or without Time-Restricted Eating in Weight Loss. New England Journal of Medicine, 386(16), 1495–1504. https://doi.org/10.1056/nejmoa2114833

[1644] Lowe, D. A., Wu, N., Rohdin-Bibby, L., Moore, A. H., Kelly, N., Liu, Y. E., Philip, E., Vittinghoff, E., Heymsfield, S. B., Olgin, J. E., Shepherd, J. A., & Weiss, E. J. (2020). Effects of Time-Restricted Eating on Weight Loss and Other Metabolic Parameters in Women and Men With Overweight and Obesity. JAMA Internal Medicine, 180(11), 1491. https://doi.org/10.1001/jamainternmed.2020.4153

[1645] Gill, S., & Panda, S. (2015). A Smartphone App Reveals Erratic Diurnal Eating Patterns in Humans that Can Be Modulated for Health Benefits. Cell metabolism, 22(5), 789-98.

1646 Trepanowski, J. F., Kroeger, C. M., Barnosky, A., Klempel, M. C., Bhutani, S., Hoddy, K. K., … Varady, K. A. (2017). Effect of Alternate-Day Fasting on Weight Loss, Weight Maintenance, and Cardioprotection Among Metabolically Healthy Obese Adults. JAMA Internal Medicine, 177(7), 930. doi:10.1001/jamainternmed.2017.0936

1647 Klempel, M. C., Bhutani, S., Fitzgibbon, M., Freels, S., & Varady, K. A. (2010). Dietary and physical activity adaptations to alternate day modified fasting: implications for optimal weight loss. Nutrition Journal, 9(1). doi:10.1186/1475-2891-9-35

1648 Catenacci, V. A., Pan, Z., Ostendorf, D., Brannon, S., Gozansky, W. S., Mattson, M. P., Martin, B., MacLean, P. S., Melanson, E. L., & Troy Donahoo, W. (2016). A randomized pilot study comparing zero-calorie alternate-day fasting to daily caloric restriction in adults with obesity. Obesity (Silver Spring, Md.), 24(9), 1874–1883. https://doi.org/10.1002/oby.21581

1649 Hoddy, K. K., Gibbons, C., Kroeger, C. M., Trepanowski, J. F., Barnosky, A., Bhutani, S., … Varady, K. A. (2016). Changes in hunger and fullness in relation to gut peptides before and after 8 weeks of alternate day fasting. Clinical Nutrition, 35(6), 1380–1385. doi:10.1016/j.clnu.2016.03.011

1650 Klempel, M. C., Bhutani, S., Fitzgibbon, M., Freels, S., & Varady, K. A. (2010). Dietary and physical activity adaptations to alternate day modified fasting: implications for optimal weight loss. Nutrition Journal, 9(1). doi:10.1186/1475-2891-9-35

1651 Heilbronn, L. K., Smith, S. R., Martin, C. K., Anton, S. D., & Ravussin, E. (2005). Alternate-day fasting in nonobese subjects: effects on body weight, body composition, and energy metabolism. The American journal of clinical nutrition, 81(1), 69–73. https://doi.org/10.1093/ajcn/81.1.69

1652 Wei, M. et al (2017) 'Fasting-mimicking diet and markers/risk factors for aging, diabetes, cancer, and cardiovascular disease', Sci Transl Med, Vol 9 (377).

1653 Templeman, I., Smith, H. A., Chowdhury, E., Chen, Y. C., Carroll, H., Johnson-Bonson, D., Hengist, A., Smith, R., Creighton, J., Clayton, D., Varley, I., Karagounis, L. G., Wilhelmsen, A., Tsintzas, K., Reeves, S., Walhin, J. P., Gonzalez, J. T., Thompson, D., & Betts, J. A. (2021). A randomized controlled trial to isolate the effects of fasting and energy restriction on weight loss and metabolic health in lean adults. Science translational medicine, 13(598), eabd8034. https://doi.org/10.1126/scitranslmed.abd8034

[1654] Gill, S., & Panda, S. (2015). A Smartphone App Reveals Erratic Diurnal Eating Patterns in Humans that Can Be Modulated for Health Benefits. Cell metabolism, 22(5), 789-98.

[1655] Stanga, Z., Brunner, A., Leuenberger, M., Grimble, R. F., Shenkin, A., Allison, S. P., & Lobo, D. N. (2007). Nutrition in clinical practice—the refeeding syndrome: illustrative cases and guidelines for prevention and treatment. European Journal of Clinical Nutrition, 62(6), 687–694. doi:10.1038/sj.ejcn.1602854

[1656] Mehanna, H. M., Moledina, J., & Travis, J. (2008). Refeeding syndrome: what it is, and how to prevent and treat it. BMJ (Clinical research ed.), 336(7659), 1495–1498. https://doi.org/10.1136/bmj.a301

[1657] Consolazio, C. F., Matoush, L. O., Johnson, H. L., Krzywicki, H. J., Isaac, G. J., & Witt, N. F. (1968). Metabolic aspects of calorie restriction: nitrogen and mineral balances and vitamin excretion. The American journal of clinical nutrition, 21(8), 803–812. https://doi.org/10.1093/ajcn/21.8.803

1658 Runcie J. (1971). Urinary sodium and potassium excretion in fasting obese subjects. British medical journal, 2(5752), 22–25. https://doi.org/10.1136/bmj.2.5752.22

1659 Hamwi, G. J., Mitchell, M. C., Wieland, R. G., Kruger, F. A., & Schachner, S. S. (1967). Sodium and potassium metabolism during starvation. The American journal of clinical nutrition, 20(8), 897–902. https://doi.org/10.1093/ajcn/20.8.897

[1660] Qian, J., Morris, C. J., Caputo, R., Garaulet, M., & Scheer, F. (2019). Ghrelin is impacted by the endogenous circadian system and by circadian misalignment in humans. International journal of obesity (2005), 43(8), 1644–1649. https://doi.org/10.1038/s41366-018-0208-9

[1661] Scheer FA et al (2013) 'The internal circadian clock increases hunger and appetite in the evening independent of food intake and other behaviors', Obesity (Silver Spring). 2013 Mar;21(3):421-3.

[1662] Thomas et al (2015) 'Usual breakfast eating habits affect response to breakfast skipping in overweight women', Obesity (Silver Spring). 2015 Apr;23(4):750-9. doi: 10.1002/oby.21049. Epub 2015 Mar 6.

[1663] Bi, H., Gan, Y., Yang, C., Chen, Y., Tong, X., & Lu, Z. (2015). Breakfast skipping and the risk of type 2 diabetes: A meta-analysis of observational studies. Public Health Nutrition, 18(16), 3013-3019. doi:10.1017/S1368980015000257

[1664] Nakajima, K., & Suwa, K. (2015). Association of hyperglycemia in a general Japanese population with late-night-dinner eating alone, but not breakfast skipping alone. Journal of Diabetes & Metabolic Disorders, 14(1). doi:10.1186/s40200-015-0147-0

[1665] Okada, C., Imano, H., Muraki, I., Yamada, K., & Iso, H. (2019). The Association of Having a Late Dinner or Bedtime Snack and Skipping Breakfast with Overweight in Japanese Women. Journal of Obesity, 2019, 1–5. doi:10.1155/2019/2439571

[1666] Azami, Y., Funakoshi, M., Matsumoto, H., Ikota, A., Ito, K., Okimoto, H., … Miura, J. (2018). Long working hours and skipping breakfast concomitant with late evening meals are associated with suboptimal glycemic control among young male Japanese patients with type 2 diabetes. Journal of Diabetes Investigation, 10(1), 73–83. doi:10.1111/jdi.12852

[1667] Rudic, R. D., McNamara, P., Curtis, A. M., Boston, R. C., Panda, S., Hogenesch, J. B., & Fitzgerald, G. A. (2004). BMAL1 and CLOCK, two essential components of the circadian clock, are involved in glucose homeostasis. PLoS biology, 2(11), e377. https://doi.org/10.1371/journal.pbio.0020377

[1668] Sonnier, T., Rood, J., Gimble, J. M., & Peterson, C. M. (2014). Glycemic control is impaired in the evening in prediabetes through multiple diurnal rhythms. Journal of diabetes and its complications, 28(6), 836–843. https://doi.org/10.1016/j.jdiacomp.2014.04.001

[1669] Basse, A. L., Dalbram, E., Larsson, L., Gerhart-Hines, Z., Zierath, J. R., & Treebak, J. T. (2018). Skeletal Muscle Insulin Sensitivity Show Circadian Rhythmicity Which Is Independent of Exercise Training Status. Frontiers in physiology, 9, 1198. https://doi.org/10.3389/fphys.2018.01198

[1670] Jamshed et al (2019) 'Early Time-Restricted Feeding Improves 24-Hour Glucose Levels and Affects Markers of the Circadian Clock, Aging, and Autophagy in Humans', Nutrients. 2019 May 30;11(6). pii: E1234. doi: 10.3390/nu11061234.

[1671] Hutchinson et al (2019) 'Time-Restricted Feeding Improves Glucose Tolerance in Men at Risk for Type 2 Diabetes: A Randomized Crossover Trial', Obesity, Volume 27, Issue 5, Pages 724-732.

[1672] Tinsley, G. M., Moore, M. L., Graybeal, A. J., Paoli, A., Kim, Y., Gonzales, J. U., Harry, J. R., VanDusseldorp, T. A., Kennedy, D. N., & Cruz, M. R. (2019). Time-restricted feeding plus resistance training in active females: a randomized trial. The American journal of clinical nutrition, 110(3), 628–640. https://doi.org/10.1093/ajcn/nqz126

[1673] Meessen et al (2022) 'Differential Effects of One Meal per Day in the Evening on Metabolic Health and Physical Performance in Lean Individuals', Front. Physiol., 11 January 2022 | https://doi.org/10.3389/fphys.2021.771944

[1674] Moro et al (2016) 'Effects of eight weeks of time-restricted feeding (16/8) on basal metabolism, maximal strength, body composition, inflammation, and cardiovascular risk factors in resistance-trained males', J Transl Med. 2016 Oct 13;14(1):290.

1675 Soeters, MR et al (2009) 'Intermittent fasting does not affect whole-body glucose, lipid, or protein metabolism', Am J Clin Nutr, Vol 90(5), p 1244-51.

1676 Varady, KA. (2011) 'Intermittent versus daily calorie restriction: which diet regimen is more effective for weight loss?', Obes Rev, Vol 12(7), e593-601.

1677 Stote KS et al (2007) 'A controlled trial of reduced meal frequency without caloric restriction in healthy, normal-weight, middle-aged adults', Am J Clin Nutr, Vol 85(4), p 981-8.

1678 Keogh, JB et al (2014) 'Effects of intermittent compared to continuous energy restriction on short-term weight loss and long-term weight loss maintenance', Clin Obes, Vol 4(3), p 150-6.

1679 Arnal, MA. et al (2000) 'Protein feeding pattern does not affect protein retention in young women', J Nutr, Vol 130(7), p 1700-4.

1680 Arnal, M.-A., Mosoni, L., Boirie, Y., Houlier, M.-L., Morin, L., Verdier, E., … Mirand, P. P. (1999). Protein pulse feeding improves protein retention in elderly women. The American Journal of Clinical Nutrition, 69(6), 1202–1208. doi:10.1093/ajcn/69.6.1202

1681 Trabelski, K. et al (2013) 'Effect of fed- versus fasted state resistance training during Ramadan on body composition and selected metabolic parameters in bodybuilders', J Int Soc Sports Nutr. 2013 Apr 25;10(1):23.

[1682] https://www.nature.com/articles/nature13236

[1683] Mulder H et al (2009) 'Melatonin receptors in pancreatic islets: good morning to a novel type 2 diabetes gene', Diabetologia. 2009 Jul;52(7):1240-9.

[1684] Azizi, F. (1978). Effect of dietary composition on fasting-induced changes in serum thyroid hormones and thyrotropin. Metabolism, 27(8), 935–942. doi:10.1016/0026-0495(78)90137-3

[1685] Chan, J. L., Heist, K., DePaoli, A. M., Veldhuis, J. D., & Mantzoros, C. S. (2003). The role of falling leptin levels in the neuroendocrine and metabolic adaptation to short-term starvation in healthy men. Journal of Clinical Investigation, 111(9), 1409–1421. doi:10.1172/jci200317490

[1686] Anita Boelen, Wilmar Maarten Wiersinga, and Eric Fliers.Thyroid.Feb 2008.123-129.http://doi.org/10.1089/thy.2007.0253

[1687] Ucci, Renzini, Russi, Mangialardo, Cammarata, Cavioli, … Verga-Falzacappa. (2019). Thyroid Hormone Protects from Fasting-Induced Skeletal Muscle Atrophy by Promoting Metabolic Adaptation. International Journal of Molecular Sciences, 20(22), 5754. doi:10.3390/ijms20225754

[1688] CARLSON, H. E., DRENICK, E. J., CHOPRA, I. J., & HERSHMAN, J. M. (1977). Alterations in Basal and TRH-Stimulated Serum Levels of Thyrotropin, Prolactin, and Thyroid Hormones in Starved Obese Men. The Journal of Clinical Endocrinology & Metabolism, 45(4), 707–713. doi:10.1210/jcem-45-4-707

[1689] Azizi F, Rasouli HA, Beheshti S. Evaluation of certain hormones and blood constituents during Islamic fasting month. Med Assoc Thailand. 1986;69:57A.

[1690] Raza, S., Unnikrishnan, A., Ahmad, J., Azad, K., Pathan, M. F., Ishtiaq, O., … Baruah, M. (2012). Thyroid diseases and Ramadan. Indian Journal of Endocrinology and Metabolism, 16(4), 522. doi:10.4103/2230-8210.98001

[1691] Burman, K. D., Smallridge, R. C., Osburne, R., Dimond, R. C., Whorton, N. E., Kesler, P., & Wartofsky, L. (1980). Nature of suppressed TSH secretion during undernutrition: Effect of fasting and refeeding on TSH responses to prolonged TRH infusions. Metabolism, 29(1), 46–52. doi:10.1016/0026-0495(80)90097-9

[1692] Azizi, F. (1978). Effect of dietary composition on fasting-induced changes in serum thyroid hormones and thyrotropin. Metabolism, 27(8), 935–942. doi:10.1016/0026-0495(78)90137-3

1693 Bakhach, M., Shah, V., Harwood, T., Lappe, S., Bhesania, N., Mansoor, S., & Alkhouri, N. (2016). The Protein-Sparing Modified Fast Diet: An Effective and Safe Approach to Induce Rapid Weight Loss in Severely Obese Adolescents. Global pediatric health, 3, 2333794X15623245. https://doi.org/10.1177/2333794X15623245

1694 Chang, J; Kashyap, SR (September 2014). "The protein-sparing modified fast for obese patients with type 2 diabetes: what to expect". Cleveland Clinic journal of medicine. 81 (9): 557–65.

1695 Palgi, A., Read, J. L., Greenberg, I., Hoefer, M. A., Bistrian, B. R., & Blackburn, G. L. (1985). Multidisciplinary treatment of obesity with a protein-sparing modified fast: results in 668 outpatients. American journal of public health, 75(10), 1190–1194. https://doi.org/10.2105/ajph.75.10.1190

1696 Friedman, A. N., Chambers, M., Kamendulis, L. M., & Temmerman, J. (2013). Short-term changes after a weight reduction intervention in advanced diabetic nephropathy. Clinical journal of the American Society of Nephrology : CJASN, 8(11), 1892–1898. https://doi.org/10.2215/CJN.04010413

1697 Isner, JM; Sours, HE; Paris, AL; Ferrans, VJ; Roberts, WC (December 1979). "Sudden, unexpected death in avid dieters using the liquid-protein-modified-fast diet: observations in 17 patients and the role of the prolonged QT interval" (PDF). *Circulation*. Dallas, TX: American Heart Association, Inc. **60** (6): 1401–1412.

1698 Chang, J. J., Bena, J., Kannan, S., Kim, J., Burguera, B., & Kashyap, S. R. (2017). LIMITED CARBOHYDRATE REFEEDING INSTRUCTION FOR LONG-TERM WEIGHT MAINTENANCE FOLLOWING A KETOGENIC, VERY-LOW-CALORIE MEAL PLAN. Endocrine practice : official journal of the American College of Endocrinology and the American Association of Clinical Endocrinologists, 23(6), 649–656. https://doi.org/10.4158/EP161383.OR

1699 Van Gaal, L. F., Snyders, D., De Leeuw, I. H., & Bekaert, J. L. (1985). Anthropometric and calorimetric evidence for the protein sparing effects of a new protein supplemented low calorie preparation. The American journal of clinical nutrition, 41(3), 540–544. https://doi.org/10.1093/ajcn/41.3.540

1700 Henry, R. R., & Gumbiner, B. (1991). Benefits and limitations of very-low-calorie diet therapy in obese NIDDM. Diabetes care, 14(9), 802–823. https://doi.org/10.2337/diacare.14.9.802

1701 Bettens, C., Héraïef, E., & Burckhardt, P. (1989). Short and long term results of a progressive reintroduction of carbohydrates (PRCH) after a protein-sparing modified fast (PSMF). International journal of obesity, 13 Suppl 2, 113–117.

1702 2015-2020 Dietary Guidelines 'Appendix 2. Estimated Calorie Needs per Day, by Age, Sex, and Physical Activity Level', Accessed Online: https://health.gov/dietaryguidelines/2015/guidelines/appendix-2/

1703 Santesso, N., Akl, E. A., Bianchi, M., Mente, A., Mustafa, R., Heels-Ansdell, D., & Schünemann, H. J. (2012). Effects of higher- versus lower-protein diets on health outcomes: a systematic review and meta-analysis. European journal of clinical nutrition, 66(7), 780–788. https://doi.org/10.1038/ejcn.2012.37

1704 Loren Cordain, Janette Brand Miller, S Boyd Eaton, Neil Mann, Susanne HA Holt, John D Speth; Plant-animal subsistence ratios and macronutrient energy estimations in worldwide hunter-gatherer diets, The American Journal of Clinical Nutrition, Volume 71, Issue 3, 1 March 2000, Pages 682–692

1705 Institute of Medicine (2005) 'Dietary Reference Intakes for Energy, Carbohydrate, Fiber, Fat, Fatty Acids, Cholesterol, Protein and Amino Acids', National Academy Press.

1706 Bilsborough, S., & Mann, N. (2006). A review of issues of dietary protein intake in humans. International journal of sport nutrition and exercise metabolism, 16(2), 129–152. https://doi.org/10.1123/ijsnem.16.2.129

1707 Layman, D. K., Anthony, T. G., Rasmussen, B. B., Adams, S. H., Lynch, C. J., Brinkworth, G. D., & Davis, T. A. (2015). Defining meal requirements for protein to optimize metabolic roles of amino acids. The American journal of clinical nutrition, 101(6), 1330S–1338S. https://doi.org/10.3945/ajcn.114.084053

1708 Campbell, W. W., Trappe, T. A., Wolfe, R. R., & Evans, W. J. (2001). The recommended dietary allowance for protein may not be adequate for older people to maintain skeletal muscle. The journals of gerontology. Series A, Biological sciences and medical sciences, 56(6), M373–M380. https://doi.org/10.1093/gerona/56.6.m373

1709 Morton, R. W., Murphy, K. T., McKellar, S. R., Schoenfeld, B. J., Henselmans, M., Helms, E., … Phillips, S. M. (2017). A systematic review, meta-analysis and meta-regression of the effect of protein supplementation on resistance training-induced gains in muscle mass and strength in healthy adults. British Journal of Sports Medicine, 52(6), 376–384. doi:10.1136/bjsports-2017-097608

1710 Hector, A. J., & Phillips, S. M. (2018). Protein Recommendations for Weight Loss in Elite Athletes: A Focus on Body Composition and Performance. International journal of sport nutrition and exercise metabolism, 28(2), 170–177. https://doi.org/10.1123/ijsnem.2017-0273

1711 Witard, O. C., Garthe, I., & Phillips, S. M. (2019). Dietary Protein for Training Adaptation and Body Composition Manipulation in Track and Field Athletes. International journal of sport nutrition and exercise metabolism, 29(2), 165–174. https://doi.org/10.1123/ijsnem.2018-0267

1712 Helms, E. R., Zinn, C., Rowlands, D. S., & Brown, S. R. (2014). A systematic review of dietary protein during caloric restriction in resistance trained lean athletes: a case for higher intakes. International journal of sport nutrition and exercise metabolism, 24(2), 127–138. https://doi.org/10.1123/ijsnem.2013-0054

1713 Aragon, A. A., Schoenfeld, B. J., Wildman, R., Kleiner, S., VanDusseldorp, T., Taylor, L., Earnest, C. P., Arciero, P. J., Wilborn, C., Kalman, D. S., Stout, J. R., Willoughby, D. S., Campbell, B., Arent, S. M., Bannock, L., Smith-Ryan, A. E., & Antonio, J. (2017). International society of sports nutrition position stand: diets and body composition. Journal of the International Society of Sports Nutrition, 14, 16. https://doi.org/10.1186/s12970-017-0174-y

1714 Helms, E. R., Aragon, A. A., & Fitschen, P. J. (2014). Evidence-based recommendations for natural bodybuilding contest preparation: nutrition and supplementation. Journal of the International Society of Sports Nutrition, 11, 20. https://doi.org/10.1186/1550-2783-11-20

1715 Stokes, T., Hector, A. J., Morton, R. W., McGlory, C., & Phillips, S. M. (2018). Recent Perspectives Regarding the Role of Dietary Protein for the Promotion of Muscle Hypertrophy with Resistance Exercise Training. Nutrients, 10(2), 180. https://doi.org/10.3390/nu10020180

1716 Martin, W. F., Armstrong, L. E., & Rodriguez, N. R. (2005). Dietary protein intake and renal function. Nutrition & metabolism, 2, 25. https://doi.org/10.1186/1743-7075-2-25

1717 Friedman A. N. (2004). High-protein diets: potential effects on the kidney in renal health and disease. American journal of kidney diseases : the official journal of the National Kidney Foundation, 44(6), 950–962. https://doi.org/10.1053/j.ajkd.2004.08.020

1718 Conn JW, Newburgh LH: The glycemic response to isoglucogenic quantities of protein and carbohydrate. J Clin Invest 15:667-71, 1936.

1719 Cederbaum A. I. (2012). Alcohol metabolism. Clinics in liver disease, 16(4), 667–685. https://doi.org/10.1016/j.cld.2012.08.002

1720 Shelmet, J. J., Reichard, G. A., Skutches, C. L., Hoeldtke, R. D., Owen, O. E., & Boden, G. (1988). Ethanol causes acute inhibition of carbohydrate, fat, and protein oxidation and insulin resistance. The Journal of clinical investigation, 81(4), 1137–1145. https://doi.org/10.1172/JCI113428

1721 Traversy, G., & Chaput, J. P. (2015). Alcohol Consumption and Obesity: An Update. Current obesity reports, 4(1), 122–130. https://doi.org/10.1007/s13679-014-0129-4

1722 Sonko, B. J., Prentice, A. M., Murgatroyd, P. R., Goldberg, G. R., van de Ven, M. L., & Coward, W. A. (1994). Effect of alcohol on postmeal fat storage. The American Journal of Clinical Nutrition, 59(3), 619–625. doi:10.1093/ajcn/59.3.619

1723 Sumi, M., Hisamatsu, T., Fujiyoshi, A., Kadota, A., Miyagawa, N., Kondo, K., Kadowaki, S., Suzuki, S., Torii, S., Zaid, M., Sato, A., Arima, H., Terada, T., Miura, K., & Ueshima, H. (2019). Association of Alcohol Consumption With Fat Deposition in a Community-Based Sample of Japanese Men: The Shiga Epidemiological Study of Subclinical Atherosclerosis (SESSA). Journal of epidemiology, 29(6), 205–212. https://doi.org/10.2188/jea.JE20170191

[1724] Purohit V. (1998). Moderate alcohol consumption and estrogen levels in postmenopausal women: a review. Alcoholism, clinical and experimental research, 22(5), 994–997. https://doi.org/10.1111/j.1530-0277.1998.tb03694.x

[1725] Emanuele, M. A., & Emanuele, N. V. (1998). Alcohol's effects on male reproduction. Alcohol health and research world, 22(3), 195–201.

Made in the USA
Monee, IL
20 November 2022

18025546R00164